big
green
purse

big
green
purse

USE YOUR SPENDING POWER
TO CREATE A CLEANER, GREENER WORLD

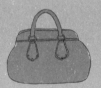

Diane MacEachern

AVERY · A MEMBER OF PENGUIN GROUP (USA) INC. · NEW YORK

AVERY

Published by the Penguin Group

Penguin Group (USA) Inc., 375 Hudson Street, New York, New York 10014, USA •
Penguin Group (Canada), 90 Eglinton Avenue East, Suite 700, Toronto, Ontario M4P 2Y3,
Canada (a division of Pearson Canada Inc.) • Penguin Books Ltd,
80 Strand, London WC2R 0RL, England • Penguin Ireland, 25 St Stephen's Green,
Dublin 2, Ireland (a division of Penguin Books Ltd) • Penguin Group (Australia),
250 Camberwell Road, Camberwell, Victoria 3124, Australia (a division of Pearson
Australia Group Pty Ltd) • Penguin Books India Pvt Ltd, 11 Community Centre,
Panchsheel Park, New Delhi–110 017, India • Penguin Group (NZ), 67 Apollo Drive,
Rosedale, North Shore 0632, New Zealand (a division of Pearson
New Zealand Ltd) • Penguin Books (South Africa) (Pty) Ltd, 24 Sturdee Avenue,
Rosebank, Johannesburg 2196, South Africa

Penguin Books Ltd, Registered Offices: 80 Strand, London WC2R 0RL, England

Most Avery books are available at special quantity discounts for bulk purchase for sales promotions, premiums, fund-raising,
and educational needs. Special books or book excerpts also can be created to fit specific needs. For details, write Penguin Group
(USA) Inc. Special Markets, 375 Hudson Street, New York, NY 10014.

Library of Congress Cataloging-in-Publication Data

MacEachern, Diane.
Big green purse : use your spending power to create a cleaner, greener world / Diane MacEachern.
p.   cm.
ISBN 978-1-58333-303-7
1. Shopping.   2. Consumer education.   3. Environmental protection—Citizen participation.
4. Green movement.   5. Countervailing power.   6. Green products.   I. Title.
TX335.M187   2008   2007049115
333.72—dc22

Printed in the United States of America
1   3   5   7   9   10   8   6   4   2

This book is printed on acid-free recycled paper. ♾

BOOK DESIGN BY TANYA MAIBORODA

Nothing in this book is intended as an express or implied warranty of the suitability or fitness of any product, service, or design. Readers wishing to use a product, service, or design discussed in this book should first consult a specialist or professional to ensure suitability and fitness for their particular lifestyle and environmental needs.

While the author has made every effort to provide accurate telephone numbers and Internet addresses at the time of publication, neither the publisher nor the author assumes any responsibility for errors, or for changes that occur after publication. Further, the publisher does not have any control over and does not assume any responsibility for author or third-party websites or their content.

To my mother, Ann MacEachern

CONTENTS

INTRODUCTION

CAN THE WAY WE SPEND OUR MONEY BRING BACK THE SNOWS OF KILIMANJARO?

In 1983, the first time I visited this iconic mountain, it sparkled with glaciers and frosty trails. By the time my husband and I took our children back in 2000, we were stunned. The ice fields capping Africa's best-known landmark had shrunk so much, the dome looked more like a minefield than the sky-high "cupcake" we'd promised the kids. Now scientists are saying the snows will be gone altogether by 2020. I've spent years urging Congress and companies to adopt policies that would reverse global warming, a key cause of Kilimanjaro's snowmelt, to no avail. I'm ready to try something new.

Shopping, anyone?

Normally, the mall would be the last place I'd go if I wanted to solve an environmental problem. After all, runaway consumerism has played a significant role in the collapse of the planet, given the energy, water, land, and other resources required to produce all the stuff people buy . . . and buy . . . and buy.

But women spend eighty-five cents of every dollar in the marketplace. According to Connie Glaser, author of *The Women's Market Rules*, between the $2.7 billion a day we collectively earn and the additional billions we manage at home, on the job, or for volunteer organizations, women's buying power exceeds the economy of Japan. When we pay for goods, manufacturers pay attention to us.

Why not use that consumer clout to pressure companies to save energy, protect forests, use safer ingredients, and otherwise become more responsible environmental citizens? "I could buy no-VOC paint so my family won't have to breathe harsh chemicals," you might say, "and I'll persuade other paint manufacturers to eliminate VOCs from their products, too." Or, "The sustainable-wood furniture I buy will not only decorate my home, it will help save forests, as well." And, "I can buy wind power not only to meet my energy needs, but also to encourage utilities to switch from the fossil fuels that cause air pollution."

Big Green Purse: Use Your Spending Power to Create a Cleaner, Greener World shows women hundreds of ways they can make their money matter and protect the planet, too.

What's at Stake?

Women's consumer spending affects virtually every aspect of the environment.

We're major purchasers of cars, electronics, tools, appliances, furniture, and sporting equipment, let alone food, clothing, and cosmetics. Even if we don't actually lay out the cash ourselves, we influence the way others in our household do. (Who among us doesn't regularly send our spouse to the store with a list?) Fifty percent of "purchasing agents" for companies now are women, which is why we're also buying fleets of vehicles, reams of paper, mountains of office supplies, and boatloads of desks and chairs.

All this consumer clout puts us in a unique position to create the world we want. Good thing, because the world we've got needs some fixing. It's not only Kilimanjaro's melting glaciers we need to worry about. Coral reefs in the tropics, wilderness in the Rocky Mountains, and agricultural croplands that define America's heartland are at risk, too. Air pollution is increasing childhood asthma rates. Mercury from power plants is contaminating our food supply. In the long run, we'll have to deal with the collapse of entire ecosystems. We're already paying more for groceries and making more trips to the doctor's office.

Tropical rain forests are disappearing at the rate of six soccer fields a minute. The annual loss amounts to an area of rain forest the size of New Jersey. Some scientific models predict that by the end of this century, the Amazon basin—which generates 20 percent of the planet's oxygen, contains 15 to 20 percent of all life on earth, and covers 2,722,000 square miles in nine countries—will have been so burned, logged, and drilled, it will look more like the parched savannas of Africa than the Eden that has allowed it to serve as the "lungs" of the earth.

Our female biology makes us extremely vulnerable to toxic exposures. When we are pregnant, the fetus is particularly susceptible to chemicals that can cause birth defects. As nursing mothers, we feed our babies dangerous compounds—like pesticides and even rocket fuel—that have accumulated in our breast milk. As we age, we face a one in ten chance of contracting breast cancer from causes that are increasingly being linked to environmental contaminants.

Millions of women hold jobs in the cleaning professions, at hair and beauty salons, and in manufacturing industries. Their exposure to poisonous industrial solvents increases their risk of cancer, reproductive failure, and other health problems. But you don't have to be a maid, janitor, professional housekeeper, or beautician to be at risk. Using household cleaning sprays and aerosol fresheners just once a week can increase your chances of developing asthma by 30 to 50 percent, according to scientists at the Municipal Institute of Medical Research in Barcelona.

Think about the places in nature that you love. Do you have a favorite forest that offers you haven? A lake that refreshes your body and soul? A meadow or marsh that reminds you how many birds there are, and the different songs they sing? Pollution, encroaching development, and resource exploitation are taking their toll here, as well.

The threats are real and the outlook is grim. No denying, we've helped make it that way. Whether we're buying too much or just enough to meet our needs, as consumers we've been part of the problem, by purchasing products that devour energy and natural resources as if there were no tomorrow—which there won't be if we all keep this up.

But manufacturers haven't been much help, either. Well-heeled industry lobbyists prevent the passage of environmental legislation that would help bring global warming and other environmental problems under control. In the political arena, public officials frequently put expedient compromises (and political campaign contributions) ahead of the health and welfare of the planet and people like you and me. As responsible ecocitizens, our first obligation is to follow the three Rs: reduce how much we buy, reuse what we have, and recycle what we can.

But the three Rs get us only so far. Whether we've been paring down our purchases for years or are greenhorns when it comes to a green lifestyle, on some level we still need to shop.

That's where our purses—and our power to protect the planet—come into play.

As much as manufacturers oppose environmental legislation and regulation, they embrace what happens in the marketplace. They have to. Consumer dollars are their lifeblood. Corporate need for profit gives consumers power. And because women spend eighty-five cents of every dollar in the retail marketplace, we have a whole planetful of power.

We've already made organic food the fastest-growing sector in the food industry. We've turned "natural" personal-care products into a booming business, too. We're transforming the clothing industry with our pesticide-free cotton and hemp purchases, and saving rain forests by buying furniture made from recycled wood.

But we have to do more. Despite the ballyhoo about organic produce, only 3 percent of food sold in the United States is grown without toxic chemicals. Fewer than 5 percent of vehicles hawked on your neighborhood car lot are highly fuel efficient. Only 2 percent of coffee is "shade grown," meaning it's raised naturally beneath a rain forest canopy that protects songbirds rather than on estates that have been clear-cut and doused with pesticides.

By intentionally shifting our spending to products and services that offer the greatest environmental benefits, we can use our purse like a bright green ring threaded through the nose of the marketplace bull—and pull that bull in a greener, more eco-friendly direction.

Does the "Big Green Purse" Work?

Consider American car companies.

Environmentalists, consumer groups, and health advocates like the American Lung Association spent decades trying to convince Congress to raise automobile fuel-efficiency standards to reduce air pollution and curb greenhouse gases. Congress was more persuaded by the car companies, who claimed higher fuel efficiency couldn't be achieved, even as evidence mounted that we had to clean up the air, reverse climate change, and relieve our dependence on fossil fuels.

Meanwhile, in 1999, along came the Honda Insight Hybrid, followed in 2000 by the Toyota Prius Hybrid. Instead of 22 or 25 mpg, these vehicles got 50 and even 60 mpg.

In just five short years, propelled by high gas prices, increasing health concerns, and the global warming crisis, hybrid car sales skyrocketed. By 2004, consumers were buying 88,000 hybrids a year; by 2007 the number had jumped to 345,000. Drivers spent so much money on these new gas-electric cars, they motivated Ford, General Motors, and Chrysler to do what they said they never could: start manufacturing hybrids themselves.

Nail polish offers another case in point. Many brands contain dibutyl phthalate (DBP). DBP increases polish flexibility but is suspected of interfering with our endocrine system, a mechanism that influences almost every cell, organ, and function of our bodies, including growth, development, and reproduction. Banned from cosmetics in Europe, the chemical is considered a reproductive toxin by the state of California. On September 5, 2006, three major nail polish manufacturers announced that they were removing dibutyl phthalate from their products. Orly International, OPI Products, and Sally Hansen all said they were reformulating their nail polishes, even though they believed the ingredient is "safe in the concentrations in which it is used."

Why the transformation?

The last couple of years, thousands of women, led by the Campaign for Safe Cosmetics, have been taking two critical steps. They've been shifting their money to options like Honeybee brand nail polish, which is dibutyl phthalate–free. And they've been urging the companies through e-mails and letters to remove phthalates from their polish or risk losing substantial market share. Bruce MacKay, a vice president for Del Laboratories, the maker of Sally Hansen nail polish, acknowledged the power of the big green purse when he attributed "changing consumer trends" to the company's decision to put a safer product on store shelves.

Women have also made a dent in the tea industry, a significant inroad considering that after water, more consumers drink tea than any other beverage in the world.

Generally, tea is grown like many other crops: under insecticide-intensive practices by farmers who are not paid a fair wage and whose children must often also labor in the fields.

Thanks to increasing organic tea sales, the number of plantations growing tea organically has ballooned. Upton, Quintessential, Numi, Choice, Tazo, and Assam are among dozens of ecologically and socially responsible brands that now compete with Bigelow and Red Rose for shelf space in major supermarkets, grocers like Whole Foods, food co-ops, and online vendors.

Demand for organic tea is so strong that it has changed practices at Lipton, one of the biggest tea suppliers on the planet. In May 2006, Unilever, the world's largest tea company and maker of the Lipton brand, announced that it would start selling tea grown according to a Rainforest Alliance regimen that treats "environment, ethics, and economics equally." To meet the Rainforest Alliance/Unilever standards, tea farmers not only must reduce pesticide use and adopt better farming techniques, they also must improve working conditions for laborers, pay decent wages, and provide access to good housing, education, and health care. Unilever's move will greatly increase the marketplace supply of tea grown with fewer pesticides, an initiative that never would have happened without consumer demand leading the way.

Even Harry Potter got into the act. In 2007, 12 million copies of the new *Harry Potter and the Deathly Hallows* were printed on almost 11,000 tons of "post-consumer waste fiber," the technical term for high-quality recycled paper. No law required Harry's finale to be bound in a socially and ecologically responsible way. The magic came from consumer demand for books printed on paper that protects forests.

Does all this ecoshopping really make a difference? Consider the lowly lightbulb. If every American home replaced just one incandescent bulb with an Energy Star compact fluorescent (as a campaign from Wal-Mart is encouraging us to do), we'd save enough energy to light more than 2.5 million homes for a year and prevent global warming gases equivalent to the emissions of nearly 800,000 cars. Every ton of recycled paper that Harry Potter used not only saved seventeen trees, it also conserved approximately four barrels of oil, offsetting additional carbon dioxide (and providing enough energy to power the average North American home for almost six months, by the way).

So What's Holding Us Back?

Despite these and other inspiring examples, we still have a long way to go when it comes to using our purse power to protect the environment. Lack of time, conflicting information, the added cost and questionable quality of some ecoproducts, and mixed messages about what's "green" versus what's being "greenwashed" all prevent women from choosing earth-friendly items over more conventional ones.

Big Green Purse will make it easier for you to overcome such obstacles, whether you want to change the world or simply make the greenest choice when you shop. This book:

- shows you how to become a savvy green consumer—or not consume at all
- focuses on twenty-five key commodity areas where your dollars can have the biggest environmental impact

- highlights standards you can use to choose the greenest option, no matter what you buy
- helps you prioritize your green spending, clarifying what's worth the premium price some green products cost, and what isn't
- lists specific companies in each category you can support (and some you should avoid)

Be One in a Million

It's one thing to push your own shopping cart. But if women know anything, it's that there's power in numbers. So imagine if one million of us collectively pledged to shift $1,000 of our annual spending on green products. We'd have an intentional marketplace impact of $1 billion a year.

Big Green Purse invites you to make this pledge.

For most women, $1,000 should be within reach. Think about the money you spend managing your family, your home, your workplace, and perhaps your volunteer organizations. You could shift $10 a week of your grocery bill—to organic apples, fragrance-free detergents, or recycled paper towels, for example—and be halfway there.

If you need guidance on what green products to choose, look for merchandise that meets certified-sustainable standards to ensure that you're getting the greenest goods available while motivating manufacturers to become greener, too. Preferring SMART lighting, furniture, and home and building products; Energy Star appliances and electronics; FSC Certified Wood; and Green-e power (all of which you'll read about in the pages of this book) will give your purse real power.

To make your pledge, go to www.biggreenpurse.com.

What's Inside *Big Green Purse*

Throughout *Big Green Purse*, I urge you to give manufacturers irresistible incentives to literally clean up their act.

Chapter 1 recaps the environmental problems you can help resolve by first reducing what you consume, then shifting your spending to commodities that offer the greatest environmental benefit. Toxins, global warming and climate change, clean air, clean water, and protection of our forests are all on the list.

Chapter 2 lays out key Big Green Purse principles to help you make the best environmental choices and avoid "greenwashing" claims by manufacturers that their products offer environmental benefits when the opposite is true. That's where you'll learn more about how useful standards can be when you're shopping or a company is making manufacturing decisions that affect the planet.

Chapters 3 through 12 spotlight important commodities and suggest where you can have a meaningful impact if you shift your spending. Those items include cars; coffee, tea, cocoa, and chocolate; cosmetics and personal-care products; clothing, accessories, and jewelry; gardening and landscaping products; cleansers; food (fruits and vegetables, dairy, meat, poultry, and seafood); lights, appliances, and electronics; furniture, paint, flooring, and fabrics; and babies' and children's products. The chapters give a thumbs up to companies that merit your money, and a thumbs-down to those that don't.

These chapters also include short columns featuring quick tips, fast facts, shopping lists, and additional resources.

 go green

GO GREEN suggests simple, immediate lifestyle changes you can make to help protect the planet, whether you shift your spending or not. For example, you'll find ten ways to save gas in the Go Green feature of Chapter 4.

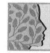 **make the shift**

MAKE THE SHIFT recommends eco-friendly products you can substitute for the conventional merchandise you're currently using. In most cases, these new choices will save you money, too.

 ecocheap

ECOCHEAP highlights ways you can save money and still live and shop green. There's no denying that many ecologically sound products are anything but wallet-friendly. Where I've figured out how to make my own green purse go a little further, I'm happy to pass those tips on to you.

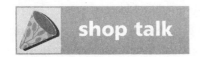 **shop talk**

SHOP TALK offers suggestions to encourage the manager of your local department store or supermarket to stock more green goods. (You can do wonders to stimulate supply simply by asking for an environmental option, even if you don't have a brand name to drop.)

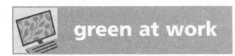 **green at work**

GREEN AT WORK provides easy ways to adapt some of the book's consumer hints to your workplace. Whether you run your company or are an employee, you can incorporate many *Big Green Purse* suggestions on the job.

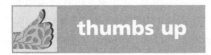 **thumbs up**

THUMBS UP indicates products, services, and practices that merit your money or time because they live up to their claims. For practical ways to benefit the environment, look for Thumbs Up.

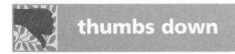 **thumbs down**

THUMBS DOWN signals companies or goods to avoid because they don't benefit the environment. It's a quick way to distinguish the "green" from the "greenwash."

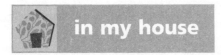 **in my house**

IN MY HOUSE volunteers a reality check. I've been living a green life for almost thirty years now, with a lot of successes and some failures. I've tried to be honest about what's worked for me and what's been a pain in the neck.

Finally, the *Big Green Purse "Little Black Book"* lists reports, websites, books, and organizations to contact for more information.

Because the green marketplace is changing so quickly, I hope you'll log on to the *Big Green Purse* website, www.biggreenpurse.com, where I continually update information and share the latest eco news. You can also download worksheets you can use to record your green expenditures on a daily or weekly basis, making it easy to watch your impact grow. While you're at it, share your shopping experiences, compare notes about what you're buying, and track the effects your purchases are having on specific commodities. Don't forget to sign up for our free Green Purse Alerts! e-newsletter for twice-a-month time- and money-saving eco-tips.

> **Sign Up for Green Purse Alerts!**
> **at www.biggreenpurse.com.**

You can read *Big Green Purse* cover to cover or thumb through it chapter by chapter. Use it to customize a shopping list on your weekly or monthly needs. Toss the book in your purse and take it to the store so you can refer to it when you stroll the aisles. Have it on your desk when you do your Internet shopping. If you find items that belong in the book's next edition or on the *Big Green Purse* website, please let us know, at info@biggreenpurse.com, so we can spread the word to other women.

If we change the way we spend our money, we'll change the world.

I'm going to be honest with you all the way through this book. So let's go back to Mount Kilimanjaro for a moment. Frankly, no matter how much we change the way we shop, we probably can't bring the snows back to the top of that mountain. We're just too late. But there are plenty of other places in the world we can save if we change our own behavior—and if we use our consumer clout to make the marketplace work for the planet, too.

We can be the world's most powerful earth-saving force, but only by buying less—and then intentionally shifting our spending to the products and services that offer the greatest environmental benefit. We have never faced a more exciting opportunity—or necessary moment—to "put our money where our mouth is." Let's get to it!

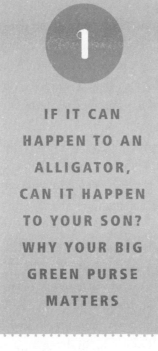

1

IF IT CAN HAPPEN TO AN ALLIGATOR, CAN IT HAPPEN TO YOUR SON? WHY YOUR BIG GREEN PURSE MATTERS

THE ALLIGATOR HAS SURVIVED IN ONE FORM OR ANOTHER FOR AT LEAST eighty million years. It has outlived the *Tyrannosaurus rex*, the mastodon, and the saber-toothed tiger. It has defied ice ages, heat waves, hurricanes, and fires. With its menacing teeth, bulging eyes, and corrugated frame, the alligator seems almost invincible.

Amazing, then, isn't it, that this fierce animal could be susceptible to a chemical designed to kill a mosquito?

After eons of adapting to natural environmental changes, it turns out that alligators are no match for pesticide runoff in the lakes where they live. Scientists studying alligators living in Florida's Lake Apopka discovered that, after years of eating fish that had absorbed the residue of DDT and other man-made chemicals, female alligators were giving birth to males whose penises were on average 25 percent smaller than normal. The males could still swim; they could wrestle a boa constrictor if they had to. Mating, however, was proving to be somewhat beyond their reach.

What does any of this have to do with us?

Like alligators, women are unwittingly exposed to environmental toxins that can build up in our bodies and affect us and our children. This chapter of *Big Green*

Purse focuses on some of the ways we encounter those chemicals and how they may reverberate not just in our sons' bodies, but in our daughters', too.

This chapter also examines global warming, the most serious environmental problem facing the world today. As the old saw goes, being forewarned is being forearmed. The more we know about what causes global warming, the more we can do to prevent it, which is one of the purposes of this book.

Because water and air impact our health and that of the planet, this chapter reviews the state of those resources. In too many ways, pollution is getting the upper hand. The chapter points out what we need to know, and sets the stage for where we should act. One important step we can take is to save our forests, the workhorses of the environment. Forests clean air, filter water, shelter animals, breed plants, and provide a great place to take a walk. We shouldn't be turning them into toothpicks and toilet paper, as I hope this chapter makes clear.

What all these issues have in common is that they determine the well-being not only of the environment, but also of you and me. What you and I have in common is that the actions we take can make a difference. By using our Big Green Purse, we can throw the full weight of our consumer clout behind efforts to protect a planet that desperately needs our help. In doing so, we protect ourselves.

Chemicals in Our Environment

In 2005 the U.S. Centers for Disease Control and Prevention (CDC) discovered 148 toxic chemicals in the bodies of "Americans of all ages." Among the ingredients that had settled into our bones and blood were:

- **Pesticides,** which have been linked to reproductive abnormalities like the kind found in the alligators.
- **Mercury,** which is particularly dangerous for women of childbearing age. Tests on schoolchildren show that kids exposed to mercury in the womb suffer from lower IQs and memory problems.
- **Phthalates,** chemicals that make plastic soft and give fragrances their "stickiness." Phthalates can lead to premature births, alter male reproductive organs, and cause premature breast development in young girls.
- **Pyrethroids,** a common farm and household insecticide that's also sprayed by public agencies to kill mosquitoes. In high doses, pyrethroids are toxic to the

nervous system. At low doses, they might affect hormones. Pyrethroids, says the CDC, exist in children's bodies in concentrations far greater than in adults, a consequence of both kids' quicker metabolism and how much more time they play on the ground.

But that's not all. Scientists at the independent Environmental Working Group found that the breast milk of American women contains the highest levels of flame retardants in the world. Flame retardants, also known as polybrominated diphenyl ethers (PBDE), are widely used in furniture and electronic equipment, among

Chemical Cocktail

Of the 48 commonly used pesticides in schools, the U.S. Centers for Disease Control says:

- 22 are probable or possible carcinogens
- 26 have been shown to affect human reproduction
- 31 damage the nervous system
- 31 injure the liver or kidney
- 41 are sensitizers or irritants
- 16 can cause birth defects

Of the 36 most commonly used lawn pesticides:

- 13 can cause cancer
- 14 cause birth defects
- 11 cause reproductive problems
- 21 are neurotoxic
- 15 are kidney and liver toxicants
- 30 are sensitizers or irritants

Source: Beyond Pesticides

other consumer products. Given their association with learning and memory problems, they're not exactly the kind of "nutrition" you'd willingly feed your child. Additional studies by the Environmental Working Group and Commonweal revealed that the umbilical cord blood in some newborn babies contained an average of two hundred industrial chemicals and pollutants. How could a newborn baby already be burdened with such an extensive chemical profile?

According to the Women's Health and Environment Network, more than 80,000 chemicals are circulating in the marketplace—and only 10 percent have been tested for safety. We come in contact with them not only through the usual questionable suspects, like fertilizers or gasoline. Every day the average American is also exposed to more than one hundred distinct chemicals from personal-care products like shampoo and deodorant. It is the unexpected toxins in these chemicals that put us at risk.

The danger stems from the fact that we're rarely exposed to just one product just one time. More often than not, we come in contact with multiple compounds over and over again. It's this chronic exposure to a legion of contaminants that creates potential problems.

It's like eating M&M's, or potato chips or ice cream sundaes. Just one won't hurt you. But eat bagfuls of candy plus chips plus sundaes and banana splits and the occasional caramel truffle for weeks on end. Before long, you'll pack on the pounds.

The difference, of course, is that you can see the weight you've gained. The chemicals accumulating in our bodies are invisible and may take decades to show up. And when they do, we can't shed them with an Atkins, Weight Watchers, or South Beach–type "lose it fast" plan.

Want to Have a Baby?

What if you wish to bear a child? Thanks to all these chemicals, it appears to be getting more difficult.

In 2007 the Medical Center at the University of California at San Francisco and the National Center of Excellence in Women's Health cohosted a Summit on Environmental Challenges to Reproductive Health and Fertility. Participants reported that, increasingly, "scientific evidence indicates that infertility . . . sperm count decline, pregnancy loss . . . early puberty . . . endometriosis, and cancers in women and men—are associated with environmental contaminants that many Americans are exposed to in their daily lives."

Professor Devra Lee Davis, head of Environmental Oncology at the University of Pittsburgh Medical Center, documented, also in 2007, that as many as one in every four couples experienced difficulty getting pregnant or having normal children. Writing in the journal *Environmental Health Perspectives*, Professor Davis noted that it is "increasingly clear" that exposure to environmental contaminants can lead to "reproductive failure, structural or functional defects, or altered expression of sex at birth."

Professor Davis's research specifically showed that men in the workplace who are exposed to certain pesticides, alcohol, lead, and solvents father fewer sons than expected, while those encountering unusually high levels of dioxin fathered only daughters. Mothers exposed to high levels of PCBs gave birth proportionally to more sons than daughters.

The work of Professor Davis reinforced conclusions shared by doctors, scientists, fertility specialists, and researchers at a groundbreaking conference convened by the University of California at San Francisco in October 2005. The group reported that as many as 7.3 million couples were experiencing difficulty conceiving or carrying a pregnancy to term. This was especially true in women under the age of twenty-five. The reason? Age, heredity, and various lifestyle factors play a part. But "increasing evidence points to environmental factors" as well.

Agreed the scientists, "Even very low doses of some biologically active contaminants can alter gene expression important to reproductive function . . . Exposures during fetal development can adversely affect health of the individual during adulthood, including reproductive health."

Environmental Health Perspectives, a scientific journal published by the National Institute of Environmental Health Sciences, observed in 2006 that in developed countries like the United States, Canada, and Great Britain, "Clues from environmental exposure assessments, wildlife studies, and animal and human studies hint [that] exposure to low-level contaminants . . . may be subtly undermining our ability to reproduce."

We Can Take Our Cues from Wildlife

A big part of the problem stems from the nature of the chemicals themselves. Many of them are considered "endocrine disruptors," man-made synthetic hormones that mimic the function of natural female hormones like progesterone and estrogen.

5

IF IT CAN HAPPEN TO AN ALLIGATOR, CAN IT HAPPEN TO YOUR SON?

When they are released by glands like the thyroid, pituitary, pancreas, and ovaries or testes, endocrine hormones control blood sugar levels, blood pressure, growth, development, aging, and reproduction. But when synthetic estrogen-like chemicals are added to the mix, they can overpower and alter our natural systems. The result?

Female alligators in Florida give birth to male babies with more feminized genitalia. Elsewhere, frogs are showing up with male and female sex organs, a quirk attributed to atrazine, a pesticide used to treat corn and soybeans. Male smallmouth bass in the Chesapeake Bay watershed were found to be carrying eggs, thanks to pharmaceutical chemicals concentrating in the water. Polar bears may be able to conquer arctic ice, but their ovaries and testicles are shrinking due to exposure to PCBs and other chlorine-based chemicals.

And for us? Some of us struggle to conceive and have a baby. Others watch as our daughters reach puberty at startlingly young ages. Many of us are on the lookout for breast cancer, which is increasingly linked to endocrine disruptors and other environmental contaminants.

Where Does It All Begin?

How do these synthetics infiltrate our bodies in the first place? If they're in the pesticide we've put on the lawn, we may inadvertently inhale them. If they're in our deodorant, body lotion, face cream, sunscreen, or lipstick, we inadvertently apply them directly to our skin. When we shower, we wash them down the drain. When it rains, runoff carries the pesticide residue into our waterways.

Few wastewater treatment plants are equipped to remove synthetic hormones from the water they treat. Over time, these chemicals get flushed into waters, including lakes and streams, where aquatic animals absorb them with occasionally devastating effects. We may not be swimming in these chemicals the way an alligator is, but given how many products we're applying to our bodies every day we may as well be.

Children are even more susceptible to environmental contaminants than we are. Pound for pound, children eat more, drink more, and breathe more than adults. The Natural Resources Defense Council points out that a bottle-fed infant consumes relatively huge amounts of water each day: when corrected for body weight, it's as if an adult were to drink seven liters of water or thirty-five cans of soda daily. If that water is contaminated by chemicals, the infant's exposure to them is disproportionately high. The consumption of breast milk is similarly large. Among the chemicals that can invade breast milk are chlordane; DDT; dieldrin, aldrin, and endrin; hexachlorobenzene; hexachlorocyclohexane (lindane) heptachlor; mirex; toxaphene; dioxins and furans; PBDEs; PCBs; lead; mercury, cadmium, and other metals; and solvents.

Who's Not Keeping an Eye Out for Us?

We're supposed to be protected from chemicals in the environment primarily by two federal regulatory agencies, the U.S. Environmental Protection Agency (EPA) and the U.S. Food and Drug Administration (FDA).

For the most part, the EPA and the FDA focus on limiting our exposure to individual chemicals but ignore the sum total of our experience. Hence, the limits they set are often inadequate to protect us from the cumulative buildup our bodies experience.

Likewise, standards set to safeguard the environment treat chemicals as if they were isolated agents rather than ingredients that, as they accumulate over time, can wield a more powerful punch. A release of a small amount of one chemical one time into a lake or stream generally has minimal impact. The constant bombardment of that chemical over months or years is far more consequential. Those alligators didn't lose their virility because their mothers ate just one fish.

One of the ways we can protect ourselves and the environment is to use our purses to choose products that are free of endocrine-disrupting and other toxic chemicals. Chapter 3 focuses specifically on aesthetic and hygienic products that offer safer alternatives to the conventional goods that may currently sit on your bathroom counter. Chapter 6 recommends pesticide-free fruits and vegetables to help minimize the contaminants you eat. Chapter 7 provides lists of phthalate-free cleaning products that will help keep you and the environment safe. Chapter 8 suggests organically grown clothes to help you find fibers that don't require significant pesticide applications to become fabrics. And Chapter 9 offers alternatives for pesticide-free care of your landscape, no matter how big or small.

The Precautionary Principle and Our Right to Know

Our mothers used to say, "A stitch in time saves nine." Today we talk about the Precautionary Principle.

The Precautionary Principle was hammered out at the historic Wisconsin Wingspread conference in 1998 by scientists, researchers, and citizens. They were concerned that industry was using the lack of absolute scientific evidence as a cover to produce products suspected of having serious consequences for human health and the environment.

The principle is grounded in the belief that we should not wait to protect ourselves or the planet until we're absolutely positive, from a scientific point of view, that certain products or activities—think dioxin, the burning of fossil fuels, or even cigarettes—can indeed do damage.

To the contrary, the principle declares: "When an activity raises threats of harm to human health or the environment, precautionary measures should be taken, even if some cause-and-effect relationships are not fully established scientifically."

We only have to look at the host of environmental problems I describe in this chapter to know that taking precautions when warning signals arise makes sense. Global warming is a prime example. A battle has raged for decades as citizens, health advocates, and a majority of scientists have argued in favor of curbing climate-changing carbon dioxide emissions, even though industry argued there was no "definitive" scientific proof that burning fossil fuels would alter the climate and create the planetary crisis we face today. Now we have to worry whether we're too late to fix a problem that could have been forestalled had we acted decades ago.

Industries use scientific uncertainty as a way to avoid cleaning up their act. They often magnify the importance of uncertainty to persuade citizens, legislators, and regulators that they, too, should delay action. At the same time, budget crunches and competing priorities mean that important studies that could document environmental impacts often are shunted aside. Meanwhile, the longer we wait to address a problem, more often than not, the greater the costs become—to the environment, to our health, and to the economy. We have enough history at this point to know that, when it comes to protecting the environment and our health, we should act sooner rather than later.

The Precautionary Principle has four tenets. First, we—consumers, governments, manufacturers—have a duty to respond to **early warnings.** Action must be taken before harm occurs, not after the fact. We don't wait for our child to get hit by a car to tell her to look both ways when crossing the street. We shouldn't need to contract cancer or asthma to use safe ingredients or control the air pollution coming out of cars.

Second, the principle pertains to **"burden of proof."** Under our current system, you and I and, essentially, the planet on which we live, have to prove that we've been harmed before the government is willing to intercede on our behalf and before industry is willing to change the way it does business. Under the Precautionary Principle, the proponents of the questionable activity would need to demonstrate safety. Can this approach work for industry? It's taken hold in Europe. Starting with chemicals already known to cause cancer and birth defects, cosmetics companies are being required to reformulate their products to contain safer ingredients. Ultimately, the goal is to replace all questionable components and make personal-care products as safe as possible. Here in the United States, the nonprofit Campaign for Safe Cosmetics is urging manufacturers to follow suit. In California, the Safe Cosmetics Act will compel cosmetic manufacturers to disclose any ingredient that causes cancer or birth defects. This approach—putting the burden of proof not on you and me but on product manufacturers—should become the law of the land.

Third, the Precautionary Principle requires us to **explore alternatives** to toxic substances and activities. What good does it do us to know, or even suspect, something will harm us if we don't choose a safer alternative? Fortunately, as *Big Green Purse* shows, we have more safe choices than ever, starting with companies that are becoming certified for achieving sustainable standards that restrict use of toxic chemicals.

Fourth, the Precautionary Principle requires **democratic participation.** The idea is to increase public participation in the decisions that affect our lives. Companies should not be allowed to decide our fate in their back rooms. It's up to us to provide guidance as well as accountability by participating in public hearings, writing letters to companies, voting on ballot initiatives, electing responsive public officials, and, of course, using our Big Green Purse in the marketplace to favor products that offer us the healthiest, safest options.

The more we participate, whether by attending a meeting or shopping online, the more informed we'll become. And in the end, information can be just as pow-

The Precautionary Principle

- Pay attention to early warnings; act *before* we get hurt.
- Shift "burden of proof" from us and the planet to manufacturers and producers.
- Develop safe alternatives to toxic substances and activities.
- Involve us—the public—in decision making.

erful as the purse in bringing about environmental change. Each of us has the **right to know** what hazards we may be exposed to, whether during an emergency or in our day-to-day lives. Federal "right to know" laws exist to provide information about chemical disasters, like the accident in Bhopal, India, in which more than two thousand people died or were seriously injured from the unexpected release of the chemical methyl isocyanate. I believe "right to know" should extend to the ingredients in our personal-care products and other consumer goods that potentially put us and the environment at risk every day.

Remember that stitch in time: as you shift your spending to greener products and services, choose sustainably certified companies that let you know what risks are involved, enabling you to take precautions to protect yourself and the planet.

Climate Change

When I first clambered around the Mendenhall glacier outside Juneau, Alaska, in 1977, the sparkling blue ice field seemed impenetrable. Last year, during a business meeting for a nonprofit organization I serve, I stopped by Mendenhall again. I was astounded. The glacier, one of Juneau's premier tourist attractions, has melted so far into the surrounding valley that I'd pretty much need a kayak to reach it. After everything that had been said and written and reported on climate change in the last thirty years, it was still very disheartening to witness such a stark example of it in person—to need, not some snazzy scientific tool to take its measure, but simply my own eyes.

How bad is global warming? It's not just melting glaciers in Alaska that are raising red flags. Hurricanes are increasing in intensity as if Mother Nature's so mad she's throwing one giant hissy fit (which, if you come to think about it, she is). Bugs and noxious plants are expanding their range and threatening all kinds of unpleasant diseases. Some people are dying from the heat. More than a thousand miles north of Mendenhall, polar ice is melting, too. As much as 40 percent of the frozen Arctic sea could be gone by the middle of the century, according to the most recent climate change projections from the National Oceanographic and Atmospheric Administration, based on greenhouse gases already in the atmosphere and those expected to be pumped out in the next two decades. There's already talk of declaring polar bears an endangered species. Will walrus, ringed seals, and other ice-dependent mammals be far behind?

Greenhouse Gas Emissions

Greenhouses always seem so delightful. How can "greenhouse gases" be dastardly enough to change the climate?

A few key human activities—burning fossil fuels like coal or oil; cutting down or burning trees; raising livestock; even producing certain chemicals—release large quantities of heat-trapping gases into the atmosphere. These gases absorb the earth's infrared radiation, preventing it from escaping back into space. Trapping heat close to the surface of the planet raises global temperatures, giving rise to what has become known as the "greenhouse effect." Carbon dioxide (CO_2) is the main greenhouse gas, though not the only one. Like a one-way filter, CO_2 lets energy from the sun pass through it, but absorbs the longer wavelength radiation emitted from the sun, creating an atmospheric greenhouse around the planet. Under normal conditions, greenhouse gases play a very useful role. If none were present, the earth would be much colder than it is now, making life as we know it impossible to maintain. But the buildup of these gases has become so great that excessive amounts of heat are being trapped.

Impact on the Environment

In April 2007 the Intergovernmental Panel on Climate Change, the international body of scientists and researchers that studies global warming, reported on the impact the hotter atmosphere was having on global systems. Their report was dire enough to make you want to park your car and get out your bicycle. Animal and fish migrations—evolutionary rites that have developed over millions of years—are occurring earlier. Birds are laying their eggs sooner in the spring, with potential impact on how many birds survive. Water temperatures in the oceans are intensifying, threatening coral reefs and ocean currents. Sea level is rising, threatening to swamp the homes of the billions of people who live near their country's coasts.

You may have noticed some of these phenomena in your own backyard. I certainly have. At my home in a suburb of Washington, D.C., the wrens that occupy the birdhouse outside the office where I'm writing this book have started returning from their winter migration to Florida a good four weeks early. As happy as I am to have their company, I can't help but worry that they're arriving too soon. Never mind the fact that the chickadees, which winter over here, usually haven't vacated the birdhouse by the time the wrens arrive.

Worldwide, the effects have been wreaking havoc for years. Warmer and drier conditions in northern Africa have shortened the growing season there, leading to crop shortages. The intensity of hurricanes Rita and Katrina, the latter of which destroyed the city of New Orleans and knocked out 10 percent of our ability to refine oil into gasoline, is attributed to climate change.

Things will probably get worse before they get better. Every continent will be affected. In North America, more snow than usual may melt in the Rocky Mountains, leading to floods in the winter and droughts in the summer. Fire may extinguish more forests—especially if they've already been weakened by the bugs and disease that thrive in drier temperatures. Fresh water stored in glaciers and snow is expected to decline, reducing water availability for more than one-sixth of the world's population. Approximately 20 to 30 percent of plant and animal species are at risk of extinction.

Overall, life may get more . . . itchy. New research shows that poison ivy today appears to be growing faster compared to earlier decades. The reason? Rising carbon-dioxide levels in the air create ideal conditions for this pesky plant, which is producing bigger leaves, tougher vines, and oil that's even more irritating. We're likely to get more mosquito and tick bites, too, as the ranges for these insects follow warming trends northward.

What About Our Health?

Climate change is also taking its toll on human health. Extreme heat waves in Paris and other cities around the world have already claimed thousands of lives. The annual Chicago marathon, normally a delightful event run on a cool autumn Sunday, had to be stopped at 11:30 A.M. on October 7, 2007, when temperatures soared to 88 degrees Fahrenheit and dozens of people collapsed from the unseasonably warm weather. In the future, cities such as Los Angeles may also experience record-setting heat, putting senior citizens at great risk. Smog, which can damage lung tissue, worsen respiratory and heart disease, and cause asthma in children, is expected to increase. Health-alert days could escalate by 68 percent over the next few decades due to the higher temperatures associated with global warming.

If you suffer from allergies, chances are you're already experiencing some global warming–related discomfort. Over the past three decades, the early spring has been bringing more than birds with it. The amount of pollen in the atmosphere has significantly increased, accelerating the onset of allergic disorders. Roughly 35 million Americans experience seasonal hay-fever allergies, and about 20 million suffer from asthma. Though the air in many cities is actually cleaner than in the past, reports *The Wall Street Journal*, hay fever has proliferated in the United States over the past few decades, a factor being attributed to climate change. In 2004, asthma affected more than 6 percent of the American population, up from a little over 3 percent in 1980, notes the U.S. Centers for Disease Control and Prevention in Atlanta.

How Will Climate Change Affect Women?

Climate change will in all likelihood cost us more money and take up more time. The Washington State Department of Ecology predicts the price of both water and milk could soar as our communities battle increasing droughts, and as dairy cattle respond to less-than-optimal higher temperatures by producing less milk.

We can also expect to make more trips to the doctor's office. If we're not taking ourselves for allergy or asthma treatments, we'll be carting our kids . . . or our par-

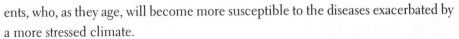

ents, who, as they age, will become more susceptible to the diseases exacerbated by a more stressed climate.

This might simply be viewed as inconvenient to women who enjoy a relatively high standard of living. But to women living in the developing world, or for those who juggle precarious situations here in the United States, climate change will become an extra burden that will make their lives more difficult. Of the twenty thousand people who died in France during the extreme heat wave that wracked Europe in 2003, significantly more were elderly women without substantial means or support networks than men.

Seventy percent of the world's poor are women—yet they're still the ones who feed their families. The more climate change takes hold, women's burdens will increase as they struggle to find cooking fuel and scavenge for food for animals. As fathers leave home to look for work, mothers will be left behind to care for children, maintain the household, and try to eke out an existence in an environment ravaged by climate change. There'll be no time for girls to go to school or women to start or run businesses if they're looking for water.

Who Else Might Be Hurt by Climate Change?

Children also bear a global warming burden. The percentage of children with asthma soared from about 4 percent in 1980 to 9 percent in 2005, according to the U.S. Centers for Disease Control, a jump that's being attributed to the increased pollen in the atmosphere due to global warming.

A report by Save the Children says up to 175 million children could be affected every year over the next decade by climate-related disasters like droughts, floods, and storms.

"Children are already bearing the brunt of climate change and there will be millions more children caught up in climate-related natural disasters every year," worries Jasmine Whitbread, head of Save the Children UK.

Business is starting to feel adverse effects, too. Financial losses from weather-related catastrophes have risen on average by 2 percent a year since the 1970s, reports risk modeling firm Risk Management Solutions. We only have to look at the ongoing devastation in New Orleans from hurricanes Katrina and Rita to appreciate how costly climate change can be.

Some of the most immediate opportunities to reduce global warming exist where we shop. In fact, by using our clout in the marketplace to favor products and services that use less energy, we encourage manufacturers to reduce the greenhouse gases they generate as well. Chapter 4 highlights fuel-efficient vehicles that save energy and emit less carbon dioxide. Chapter 6 suggests food choices that can have a positive climate impact. Chapter 9 reviews lawn-care equipment that minimizes emissions and reduces water pollution, too. And Chapter 11 focuses on energy-saving appliances that will help you use energy more efficiently at home.

Water

Did you make a cup of tea or throw in a load of laundry before starting to read this book? You probably could have, given the easy access most of us have to clean water.

One person of every three on the planet today isn't nearly so fortunate, according to the International Water Management Institute, given their lack of reliable access to fresh water or, in the case of some 2.6 billion people by World Health Organization estimates, proper latrines. Even here in the United States, the federal Government Accountability Office reported in 2003 that "water managers in thirty-six states anticipate water shortages locally, regionally, or statewide within the next ten years." The rest of the world looks equally thirsty. By 2025, worries the Water Management Institute, all of Africa and the Middle East, and almost all of South and Central America and Asia, will either be running out of water or unable to afford its cost.

They'll also be contending with its safety. "Every day more children die from dirty water than HIV-AIDS, malaria, war, and accidents all put together," says Maude Barlow, national chair of the Council of Canadians, a citizens' advocacy group, and coauthor of *Blue Gold: The Battle to Stop the Corporate Theft of the World's Water.* According to a 2003 survey by the European Environment Agency, nitrates, toxins, heavy metals and/or harmful microorganisms contaminate groundwater in nearly every European country and former Soviet republic.

In America, given how easy it is to turn on the tap and enjoy the water that comes gushing out, it's hard to believe a global struggle over water is being waged. If today is an average day, you'll probably use about ninety gallons of water, which amounts to about 107,000 gallons for the year—enough to fill your bathtub almost 3,000 times. We use water to grow lawns, wash dishes, rinse food, shower and shave, and let the tap run when we brush our teeth. About 14 percent leaks down the drain. Our older toilets waste more clean water in a single flush than many Africans use in an entire day. But that doesn't change the facts: only 1 percent of all the world's water can be used for drinking. Nearly 97 percent of the world's water is salty and otherwise undrinkable. The other 2 percent is locked up in the ice caps and glaciers. There is no such thing as "new" water. We are essentially drinking the same water Cleopatra drank two thousand years ago.

In the United States, we count on our tap water to be safe, and for the most part it is. The EPA sets standards for approximately ninety contaminants in drinking water. Outbreaks from microbial contamination—the kind that give you a stomachache or diarrhea—are rare, given how many people are serviced by the public drinking water system. The bigger issue may revolve around chemicals that wastewater treatment facilities weren't designed to remove. The common fertilizer ingredient nitrate, for example, can seep into drinking water through runoff from lawns, gardens, and agricultural fields, causing "blue baby syndrome" if it depletes a newborn baby's hemoglobin. Pregnant and nursing women and the elderly should also avoid water that's high in nitrate content.

Bottled water won't be the solution. Since so much "bottled" water is actually tap water, there's no guarantee there'll be enough to go around (remember, we can't make water). Plus, as you'll read in Chapter 2, packaging bottled water creates a whole host of environmental problems that are better left alone.

Pharmaceuticals—including painkillers, depression medication, and birth control drugs—and endocrine-disrupting chemicals from deodorants, shampoos, body soaps, and lotions are also roiling America's freshwater supplies. The cumulative effect of trace amounts of these chemicals has the EPA concerned, given their links to behavioral and sexual mutations in fish, amphibians, and birds. Part of the problem is that consumers flush old and unwanted drugs down toilets or drains. Another factor is the sheer volume of pharmaceuticals and personal-care products entering our waterways. More Americans, especially aging baby boomers, are taking—and discarding—more drugs than at any time since probably the sixties. In a U.S. Geological Survey/EPA study of 139 streams in 30 states, pharmaceuticals were found in 80 percent of the samples taken.

Possible effects of this medicinal runoff are showing up among the fish in the Chesapeake Bay watershed, a region that drains Pennsylvania, Virginia, Maryland, Delaware, and Washington, D.C. Smallmouth bass in the Potomac and Shenandoah rivers have turned up sporting both male and female sex organs . . . on the same fish. The suspected causes include "previously banned compounds . . . such as DDT and chlordane, natural and anthropogenic hormones, herbicides, fungicides, industrial chemicals" and other compounds that might act as endocrine disruptors, according to a 2006 summary of the various studies prepared by the U.S. Geological Survey.

The National Academy of Sciences is worried, too. Its list of "naturally occurring and man-made contaminants in drinking water [that] are of concern to all of us" includes: arsenic, perchlorate (a component of rocket fuel and fireworks), copper, and methylmercury, the scourge of parents anxious about learning disabilities and developmental disorders in their kids.

Evidence is growing that trichloroethylene (TCE), a solvent widely used as a degreasing agent, is contaminating air, soil, and water at several military installations and hundreds of waste sites around the country. Research suggests that TCE may cause kidney cancer and other kidney problems, reproductive and developmental problems, impaired neurological function, and autoimmune disease. Meanwhile, work by the National Research Council, the research arm of the National Academy of Sciences, has strengthened the evidence of a link between bladder and lung cancer and exposure to arsenic in drinking water.

The ocean's misfortune is also our own, for reasons that have to do with some factors we've already discussed, like climate change and chemical pollution. Twenty percent of coral reefs and 35 percent of mangroves have been lost since 1980, along with their capacity to buffer coastal communities from storms. With nearly half the world's cities located within 50 kilometers of a coast, people are more vulnerable than ever before to extreme weather events, like the Asian tsunami and hurricane Katrina. Over half of the synthetic nitrogen ever used to fertilize American farmland has been applied in the last two decades. As much as 50 percent of it has run off, creating dead zones in great aquatic cauldrons like the Gulf of Mexico that make short shrift of those shrimp you like to serve for dinner.

As hopeless as all this sounds, there are dozens of meaningful ways you can use your purse to protect water. Chapters 3 and 9 will help you find makeup, deodorant, shampoo, and lawn and garden chemicals that won't pollute the water supply or turn male fish into females. Chapter 6 suggests opportunities to buy organically grown food; Chapter 8 focuses on organically grown cotton and other fibers. Both highlight the benefits of organic agriculture in protecting water quality. Chapter 7 lists cleansers for your bathroom, kitchen, and living room that provide good alternatives to more-industrial solvents.

Forests

Your morning coffee. A chocolate truffle. The Sunday paper.

You think of these treats as life's essential pleasures. What they have in common is that they are all products of a forest.

Coffee and chocolate both derive from plants that grow naturally in rain forests, as do one-quarter of the medicinal drugs prescribed in the United States. Paper is made from forests found in many parts of the world, tropical and temperate alike. Toothpicks and toilet paper? They were once trees, too.

Let's talk about rain forests first. Half of all plant and animal species in the world live in rain forests. Yet it's been said that we know more about some areas of the moon than we do about these great tropical jungles. In a typical four-square-mile patch, the National Academy of Sciences has found as many as fifteen hundred species of flowering plants and at least seven hundred fifty kinds of trees, plus hundreds of different species of mammals, birds, reptiles, amphibians, and butterflies. Imagine a treasure chest brimming with not just the jewels you know, but also gems you've never even heard of. That's what the bounty in the rain forest is like.

Despite this abundance rain forests are disappearing at the rate of six soccer fields a minute. If deforestation continues unabated, these ecological riches will be lost forever.

Why are the forests vanishing? In the tropics, trees are being burned for fuel and chopped up for building materials. Mahogany and other rare tropical hardwoods are recast as living room furniture. Teak ends up as patio lounge chairs. Forests are also decimated to clear acreage for cattle ranching and coffee estates. Forty percent of Central American rain forests have been converted into pastures for beef production, 90 percent of which is exported to the United States primarily for use in the fast-food market or in pet food. Increasingly, rain forests are being razed to grow soybeans for animal feed and to plant sugar cane to fuel Brazil's booming ethanol industry.

What about the forests closer to home? The United States is losing 1 million acres of forests—an area larger than all of Rhode Island—to housing development annually, according to the U.S. Forest Service. Thirteen million acres, an area almost the size of West Virginia, have been lost since 1992.

Trees are also being chopped, pulped, and bleached so they can become paper. Astoundingly, nearly half the trees cut in North America are used to make paper.

According to the Center for a New American Dream, U.S. paper consumption is the world's highest, devouring 12,430 square miles of forests each year. All the notepads, paper bags, reams of computer paper, and wrapping paper you use? It really adds up: each American on average consumes upwards of 730 pounds of paper each year, an amount when all of us are counted together that requires more than 535 million trees and twelve billion gallons of oil to produce.

Not only is the U.S. paper industry the country's largest single consumer of wood, the industry also ranks first in use of industrial process water, third in toxic chemical releases, and fourth in emissions of the air pollutants that cause respiratory problems. Overall, pulp and paper manufacturing is the third-most-polluting industry in North America and one of the largest and most-polluting enterprises in the world. Little wonder that recycling is so ecologically appealing: producing recycled paper generates 74 percent less air pollution and 35 percent less water pollution than producing paper from trees, while creating five times the number of jobs.

In addition to preserving life-giving species, forests regulate the flow of water on earth. Like a gigantic sponge, they soak up rainwater, then release it slowly and steadily, providing a constant supply for people and farmers living hundreds, even thousands of miles away. Forests also play a central role in the global recycling of carbon, another process that can affect global warming. Trees absorb carbon dioxide as they grow. But when they are burned or logged, the carbon they contain, as well as some of the carbon in the underlying soil, goes back into the air, adding to a carbon dioxide buildup that is weaving a blistering atmospheric blanket around the entire globe. According to Environmental Defense, the burning of tropical forests accounts for at least 10 percent of the greenhouse effect.

In the world's drier tropical regions, deforestation brings other dangers. As forests recede, deserts expand. In fact, desertification commonly follows deforestation because water runs off bare hills too quickly, carrying topsoil with it and disturbing the water balance. As crops fail, domestic animals die, water sources dry up, and fuel wood becomes scarcer, prospects for survival by person or beast dwindle. Thirty-five million people in Africa alone have been threatened by drought, in part as a result of increasing deforestation. Trees can intercept rainfall and allow soil to absorb much of the water before it runs off, keeping an area moist, preventing drought and desertification, and staving off erosion.

Intact forests can be literal lifesavers. A study of mangrove forests in Sri Lanka after the tsunami of 2004 showed that healthy trees that bore the brunt of the waves' force were not uprooted, mitigating the floodwaters' impact on the shores behind them. In areas where the mangroves had been even slightly disturbed, however, impact on the coast was more devastating.

Chapter 5 points out the value of growing crops like coffee and cocoa in the understory of the rain forest—rather than on land cleared of trees—as a way of protecting natural habitat. Chapter 6 focuses on ways to trim meat from your diet as a way of protecting rain forests from the grazing that leads to their destruction. Chapter 12 suggests opportunities to use your purse to support and expand the growing sustainable furniture industry by furnishing your home in ways that sustain the rain forest, too.

Air

Perhaps even more than living in a climate that doesn't change or having access to a forest full of trees, we feel entitled to breathe clean air. And no wonder. When women respire the polluted air that's common in many cities, we also increase our risk of heart disease.

Air pollution is made up of minuscule particles of dirt, dust, soot, and grit that come from burning fuel at power plants, industrial facilities, and cars. When we inhale dirty air, these "particulates" can get stuck deep inside our lungs. If our lungs become inflamed as a result, we could have a heart attack or stroke. According to a University of Washington study, women are more susceptible than men to air pollution and the heart problems it causes because, among other reasons, our blood vessels are smaller than men's.

Both women and men are vulnerable to increased ailments like asthma when the air is bad. The Environmental Protection Agency estimates that the two sexes may suffer as many as 554,000 asthma attacks each year due to air pollution. Carbon monoxide, a colorless, odorless, poisonous gas created by cars and power plants, poses another significant risk, especially to heart patients. Carbon monoxide reduces the amount of oxygen available to body tissues and weakens heart contractions, reducing blood flow from head to toe.

Though much pollution occurs when cars and industrial plants burn fossil fuels, the Union of Concerned Scientists warns that other highly toxic air pollutants also pose serious health risks. These include pesticides that evaporate from fields or our gardens and emissions from chemical plants and sewage-treatment facilities. Acid rain is caused by emissions of sulfur dioxide and nitrogen oxides. Each year, almost twenty-five million tons of sulfur dioxide are pumped into the sky, primarily from furnaces run by coal-burning utilities and certain metal smelters. Nitrogen oxides come principally from motor vehicle exhaust and stationary sources like electric utilities and industrial boilers that burn coal or oil. Ground-level ozone, the main component of smog, forms when sunlight combines with nitrogen dioxide and hydrocarbons. Not only does it retard crop and tree growth and limit visibility, it can also send asthmatics into a coughing, wheezing, or breathing frenzy.

At least 2.4 billion pounds of dangerous pollutants are released into the air each year from every state. The chemical industry spews the most, but any factory that burns coal or oil does its part. Some 225 U.S. counties, including much of the urban Midwest and East, violate minimal air-quality standards, suffering from more air pollution than is legally permitted under the federal Clean Air Act and endangering the lives of more than 100 million Americans. The American Academy of Pediatrics believes that as many as twenty-eight million children have been put at risk because the air is too dirty to breathe safely.

Unfortunately, the science lessons we learned in middle school are still true: what goes up must come down. At least 80 percent of the toxic pollution in Lake Superior and up to 50 percent of the toxic pollution in Lakes Michigan and Huron comes from the atmosphere. More than eight hundred toxic chemicals, some from as far away as Central America and Asia, have been found in the water, fish, and wildlife of the Great Lakes. It also explains why, if you're pregnant or planning to have a baby, the EPA says you should avoid eating tuna and swordfish. In all likelihood, these fish have absorbed mercury that was spewed into the sky from a coal-fired power plant, then fell into a lake or sea before being inadvertently concentrated in their meat.

If these compounds fall on the land, they may return to earth as toxic rain, snow, fog, or dust. When the environment cannot neutralize the components, damage occurs. Thousands of acres of woodlands have been chemically stripped on hills and mountaintops stretching from Maine to Georgia, from the Rocky Mountains to the Sierra Nevadas, leaving behind a swath of ghostly forests spiked by withering trees.

As a consumer, you can make the biggest difference to air quality in the way you use energy and in the products you buy that have been produced in the least energy-intensive way. Chapter 4 highlights vehicles that reduce air pollution. Chapter 6 will help you buy organically grown food that didn't contribute to airborne pesticides. Chapter 11 focuses on how you can save energy at home by using appliances more efficiently and adopting alternative sources of energy.

Make Your Money Matter

You've all heard the expression "Money talks." But have you ever wondered "Who's listening?" As it turns out, manufacturers of the products you buy are paying close attention to your every purchase. When you shift your spending to goods and services that protect you from dangerous chemicals, slow climate change, safeguard the air you breathe and the water you drink, and restore our forests, you're as good as talking directly to industries. And what are you saying? Protect the planet, don't pollute it—or us. As the rest of *Big Green Purse* makes clear, there's no sense whispering about that, is there?

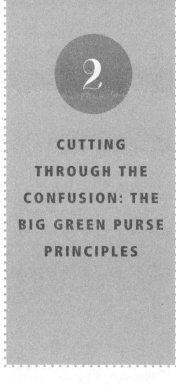

2

CUTTING THROUGH THE CONFUSION: THE BIG GREEN PURSE PRINCIPLES

WHEN SHOULD YOU SPEND YOUR MONEY TO PROTECT THE PLANET—AND when should you keep it in your purse?

Given the thousands of green products being introduced these days and the vague marketing claims used to sell them, you don't want to blow your budget just to keep up with the newest "eco," "herbal," or "biodegradable" fad. Consider Crest "Natural" toothpaste. Sure, it's flavored with mint and lemon, but does that make it more natural than any other toothpaste on the shelf? Or is the company simply trying to exploit your hankering for green goods to extract the greenbacks from your bag?

On the other hand, genuinely earth-friendly products do help minimize your environmental impact. Every organic cotton T-shirt you buy, for instance, helps reduce the use of toxic agricultural chemicals, protecting the air and water. Moreover, that same tee waves like a bright green flag in front of conventional cotton producers, reminding them that your money is filling their organic competitors' coffers. Using your Big Green Purse to favor companies whose goods protect the climate, eliminate toxins, keep the air and water clean, and safeguard forests and other natural places creates a powerful incentive for their rivals to follow suit.

The challenge is in knowing how to avoid the "greenwash" so you can promote more green. A few clear principles will help you distinguish an ecobargain from a rip-off, while getting manufacturers to transition as quickly as possible to the most earth-friendly practices available.

THE BIG GREEN PURSE SHOPPING PRINCIPLES

1. Buy less.
2. Read the label.
3. Support sustainable standards.
4. Look for third-party verification.
5. Choose fewer ingredients.
6. Pick less packaging.
7. Buy local.

❶ Buy Less

Okay, let's get the "sacrifice" message out there in the open first. If we really want to protect the planet, we have to stop consuming so many resources and producing so much waste. There's a reason "reduce" is the first R in the environmental mantra "Reduce, Reuse, Recycle." Between 1972 and 1987, the U.S. population grew by only 16 percent—but the amount of garbage we generated increased by 35 percent. Right now, according to the U.S. Environmental Protection Agency (EPA), each one of us throws away three-quarters of a ton of garbage every year. All together, that's enough trash to fill the Louisiana Superdome twice a day, every day. If we each cut waste by only 5 percent, we could collectively "lose" more than 20 billion pounds of trash every year. Talk about a diet worth sticking to!

What else do we have to gain if we reduce?

Environmental domino effect. Using less scales back manufacturing, which prevents pollution, helps curtail global warming and climate change, and protects air, water, and wildlife.

Money in the bank. Using less leads to buying less, which leads to money in the bank that can be saved for retirement or spent on items with minimal eco-impact, like kids' college tuition or extra mortgage payments.

Less stuff, more fun. Buying less leaves more time to enjoy friends and family, explore the outdoors, read, listen to music, play, exercise, garden, learn a new skill, perfect an old skill, resume a hobby, and simply get more out of life. Americans on average spend six hours each week shopping for goods that may not even be necessary. According to polls, about 53 percent of grocery and 47 percent of hardware store purchases are spur of the moment; only 25 percent of shoppers shop for specific items. Rather than hassle with traffic, long cashier lines, strip malls, and online shopping sites, wouldn't you rather pursue activities that enrich your life rather than deplete your pocketbook as well as the planet?

Does buying less mean you need to do without? Not at all. Remember the mantra. In addition to reduce, "reuse" and "recycle" play important roles.

"Free" Trade. Thanks to the Internet, active opportunities exist for donating, bartering, and trading your goods. For example, the online Freecycle Network connects people who want to give or get stuff for free in their own towns. Whether you need to dispose of an item you no longer want—like a chair, a fax machine, a piano, or a bicycle—or get something "new" yourself, e-mail your local Freecyclers (www.freecycle.org). Craigslist (www.Craigslist.org) provides another opportunity to barter, exchange, donate, and cheaply buy used goods.

Neighborhood Listserv. You can create your own version of Freecycle by establishing a neighborhood Listserv. I've saved hundreds of dollars on garden plants, kids' toys and clothes, books, DVDs, fitness equipment, cookware, home appliances, and other items by "shopping" the free postings that appear on my neighborhood Listserv. I reciprocate by posting my own offerings. Websites like Yahoo! groups make it easy to launch community Listservs.

Thrift shop/yard sales. Buy gently used items at bargain basement prices from thrift shops and yard sales. Make some extra cash yourself (or let the kids earn spending money) by cleaning out closets and selling clothes and toys at the local consignment shop or at an annual yard sale hosted by your family or others in the neighborhood.

Rent, borrow, or share. Renting or borrowing equipment is more eco-friendly than buying items you may use only once or a few times a year. Some of the most commonly rented items include trailers, carpet shampooers, lawn-care equipment, folding tables and chairs, ladders, power tools, tents, and tree trimmers. If you need a big-ticket item like a snowblower or a leaf shredder, share with a neighbor. Borrow appliances and tools that you only need occasionally, and lend yours just as freely.

Just buy one. Instead of many different types of products, use one for several purposes. Cleansers are a perfect example. There seems to be a different cleaner for every surface in your house: windows, countertops, bathtubs, floors, walls, doorknobs, and more. Why not buy one general-purpose cleaner you can use on most surfaces? You'll reduce the number of containers you throw away, save money buying so many different products, minimize your exposure to all the different chemicals those products contain, and reduce the amount of time you spend shopping.

Save paper. The Center for a New American Dream estimates that recycling one ton of paper saves 17 trees, 7,000 gallons of water, and 380 gallons of oil—enough energy to heat the average home for six months. Buy recycled paper, then recycle the paper you use. Print only final drafts of documents, and print on both sides to cut paper consumption in half. Find other ways to use less paper at www.big greenpurse.com.

Get a library card. Enjoy books, CDs, and DVDs from your local library. For years, my community also maintained a tool library, providing easy access to a saw, lawn mower, weed and grass trimmer, and other expensive or unusual equipment without having to buy or maintain it.

Use the Internet. Currently, less than 5 percent of paper consumed to produce magazines is recycled, and most DVD and CD cases are made from hard-to-recycle PVC plastic or polystyrene, reports green blog Ideal Bite. Read newspapers and magazines online—you may still pay for the subscription, but you'll be saving paper, energy, and other natural resources. For the same reason, download music, videos, TV shows, and movies (legally, of course) rather than buy the CD or DVD. Get updates to this book online at www.biggreenpurse.com.

Close the loop. Not only use less yourself, but also ask product manufacturers to reduce the natural resources they consume by incorporating more recycled materials into the goods they make. If your community offers curbside recycling, join in. Otherwise, locate the nearest recycling center by checking www.earth 911.org. Donating books to libraries, hospitals, shelters, and schools helps minimize their need to buy new, too. Selling your books to used bookstores and the "buy back" programs cropping up at airports keeps the same books circulating among many readers.

② Read the Label

We've learned to read food labels to avoid trans fats, sugar, and salt. Why not read labels on the cleansers, personal-care products, furniture, clothing, and home-improvement goods we buy so we can more easily shift our spending to those that offer the greatest environmental benefit? Look for the following clues so you can beware of "greenwashing" and be a savvy shopper:

- Products labeled "natural" may contain some biological ingredients, but they may also include synthetic dyes and fragrances.
- "Hypoallergenic" has no medical meaning. The word was invented by advertisers who used it in a cosmetics campaign in 1953. Says the FDA, "There are no federal standards or definitions that govern the use of the term hypoallergenic. [It] means whatever a particular company wants it to mean."
- "Biodegradable" should mean that, when a product is exposed to air, moisture, bacteria, or other organisms, it will break down and return to its natural state within a reasonably short time. However, no government entity verifies the accuracy of a biodegradable claim; the term is often used simply to provide a marketing edge to a product that otherwise has no real environmental attributes.
- "Free range" implies that a meat or poultry product, including eggs, comes from an animal that was raised in the open air or was free to roam. But a vendor can give his livestock as little as five minutes of fresh air and still make the claim. Free range . . . or free rein to greenwash you, the concerned ecoshopper?
- "Fragrance-free" suggests a product has no perceptible smell; however, synthetic ingredients may have been added to mask odors.

Since no government standards define specific "eco" terms, companies can use these words to gain a marketing advantage regardless of their accuracy. The Federal Trade Commission (FTC) prohibits deceptive advertising and has issued guidelines encouraging manufacturers to substantiate environmental claims, but the agency rarely enforces its own rules.

Product names, too, can be misleading. Take Clairol's Herbal Essences shampoo. It sounds like something Mother Nature might have concocted herself. But consider the ingredients: water, sodium laureth sulfate, sodium lauryl sulfate, cocamido propyl betaine, sodium chloride, citric acid, sodium citrate, fragrance, passiflora incarnata flower extract, anthemis nobilis flower extract, aloe barbadensis flower extract, PEG-60 almond glycerides, cocamide MEA, sodium benzoate, tetrasodium EDTA, guar hydroxypropyltrimonium chloride, linoleamidopropyl pg-dimonium

Words That Make You Buy but May Not Mean a Thing

Biodegradable	Environmentally safe
Cruelty-free	Free range
Dermatologist tested	Green
Earth smart	Natural, nature's friend
Ecosafe	No additives
Environmentally friendly	Nontoxic

chloride phosphate, sodium xylene sulfonate, methylchloroisothiazolinone, methylisothiazolinone, yellow 5, orange 4, ext. violet 2. Does that sound like the "essence of herbs" to you?

Don't be fooled by a label or name that sounds green or healthy but fails to deliver specific environmental and health benefits.

Focus on energy. Given the critical need to reverse global warming, we need to do everything possible to use less energy, particularly fossil fuels. Yet trying to buy products that minimize climate change specifically is a challenge. No labels—yet—list a product's "carbon content" or "climate impact" so you can tell how much that product contributes to the warming of the earth's atmosphere. The Climate Counts website (www.climatecounts.org) ranks dozens of consumer companies for effectiveness in curbing climate change. The rankings are available online and by cell phone so you can access a company's score while you're shopping. Two labels—EPA's Energy Star, see page 31, and the Energy Guide for appliances you'll read about in Chapter 11—make it easy to figure out how much energy most electronics and household appliances consume. The Green-E label, described on page 32, showcases companies that use renewable energy like wind to avoid contributing to global warming.

Check for signal words. The words "caution," "warning," "danger," and "poison" indicate the level of hazard a given product poses, in that order. Always choose the least hazardous product to do the job.

Tune in to specifics. A paperboard package composed of "50 percent recycled fiber" is a more reliable ecobuy than one vaguely marketed as "made from recycled paper." A "biodegradable" lawn fertilizer is iffy compared to one that "biodegrades in forty-eight hours, leaving by-products completely safe for birds and insects."

③ Support Sustainable Standards

You could avoid greenwashing traps and label ambiguities altogether if more companies adopted comprehensive standards guaranteeing that their products were fully "sustainable": that they protected public health and the environment throughout their entire commercial "life cycle," from the extraction of raw materials through their manufacture and use to final disposal or reuse in a new product.

SMART Certified (http://mts.sustainableproducts.com/standards.htm), a program of the Institute for Market Transformation to Sustainability (MTS), rates building products, fabrics, apparel, textiles, and flooring by considering the product's complete life cycle. It evaluates a manufacturer's success in reducing more than thirteen hundred pollutants; in using renewable energy as well as postconsumer recycled or organic materials; and in reusing materials to save energy, water, and other resources. Through this life-cycle analysis, SMART encourages industries to achieve ambitious environmental goals that benefit society and the economy, too.

For example, if just one 100,000-square-foot building adopted the SMART standards, it could save:

- $80,000/yr in energy costs through the use of ten different efficiencies
- $93,000 through waste reduction, keeping 186 tons out of the landfill
- $44,000/yr for avoided wastewater treatment from water-conserving equipment
- $53,368/yr through the use of energy-efficient appliances and lighting

Right now, SMART certification covers sustainable lighting; furniture, home, and building products; apparel, fabric, and textiles; and carpet. The California Gold standard duplicates the SMART standard for sustainable carpet. You can find a list of many of the companies that have achieved sustainable certification at http:mts.sustainableproducts.com/standards.

---

① Look for Third-Party Verification

In the absence of universal sustainable standards, if a company says it's good for the earth, your first question should be, "Who else says so?"

Increasingly, reliable ecoproducts are being backed up by an independent institution or nonprofit organization that has investigated the manufacturer's claims so you don't have to. These third-party certifiers apply meaningful criteria consistently to all products on which a particular label is used. Here are some of the certifications you are likely to see:

LABELS TO LOOK FOR

Green Seal (www.greenseal.org) provides science-based environmental certification standards for hundreds of products and services ranging from coffee and paint to windows and sticky notes. To earn the Green Seal, a product must meet rigorous evaluation and testing objectives, as must the plant where it is manufactured.

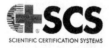

Scientific Certification Systems (www.scs1.com); SCS certifies environmental claims related to recycled content, certified organic ingredients, water efficiency, and sustainable forestry. (Many products in Home Depot's Eco Options line have been certified by SCS.) SCS certifications meet international environmental labeling standards as well as guidelines issued by the U.S. Federal Trade Commission for responsible environmental marketing.

The Forest Stewardship Council (http://fscus.org); the FSC accredits other organizations to certify wood from responsibly managed forests. In the United States, Scientific Certification Systems (see above) and the Rainforest Alliance's **SmartWood** (www.rainforest-alliance.org/programs/forestry/smartwood/) **program,** among others, have been accredited by the FSC to evaluate claims that forests are being managed in an environmentally responsible way. Once certified, flooring, furniture, paper, and construction materials can carry the FSC logo.

 The Leadership in Energy and Environmental Design (LEED®) Green Building Rating System is the nationally accepted benchmark for the design, construction, and operation of high-performance green buildings. A program of the U.S. Green Building Council (www.usgbc.org), LEED promotes a whole-building approach to sustainability by recognizing performance in five key areas of human and environmental health: sustainable site development, water savings, energy efficiency, materials selection, and indoor environmental quality.

  Chlorine Free Products Association (www.chlorine freeproducts.org) certifies paper mills for chlorine-free and processed chlorine-free production. **Processed Chlorine Free** certification indicates recycled content paper that has not been rebleached with chlorine-containing compounds. A minimum of 30 percent post-consumer content is required. **Totally Chlorine Free** certification indicates papers that do not use pulp produced with any chlorine or chlorine-containing compounds as bleaching agents. Wood from virgin forests cannot be used to make paper that carries either label.

 Energy Star (www.energystar.gov), a joint program of the U.S. Environmental Protection Agency and the U.S. Department of Energy, certifies energy-saving products and practices. Energy Star homes and buildings, appliances, computers, lightbulbs, copiers, printers, furnaces, and many other products meet strict energy-efficiency guidelines that help save energy and money and protect the environment.

 The **VeriFlora** label (www.veriflora.com), developed by SCS, is awarded to flower growers who do not use "extremely hazardous" or "highly hazardous" agrochemicals. The VeriFlora label also indicates that growers are converting to organic and sustainable crop-production practices. The standard contains extensive water and ecosystem protection measures to ensure that farmers are not damaging surrounding wildlife or habitats. In addition, it requires growers to provide a fair, equitable, and safe workplace.

Fair Trade Certified (www.fairtradecertified.org) is the label issued by Trans Fair USA to demonstrate that the farmers and workers behind Fair Trade goods were paid fair wages and have opportunities for better health care, housing, and education. The program also supports community development and environmental stewardship. The Fair Trade label is attached to coffee, chocolate, cocoa, tea, fruit, rice, sugar, and spices produced in developing countries.

Certified Humane Raised & Handled (www.certifiedhumane.org) provides independent verification that the care and handling of livestock and poultry on farms enrolled in the program meet high-quality, humane animal-care standards. These include access to clean and sufficient food and water; sufficient protection from inclement weather; and enough space to move about naturally.

Leaping Bunny (www.leapingbunny.org) is the certification program of the Coalition for Consumer Information on Cosmetics. The mark certifies that companies have not tested their products on animals during any stage of development. The company's ingredient suppliers make the same pledge, resulting in a product guaranteed to be 100 percent free of new animal testing. The Leaping Bunny label can be found on cosmetics and personal-care, household, and cleaning products.

Marine Stewardship Council (www.msc.org) provides an eco-label for fish that come from certified sustainable and well-managed fisheries. Any fish bearing the MSC eco-label can be traced to an independently certified sustainable fishery. Wal-Mart plans to purchase all of its wild-caught fresh and frozen fish for the North American market from MSC-certified fisheries within the next three to five years.

Green E (www.green-e.org), administered by the Center for Resource Solutions, identifies companies that generate at least 50 percent of their power from renewable sources like wind and solar energy.

big green purse

For information on more labels, or to verify a specific eco-label claim, see the Consumers Union Guide to Environmental Labels, www.eco-labels.org.

Certified Organic Products

One eco claim that has been validated after years of public debate is "certified organic."

According to the USDA's national organic standard, (www .ams.usda.gov/NOP/Consumers/Consumerhome.html), products labeled **"100 percent organic"** must contain only organically produced ingredients. Products labeled **"organic"** must consist of at least 95 percent organically produced ingredients. Products meeting the requirements for "100 percent organic" or "organic" may display the USDA Organic seal.

Processed products that contain **at least 70 percent organic ingredients** may use the phrase "made with organic ingredients" and list up to three of the organic ingredients or food groups on the principal display panel. For example, soup made with at least 70 percent organic ingredients and only organic vegetables may be labeled either "made with organic peas, potatoes, and carrots" or "made with organic vegetables." The USDA seal may not be used anywhere on the package.

Processed products that contain **less than 70 percent organic ingredients** may not use the term "organic" other than to identify the specific ingredients that are organically produced in the ingredients statement.

Note: Organic standards for pet foods, fabrics, cosmetics and personal-care products, over-the-counter medications, dietary supplements, fertilizers, and soil amendments have not been as rigorously developed as have the standards for food. If you have any question about the organic claims a company is making, contact the Organic Trade Association (www.ota.com) for guidance.

Despite the success of the organic label, some corporations and members of Congress are trying to weaken the USDA's organic standards and allow conventional chemical-intensive and factory farm practices on organic farms. In September 2007, Aurora Organic Dairy was forced to remove the organic label from some of its milk for violating federal organic regulations. Support efforts by the Organic Consumers Association and others to maintain and strengthen organic standards. You can get more information at www.organicconsumers.org.

⑤ Choose Fewer Ingredients

Generally speaking, the fewer ingredients a product contains, the less hazardous it is likely to be. This is especially true for personal-care and cleaning products, where a long ingredients list often indicates the presence of questionable chemicals.

Compare the ingredients in two similar hand lotions:

Organic Essence Lotion to Go
Certified organic beeswax, certified organic safflower oil, certified organic shea butter, certified organic cocoa butter, certified organic lemongrass oil, and certified organic rosemary extract

L'Occitaine Harvest Ice Hand Cream Gel Verbena
Water, alcohol denat., tapioca starch, cyclomethicone, glycerin, glyceryl polymethacrylate, menthyl lactate, ammonium acryloyldimethyltaurate/vp copolymer, lippia citriodora flower extract, PPG-26 buthet-26, PEG-40 hydrogenated castor oil, chlorphenesin, fragrance, butyl/ethyl/methyl/propylparaben, ethyhexyl methoxycinnamate/octinoxate, butyl methoxydibenzoylmethane/avobenzone, cyclohexasiloxane, ethylhexyl salicylate/octisalate, tetrasodium edta, propylene glycol, cyclopentasiloxane, gardenia florida extract, citral, limonene, geraniol, hexyl cinnamal, benzyl benzoate, linalool, benzyl alcohol, citronellol

Or

Burt's Bees Farmer's Friend Hand Salve
Sweet almond oil, olive oil, beeswax, tocopheryl acetate, tocopherol (vitamin E), comfrey root extract, rosemary oil & leaf extract, lavandin oil & flower extract, eucalyptus oil

Neutrogena Visibly Younger Hand Cream
Octinoxate 7.5%, Avobenzone 3%. Inactive ingredients: water, glycerin, glycolic acid, glyceryl distearate, dimethicone, cetearyl alcohol, stearyl alcohol, ceteareth 20, steareth-10, ammonium hydroxide, cholesterol, ascorbic acid, BHT, camellia oleifera leaf extract, tocopherol, calcium pantothenate, retinol, polysorbate 80, eth-

ylhexyl hydroxystearate, trimethylolpropane triethylhexanoate, butylene glycol, polysorbate 20, disodium EDTA, acrylates/C10-30 alkyl acrylates crosspolymer, methylparaben, phenoxyethanol, propylparaben, fragrance

According to the Safe Cosmetics Data Base maintained by the nonprofit Environmental Working Group, both Burt's Bees and Organic Essence pose no or a low health hazard to consumers. The sheer number of ingredients in the Neutrogena and L'Occitaine products increases the likelihood that at least some of the chemicals used pose risks to the environment and human health. You can compare these and other lotions using the EWG's Skin Deep cosmetics safety database (www.cosmeticsdatabase.com).

Now compare two countertop cleansers, courtesy of the National Institutes of Health Materials Safety Data Base (MSDB):

Baking Soda
Sodium bicarbonate

Comet Cleanser with Chlorinol
Fragrance(s) perfume(s), sodium carbonate, calcium carbonate (limestone), quartz, sodium dichloroisocyanurate dihydrate, colorant/pigment/dye(s), quality control agent(s)

It's not clear in the MSDB what additional chemicals make up the "fragrance(s) perfume(s)," "colorant/pigment/dye(s)," or "quality control agent(s)"; as you'll read in Chapter 3, "fragrance" usually consists of phthalates, chemical compounds that can harm fish and frogs and that have been linked to reproductive abnormalities in people. Neither is it known from the MSDB listing what chemicals comprise the other ingredients, though it is fair to say that you and the environment are exposed to more chemicals using Comet than you are using mere sodium bicarbonate.

When you have a choice between two products, other factors being equal, choose the one with the fewest ingredients.

⑥ Pick Less Packaging

When I ask women what annoys them most after a shopping experience, many respond, "All the plastic and paper wrapping I have to throw away!"

Obviously, some packaging is necessary. It protects food from contamination or getting spoiled. It prevents damage during shipping. Packaging can also provide useful information. Plus, some products need packaging that is tamperproof and child-resistant.

But packaging often serves as nothing more than an advertising ploy to get you to buy. According to the EPA, during the past thirty-five years, the amount of waste each person creates has almost doubled, from 2.7 to 4.4 pounds per day. One out of every eleven dollars we spend at the store pays for packaging. The frozen dinner is a good example. When you buy a meal in a box, you pay not only for supper but for the outer paperboard, the plastic or foil tray that holds the meal, and the plastic wrap covering the food. What you eat pales in comparison to what you throw away. No wonder, when all packaging is accounted for, it adds up to about one-third of the trash that we generate.

Your alternatives?

- Cleaning and personal-care products with sealed, tamperproof bottle tops and lids but sold without extra paperboard, plastic wrap, or other type of secondary packaging.
- Detergents, bleaches, cleansers, and fabric softeners in "ultra" or concentrated forms (the smaller containers require fewer materials for manufacture and shipping).
- Fresh fruits and vegetables sold in bulk; packaged meals sold in one box or bag rather than a tray plus liner plus wrapper.
- Create the "one trash can" rule: in our house, we aim to fill no more than one can of trash every week. We manage it easily when we compost our kitchen waste; recycle paper, packaging, bottles, and cans; give away clothes, toys, tools, and household items, rather than trash them; and avoid excessively packaged products when we shop.

big green purse

More Smart Strategies

Buy in bulk and "refills." When practical, buy the economy size of a product rather than single servings. Not only will you reduce packaging; you'll save money, too. You pay nearly twice the price for the same weight when you buy the individually wrapped product. Fabric softener, laundry detergent, cleanser, hand soap, dish soap, shampoo, and even pet food are good examples of products you can buy in bulk sizes to refill a smaller container at home.

Reuse or recycle as much packaging as possible. Know what you can recycle in your community and where: curbside programs pick up most cans, bottles, and jars as well as laundry detergent boxes and bottles if they're #1 or #2 plastic (check the bottom). Grocery items will vary: you'll be able to recycle an empty can of coffee but not an individually wrapped, single-serve coffee packet. Most grocery stores now take back plastic bags.

Choose concentrates. Juice sold as a concentrate in a small container can be reconstituted with water in your kitchen. Many laundry detergents and liquid cleansers come in concentrated forms that reduce packaging and save energy.

BYOB. Instead of paper or plastic, bring your own bags when you shop. Invest in a supply of canvas bags, or bring back the bags you used on your last shopping trip for a refill.

Avoid styrene. White foam polystyrene (like Styrofoam) in blocks protects hard goods (like appliances and electronics); "peanuts" cushion smaller items that are shipped; and food-grade styrene goes into soup cups. While more facilities are beginning to accept block foam and peanuts for recycling, the food foam can't be recycled or reused after it's been tainted by coffee, a cup of noodles, or Chinese takeout. Why avoid styrene? It's classified as a possible carcinogen by the U.S. Department of Health and Human Services, and presents serious health risks to the people who make it. Because it's not biodegradable, it persists in the environment, potentially for hundreds of years. Furthermore, foam packaging is made from non-renewable petroleum products rather than renewable or recycled materials.

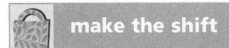
make the shift

Instead of Polystyrene . . .

- Buy products sold in reusable and recyclable containers in packaging made from recycled material that can be recycled again when you're finished using it.
- Choose alternatives to products like instant soup that are packaged in foam cups or bowls. Instead, buy fresh ingredients or quick mixes in cellophane packaging.
- Purchase meat directly from the butcher wrapped in paper to avoid foam meat trays.
- Choose recyclable paper or plastic egg cartons rather than foam trays.
- Bring your own reusable container for leftovers when you eat out.
- Carry a reusable mug or cup for coffee, juice, soda, or smoothies.

But it's so convenient . . .

The more pressed for time we are, the more trash we create. It's so much easier and faster to buy the pineapple already cored, chopped, and packed in a throwaway plastic tub than to have to tackle a fresh pineapple yourself. One of the best ways to reduce our environmental impact overall is to take a little more time to live our lives, rather than race to keep up with them. Try slowing down at least one day a week. Buy fresh food you have to chop for meals you actually have to cook rather than zap in the microwave. Eat dinner around the kitchen or dining room table rather than on the run. Unplug—from the computer, the telephone, the television—and tune in—to nature, other people, and your own inner self. In simplifying your life, you'll simplify the impact you have on the world around you.

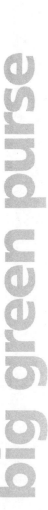
big green purse

CHOOSE THIS . . . NOT THIS	
Choose This	*Not This*
Bulk or concentrated options	Individually wrapped packages
Recyclable or reusable products	Throwaways
Whole fruits and vegetables	Shrink-wrapped fruit or vegetables on plastic or polystyrene trays
Your own shopping bags	Plastic or paper bags

Post-consumer and Pre-consumer Waste

"Post-consumer" refuse has been used, discarded, collected through recycling efforts, and sold to manufacturers for fabrication into new items. Post-consumer waste shows up most frequently in paper and plastic products, and to a lesser degree in fabrics, furniture, and construction materials. For instance, paper made from post-consumer waste has been manufactured from other paper that's been thrown away rather than from trees that have been cut down to make new paper. By purchasing products with the highest percentage of post-consumer waste available, you help save forests, energy, water, and other resources. You also bolster the recycling market by increasing demand for recycled materials.

"Pre-consumer" refers to waste that's generated during manufacturing. It can include damaged products, material trimmings, or production overruns. Manufacturers reuse pre-consumer waste to save money, reduce trash, and minimize the amount of raw materials needed to create their products.

Every time you use your purse to buy merchandise made from pre-consumer and especially post-consumer waste, you protect natural resources, save energy, and reduce pollution.

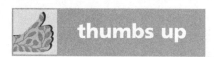

Pared-down Products at Wal-Mart

America's largest retailer has asked its 60,000 worldwide suppliers to help the company reduce its overall packaging demands by 5 percent. Don't think that sounds like much? Think again. Initially, Wal-Mart focused on the packaging of around three hundred toys manufactured for its Kid Connection toy line. By reducing the toys' packaging, Wal-Mart saved 3,425 tons of corrugated materials, 1,358 barrels of oil, 5,190 trees, 727 shipping containers, and $3.5 million in transportation costs in just one year. By expanding its initiative storewide, Wal-Mart hopes to prevent millions of pounds of trash from reaching landfills and keep 667,000 metric tons of carbon dioxide out of the atmosphere—the equivalent of taking 213,000 trucks off the road annually, or saving 323,800 tons of coal and 66.7 million gallons of diesel fuel from being burned.

Want to Recycle Plastic? Do It by the Number

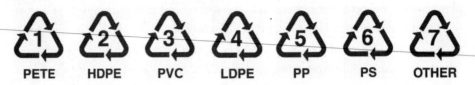

A number system ranging from 1 to 7 differentiates which plastic you can recycle, and which you'll have to trash. Here's what the numbers mean:

Easiest Plastics to Recycle

#1: Polyethylene terephthalate (PETE/PET), the most commonly recycled plastic, includes soda and water bottles, medicine bottles, some egg cartons, and other food containers. Once it has been processed at a recycling facility, PETE can become fiberfill for winter coats, sleeping bags, vests, life jackets, beanbags, rope, car bumpers, tennis ball felt, combs, cassette tapes, sails for boats, furniture, and other plastic bottles.

#2: High-density polyethylene (HDPE) plastics include heavier containers like those that hold laundry detergent, bleach, milk, shampoo, and motor oil. Number 2 plastic may be recycled into toys, piping, plastic lumber, and rope. It is usually accepted in curbside recycling programs and at recycling centers.

Plastics Recycled at Dedicated Locations

#4: Low-density polyethylene (LDPE) is found in wrapping films, grocery and sandwich bags, and some containers. It cannot be easily recycled in curbside recycling programs. Plastic grocery bags can be taken back to the grocery store.

#6: Polystyrene (Styrofoam) (PS) from coffee cups, soup cups, and meat trays that have been used cannot be recycled; some packing facilities and mailing houses will accept Styrofoam "peanuts" and hard foam bricks for recycling. Call the Alliance of Foam Packaging Recyclers at 410-451-8340 or visit www.earth911.org to find a recycling center in your area that accepts foam packaging.

Most Difficult Plastics to Recycle

#3: Polyvinyl chloride (PVC) is commonly used in plastic pipes, shower curtains, medical tubing, vinyl dashboards, and even some baby-bottle nipples. Few municipal centers will accept number 3 plastic.

#5: Polypropylene (PP) is used in Tupperware, yogurt containers, syrup bottles, diapers, and plastic bottle tops. It is usually not recycled.

#7: Plastic that consists of several layers or composites of different plastics is usually not accepted at most recycling centers.

Buy Local

As you shop, look for products made as close to your community as possible. Why?

Environmental benefits. Since it reduces the amount of energy needed to transport goods to market, buying local helps reduce global warming and air pollution.

Economic benefits. Buying local keeps money local. According to a study by London's New Economics Foundation, a dollar spent on locally made goods generates twice as much income for the local economy as money spent on imported goods.

Health and safety benefits. Supporting local entrepreneurs and businesses also increases the likelihood that U.S. environmental laws and regulations will be followed. This point was driven home in the summer of 2007, when the U.S. Consumer Product Safety Commission recalled thousands of toys made in China because they were decorated with lead paint, a toxin that causes a wide variety of serious illnesses in children. Small American toy companies that rely on safe paints and nontoxic materials quickly became the manufacturers of choice for parents and many toy stores alike.

Buying locally grown food offers another example of the benefits you can enjoy by supporting neighborhood entrepreneurs. Food raised and sold locally may travel one hundred fifty to two hundred miles from the farm gate to your kitchen plate. Compare that to the "average" food item which, according to the Worldwatch Institute, travels from 1,550 to 2,480 miles to become your dinner; is doused with pesticides to protect it from spoiling during its journey; and requires heavy packaging to prevent damage.

As important as buying local is, don't ignore the other Green Purse Principles, which together are intended to help you purchase the most environmentally benign products available. The first hybrid vehicles were made in Japan. If the hundreds of thousands of Americans who bought them had stuck with American cars, U.S. manufacturers would never have felt the pressure to improve the fuel efficiency of their own models.

Is Bottled Water Better?

In a word, NO.

- *Bottled water guzzles oil.* Approximately 1.5 million barrels of oil, enough to run 100,000 cars for a whole year, are needed to make plastic water bottles, not to mention the amount of oil required to transport bottled water all over the world.

- *Bottled water is rarely healthier than tap water.* Despite slick advertising campaigns designed to portray bottled water as fresh and pure, tap water is actually held to a higher health standard than bottled water. In fact, some brands of bottled water may be nothing more than tap water packaged behind a fancy label.

- *Bottled water wastes water.* To add insult to injury, in addition to the millions of gallons of water used in the plastic-making and water-bottling process, two gallons of water are wasted in the purification process for every gallon that goes into the bottles. What's more, only about 10 percent of water bottles are recycled. The rest end up in landfills, along the side of the road, or bobbing in our lakes and rivers, where they could take thousands of years to decompose.

The solution? Carry your own reusable bottle. (Find options at www .biggreenpurse.com (search: reusable bottle). At home, if you don't like the taste of your tap water, you can get an inexpensive filter online or at most supermarkets, drugstores, and hardware stores to improve the quality. If you must buy water, choose cans or glass over plastic bottles; recycle any container you buy.

To keep kids from losing their reusable bottles . . .

- Give them a nickel or dime to save every day they bring the bottle back (just like the "deposit" on a returnable soda bottle); that's much cheaper than the dollar or more it costs you to buy a bottle of water. At the end of the school year, the kids can use the money to buy something of value, donate to their favorite charity, or bank for the future.

- Put your last name and address or phone number on the bottle so it can be returned to you if it is lost.

In eleven states, deposit laws require retailers to give consumers five or ten cents back for every soda and beer bottle they return to the retailer. Several of those states are trying to expand those laws to include water bottles, as well as juice and sport drinks. Support any initiative in your community to expand recycling of plastic drink bottles or to include them in a deposit/return program.

Putting the Principles to Work

Hopefully, the principles laid out in this chapter will make it easy to use your purse to protect the environment no matter what you buy. The remaining chapters of *Big Green Purse* focus on specific commodities where your purchases can make the biggest environmental impact. Don't forget to sign up for the One in a Million Campaign at www.biggreenpurse.com to show your results, share your successes with others, and join a million other women who are using their purses to get the world they want.

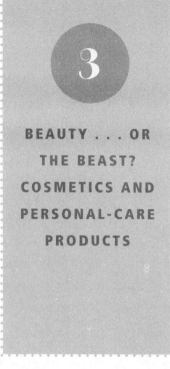

3

BEAUTY . . . OR THE BEAST? COSMETICS AND PERSONAL-CARE PRODUCTS

IF EVER THERE WERE AN INDUSTRY WHERE WE WOMEN REALLY NEEDED TO spend our money to make a difference, this is it.

Cosmetics and personal-care products literally touch every part of our bodies. We've been convinced that they'll make us beautiful. They often make us feel better. But evidence is emerging that the cumulative use of these products may be contributing to asthma, the onset of puberty in girls as young as three years old, and even the feminization of baby boys. Their notorious overpackaging helps fill the bags of trash we throw away every week and adds to the mountains of garbage clogging our landfills. And, because cosmetics, soaps, and shampoos are washed down the drain, they get into our water system, where they're wreaking havoc on wildlife.

Despite these concerns, lipstick, nail polish, shampoo, perfume, deodorant, and the other concoctions we liberally apply to our faces, lips, eyes, noses, nails, heads, necks, legs, armpits, and vaginas are among the least-regulated substances in the marketplace.

That's because the makers of cosmetics and personal-care products are not required to meet specific federal standards that guarantee our personal health or safety. The FDA requires manufacturers to put a warning statement on the front of products that have not been tested that reads, "WARNING—The safety of this product has not been determined." Not many of them do.

Cosmetics companies are not held responsible for the environmental consequences their products have once they escape into the environment. Only one state, California, requires cosmetics manufacturers to disclose any product ingredient that is on state or federal lists of chemicals that cause cancer or birth defects.

According to the FDA's Office of Cosmetics and Colors, which oversees the industry, "a cosmetic manufacturer may use almost any raw material as a cosmetic ingredient and market the product without an approval from the FDA."

That really makes you want to put your lipstick on, doesn't it?

The industry claims to regulate itself through a board called the Cosmetic Ingredient Review panel. But a report titled "Skin Deep" by the Environmental Working Group (EWG), a nonprofit research institute based in Washington, D.C., showed that 89 percent of 10,500 ingredients used in lipstick, nail polish, hair coloring, soap, and other personal-care products have not been evaluated for safety . . . 89 percent.

Of the thirty-six different ingredients in just one lipstick brand, Revlon ColorStay, thirteen have not been assessed for safety by the cosmetics industry, according to the EWG's analysis. Many of the chemicals used in this product have been linked to specific health concerns, like potential impact on the immune system and breast cancer.

While there's no specific connection between any one product and breast cancer, scientific evidence is growing that women face some risk of contracting the disease due to their cumulative exposure to the chemicals in cosmetics and personal-care products.

"Is there a direct connection we can make between the use of these products and breast cancer?" asks Dr. Julia Smith, the director of breast cancer screening and prevention at the Lynne Cohen Breast Cancer Preventive Care Program at the NYU Cancer Institute and Bellevue Medical Center, in New York City. "No. But there are strong scientific suspicions that some of the chemicals found in the environment, including those used in cosmetics and other personal-care items, might increase the risk, especially if there is heavy exposure before the age of twenty-five."

Dr. Smith, in a lengthy interview in WebMD, says this is because these are the years when breast tissue is developing and most susceptible to outside influences. Dr. Smith is concerned that multiple exposures could create a cumulative or "domino effect" that could ultimately result in the disease.

Only 10 percent of breast cancers have been linked to known risk factors like smoking and heredity. With so little known about what triggers the other 90 percent, the chemical cocktails that make up our lotions and deodorants have drawn increased scrutiny from doctors and scientists looking for answers.

The majority of researchers agree that it's difficult to link these chemicals—and other environmental factors—with certainty to health disorders. Janet Gray, Ph.D., a professor of neuroscience at Vassar College, worked with experts from the University of Pittsburgh Cancer Institute to compile a report on what is known to date about the environmental links to breast cancer. Gray says that while there may be no "smoking gun" that implicates any one chemical, the evidence is starting to mount indicating that steady, personal exposure to low levels of lots of different chemicals does matter.

"A compilation of epidemiological studies, cell culture studies, and animal data . . . are all consistent and I believe are coming together to show us that some of what women are exposed to every day may be increasing their risk of breast cancer," Professor Gray also told WebMD. "What's really new in this field," she adds, is that "finally people are starting to look at interactions—and the fact that exposure to low doses of lots of different chemicals may yield a result similar to a high-dose exposure to one chemical."

While we can't change our genetics, experts say we can, to some extent, control our environment.

You might think this means avoiding carcinogens, chemicals known to cause cancer. But experts say when it comes to breast cancer, of far greater concern is exposure to what are called "endocrine disrupters." These are chemicals and by-products that, when inhaled, ingested, or absorbed through the skin, can either mimic the effects of estrogen in the body or cause estrogen to act in a way that isn't normal.

Since estrogen can spark the growth of tumors, Gray says anything that interferes with estrogen metabolism could cause harm.

"These chemicals cause a 'triple whammy'—they increase levels of estrogen, alter cell metabolism, and influence the pathways that increase the risk of cancer," says Gray.

Elizabeth Ward, Ph.D., a spokeswoman for the American Cancer Society, told WebMD that "no strong evidence has emerged of a relationship [between breast cancer risk] and exposure to environmental contaminants."

NYU's Dr. Smith offers this advice: "You have to accept in life that there is a great deal we don't know—and just stay as close as possible to a natural state of living. Cut down where and when you can and minimize risks when and where you can in all areas of your life."

We can also use our consumer clout to pressure cosmetic manufacturers to reduce their use of harmful chemicals.

The Good News

Every year, we spend $50 billion on cosmetics and personal-care products. Individually, that amounts to between five hundred dollars and fifteen hundred dollars that each of us could shift to beauty products and toiletries that are healthier for us and better for the planet.

Even a small change can make a big difference when you're trying to get an industry's attention. Remember the story in the introduction about consumers who objected to dibutyl phthalate, the chemical linked to reproductive abnormalities in baby boys? They managed to persuade major nail polish manufacturers to remove the chemical from their product by spending their money on phthalate-free alternatives.

This chapter focuses on many additional ways we can alter our cosmetics spending to create a cleaner, greener world. It includes profiles of some of the key chemical ingredients we should try to avoid. Cosmetics and personal-care products contain hundreds of substances. *Big Green Purse* recommends four we can shift our spending on right now: fragrances, phthalates, parabens, and triclosan.

This chapter also lists several companies that merit your attention for their efforts to reduce harmful ingredients and minimize wasteful packaging. I hope the message is clear: *If you want to change a company's behavior, spend your money on a competitor's more desirable offerings.* The good news is that the number of green and clean options we have in the marketplace is growing. These pages direct you to some of the best alternatives and companies available in store aisles and on websites while giving you the tools you need to find more on your own.

You can also *choose not to spend your money at all.* To send a message to manufacturers that their products don't meet your standards, this chapter suggests priorities for cutting back on certain beauty aids. Think about it: Do we really need to slather our bodies with ten or fifteen products every day? Or have the manufacturers of these commodities simply convinced us that we do? If you keep reading, you'll find recommendations for ways to reduce what you consume, putting you—not manufacturers—in charge of what goes on your body. In addition to the health and environmental benefits, you'll save money, too.

Because manufacturers are creating more salon-type products for men, we've highlighted some items that could be of particular concern to the guys in your life. And if thinking of guys gets you thinking of sex, you'll want to read the information on biodegradable condoms and other earth-friendly birth control methods.

Throughout, I refer to additional sources of information: studies on health and safety risks associated with chemicals in cosmetics; links to alternative products you might want to try; and books that offer recipes for making your own cosmetics sans the chemical cocktails worked up in industrial labs.

After reading this chapter, drop in on www.biggreenpurse.com. That's where you can find a worksheet to help you calculate what you're already spending and keep track of the "one in a million" pledge you make to shift your money to cosmetics that contain the safest possible ingredients. The amount you decide to move is up to you (you may be surprised at what you're spending now!). Keep in mind that if this year a million of us spent just $1,000 on safer cosmetics and personal-care products, we'd have a *$1 billion impact* on this industry. That's not the kind of shopping "spree" any manufacturer can afford to ignore.

How Much Do You Use? It All Adds Up

The cosmetics and personal-care products industry says you don't need to worry about the ingredients in your products because they're present in such small amounts. But since we use so many products every day, our exposure to all these chemicals really adds up.

How many personal-care and beauty aids do you apply in a single day?
Check all that apply:

__ skin cream	__ makeup remover	__ sunless tanning lotion
__ body lotion	__ permanent waves	__ antiaging cream
__ perfume	__ hair straightener	__ vaginal deodorant
__ lipstick	__ hair dye	or douche
__ lip gloss	__ shampoo	__ body wash
__ fingernail polish	__ conditioner	__ body deodorant
__ cuticle creme	__ hair gel	__ shaving cream
__ nail polish remover	__ mousse	__ blush
__ eyeliner	__ hair spray	__ powder
__ eye shadow	__ toothpaste	__ foundation
__ mascara	__ whitening strips	__ acne treatment
__ eyebrow pencil	__ suntan lotion	__ insect repellent

If you have children, on any given day you might be exposing them, too. Many mothers readily pour, lather, or spray some combination of shampoo, lotion, diaper cream, powder, insect repellent, and sunscreen on their skin.

Most of us use these products without giving them a second thought. Because they're available over the counter, we believe that the government must certainly be policing the safety of the mixtures found in these myriad containers. But we're wrong. The government does not require health studies or premarket testing for these items before they are sold. And because these products together contain more than a hundred different ingredients, their chemical components are causing concerns for human health as well as for the impacts they may have on wildlife, rivers, and streams.

A product-use survey of twenty-three hundred men and women conducted by the Environmental Working Group in 2004 showed that more than a quarter of all women and one of every hundred men use at least fifteen products daily. Yet the Cosmetic Ingredient Review, the safety panel for the personal-care products industry, approaches each safety analysis as if consumers are exposed to just one product—one chemical—at a time. It treats each product like it is the only source of exposure for each chemical being considered.

"By considering the human body to be a 'clean slate' free of background contamination, free of related chemicals linked to common health harms, and free of exposures from other kinds of consumer products," says the EWG, "the industry's panel will every time underestimate the potential for a particular personal-care product ingredient to harm human health."

The impact in the natural environment may be underestimated to an even greater degree. When personal-care products are washed down the drain, wastewater treatment systems cannot remove many of the chemicals they contain. The discharge ends up contaminating streams and rivers with substances that affect frogs, mussels, and other wildlife.

Reproductive abnormalities found in fish and frogs in recent years show that these chemicals should not be ignored, and not just for the animals' sake. When male fish start sporting egg sacs or male frogs develop both male and female genitalia, scientists worry whether humans, too, may be at risk. Threats to people are harder to pinpoint because we are subject to so many different environmental and genetic variables. However, minute levels of phthalates, which are used in drug capsules, cosmetics, and perfumes, have been statistically linked to sperm damage in men and genital changes, asthma, and allergies in children, reported *The Wall Street Journal* in 2005. And one thing we do know: some groups are exceedingly vulnerable to the effects of toxins. A developing fetus, an infant, or a person with a compromised immune system is more vulnerable than someone who is healthy.

Time has shown that we need to pay attention to early warning signs if we are to prevent later problems to our health and the environment. This is the foundation for what's known as "the Precautionary Principle" (see more extensive explanation in Chapter 1). When we suspect harm is being done, even if we lack conclusive scientific evidence, the Precautionary Principle encourages us to act to prevent possible consequences.

Remember the old saw "an ounce of prevention is worth a pound of cure"? It applies to the environment and our health in spades. Preventing dangerous chemical buildup in the environment is far more economical and ecological than trying to remove the chemicals once they're entrenched.

Use Your Big Green Purse

Cosmetics and personal-care products offer dozens of opportunities to change the marketplace, improve your choices, and protect the planet and yourself.

- Give your body a break
- Focus on ingredients
- Shop for safer products
- Send companies a message
- Choose less packaging

Give Your Body a Break

The most immediate way to let cosmetics manufacturers know you're concerned about the impact their goods could have on your health and the environment is to cut back on what you buy. Inventory all the cosmetics and personal-care products you use on an average day. How many of them do you really need? How many of them do you apply because manufacturers have swept you up in an irresistible marketing campaign?

Manhattan dermatologist Fran Cook-Bolden told *The New York Times,* "Just two products, a gentle cleanser and a good sunscreen, are enough daily skin care for most people." Dr. Sarah Boyce Sawyer, an assistant professor of dermatology at the School of Medicine at the University of Alabama at Birmingham, also featured in the *Times,* concurs. Not only could it be better for your skin, it will also save you money. Dr. Sawyer advises her patients to ". . . cut down on skin-care products and cut your skin-care budget."

"We have good medical evidence on prescription products," Dr. Sawyer says. "But the science is fuzzy with a lot of cosmetics." Given that many beauty claims cannot be substantiated, pay attention to the potential health risks. Save your money—as well as your skin.

Check shampoos, conditioners, crème rinses, and soaps. Since you rinse them off, they are probably of secondary concern to your personal health. However, you're still washing their contents down the drain and into the environment, so take care. Can you shampoo your hair every other day rather than daily? Can you limit yourself to one soap in the shower rather than multiple soaps and gels?

By the way, give your kids a break, too. They don't need dozens of personal-care products any more than you do. Reserve the antibacterials for scrapes and cuts, apply sunscreen when they go out to play, and choose soaps and shampoos with the fewest ingredients.

Give Your Body a Break: Cut Back on These Products First

PRODUCT	ACTION
Nail polish	Limit to special occasions
	Apply in well-ventilated room
	Use phthalate-free and self-peeling polish
	Polish toes; skip fingernails
Hair dye	Avoid dark, permanent hair dyes
	Don't begin dyeing hair until graying occurs
	Use "color gray" color sticks to treat roots to avoid redyeing whole head
	Avoid hair dyes that contain lead and coal tar
Antibacterial soaps, lotions, shampoos	Use plain soap and water for hand washing
	Avoid products with triclosan and other antibacterial agents
Perfume	Limit to special occasions
	Apply in well-ventilated room
	Don't pour ingredients down sink or into toilet
	Use phthalate-free products
	Make your own using essentials oils, herbs, flowers
Eye makeup	Limit to special occasions
	Choose products with the fewest ingredients
Body lotion	Choose products with the fewest ingredients
	Choose "no added fragrance" or "fragrance free" products
	Avoid phthalates, parabens, triclosan (see descriptions pages 56–59)

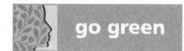

go green

Give Your Body a Cosmetic Breather

- Use fewer or no cosmetics on days you don't go to work.
- Reduce the number of products you use overall by three.
- Pick one weekend a month to "go natural"—apart from washing your face and brushing your teeth, just leave your body alone.
- What else can you do to take a break?

thumbs down

Don't Douche!

Now here's a product that causes more trouble than it's worth.

It's a "douche," a wash for the vagina. It usually consists of prepackaged mixes of acidic ingredients, like water and vinegar, sold in a bottle fitted with a tube or nozzle so you can easily squirt the liquid and throw everything away when you're done. The U.S. Department of Health and Human Services estimates that between 20 and 40 percent of women aged fifteen to forty-four douche regularly, even though the practice appears to do more harm than good. Contrary to popular belief, douching does not dissipate vaginal odors, help a woman avoid sexually transmitted diseases (STDs), or prevent pregnancy. Instead, says the American College of Obstetricians (ACOG), women who douche suffer more vaginal irritation and pelvic inflammatory disease, an infection of the uterus, fallopian tubes, and/or ovaries. ACOG suggests we avoid douching completely.

If you're concerned about your vaginal vitality, do what Mother Nature does. Let your vagina clean itself naturally, which it does by producing mucus that washes away menstrual blood, semen, and other vaginal discharges. Otherwise, warm water and mild soap during baths and showers will keep your nether regions clean and healthy. Of course, if you are experiencing ongoing pain or extreme discharge, seek medical attention. But note: even healthy, clean vaginas may have a mild odor—one your playmate might find sexy!

Doctors bolster some other advice you'll see throughout these pages: avoid fra-

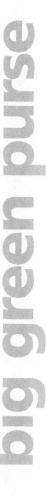

big green purse

grances, specifically scented tampons, pads, powders, and sprays. The chemicals in these products irritate skin and may increase your chances of contracting a vaginal infection.

Focus on Ingredients

A given product could consist of two dozen or more ingredients, most of whose names are so complicated you'll never remember what to look for. Start with these four, which are found in at least 50 percent of the standard cosmetics and personal-care products you normally purchase. You'll find them listed on the product's label.

1. Fragrances
2. Phthalates
3. Parabens
4. Triclosan

Fragrances

Fragrances and preservatives are the main ingredients in cosmetics. As it turns out, fragrances are also the most common cause of skin problems, like contact dermatitis. More than five thousand different kinds of fragrances are used in products ranging from makeup to shampoo to soap, as well as plastics, house paints, cleansers, and some pesticide formulations. Fifty percent of all personal-care products on the market contain added fragrance.

Fragrances don't just make us itch. They've been increasingly cited as a trigger for asthma, allergies, and migraine headaches.

Writing in *Flavour and Fragrance Journal,* author Betty Bridges reports: "Asthma rates have soared since the 1970s. It is important to look at changes that have taken place during this time period that might contribute to the rising rates. In the past three decades fragrance has gone from 'special occasion' to use of multiple scented products on a daily basis. According to fragrance industry demographics, blacks and Hispanics are more frequent users of fragrance than other segments of the population. They are also more likely to suffer from the effects of asthma. While these things are not proof of the impact fragrance has had on asthma, they certainly support the need for further and more extensive examination of respiratory effects of fragrance."

Some fragrance ingredients have been detected in breast milk—though we're not sure what the long-term consequences of this will be. Other fragrance chemicals may mimic the body's own hormones, disrupting our endocrine system and the way it regulates growth and reproduction. Because fragrances are volatile compounds, they can contribute to both indoor and outdoor air pollution. Safety testing by the fragrance industry focuses primarily on skin effects; it does not take into account the impact these chemicals can have on our respiratory and neurological systems, let alone fetal development.

Overall, the vast majority of fragrance chemicals have not been assessed for their effects on us body-wide. The long-term impacts simply are not known. In fact, it could be years before the problems are felt. Until they are, your smartest bet is to shop for fragrance-free or no-fragrance-added cosmetics and personal-care products.

Phthalates

Phthalates, industrial compounds that soften plastic, give perfume its slightly oily texture, and put the volatile oomph in hair sprays, are also found in nail polish, toothpaste, and hundreds of other personal-care products. In May 2005, researchers identified for the first time that some women who are exposed to phthalates in the normal course of everyday life give birth to male babies with abnormal genitals.

The study was just the latest in a string of investigations into the impact that phthalates can have on human health. In August 2000, Puerto Rican scientists found a relationship between exposure to phthalates and premature breast development in girls as young as thirty-one months old. Between 2002 and 2003, three additional studies linked phthalate exposure to lower semen quality, including DNA damage in sperm. In June 2003, the American Academy of Pediatrics recommended that research on phthalates and their effects on fetuses and infants be undertaken, especially in light of animal research from the U.S. Centers for Disease Control that clearly documents harm.

These studies have been enough for Dr. Devra Davis of the University of Pittsburgh's Center for Environmental Oncology, as well as many other scientists, public health advocates, and environmental organizations, to recommend that phthalates be removed from cosmetics and personal-care products. But because the industry regulates itself, no formal action has been taken.

Cut Back on Fragrances and Phthalates

- According to the FDA, fragrances are the most common cause of skin problems.
- Phthalates, a common ingredient in hundreds of personal-care products, appear to feminize the reproductive organs of baby boys, according to studies conducted for the U.S. Centers for Disease Control.
- Fragrances may trigger asthma and other respiratory conditions, according to the American Lung Association.
- Wastewater is often contaminated with fragrance that cannot be removed when it washes down the drain. The fragrance ends up in streams and rivers, where it's absorbed by wildlife. Researchers at Stanford University have shown that mussels lost their ability to clear their bodies of poisons when exposed to minuscule levels of common fragrance musks.

Parabens

Like phthalates, parabens, one of the most common cosmetic preservatives, cause problems like allergic dermatitis and skin rashes. Even more alarming, evidence published in the *Journal of Applied Toxicology* indicates that parabens, which are usually added to deodorants, mascara, and other personal-care products, can be detected in human breast tumors.

Dr. Philippa Darbre, a researcher at England's University of Reading, is leading a research project there to study the link between parabens and breast cancer. "Parabens are used as preservatives in thousands of cosmetic, food, and pharmaceutical products but this is the first study to show their accumulation in human tissues. It demonstrates that if people are exposed to these chemicals, then the chemicals will accumulate in their bodies," she says.

Whether these ingredients actually cause breast cancer still remains to be proven. The National Institutes of Health notes that estrogen may cause breast cancer tumors to grow. Meanwhile, "parabens have been shown to mimic the action of estrogen," Dr. Darbre maintains.

"It would therefore seem especially prudent to consider whether parabens should continue to be used in such a wide range of cosmetics applied to the breast area [including antiperspirants/deodorants]," says Dr. Darbre, especially when alternatives exist.

Triclosan

Antibacterial soap used to be dispensed primarily in doctors' offices and hospitals, arenas designed to wage battle with health-threatening bacteria. No more. The latest marketing craze is trying to convince us that dangerous "super germs" lurk on every surface and in every space. One antibacterial in particular, triclosan, is being added to products as harmless as toothpaste, hand lotion, and body wash.

What are the consequences to us and the environment of using bacteria-fighting products so liberally and every day?

Many health-care professionals worry that the more than seven hundred products on the market labeled "antibacterial" are promoting resistance among some of the very bacteria they're designed to fight. In fact, the more antibacterials we use, doctors say, the more resistant bacteria grow. We've all heard of "staph infections." Resistance to dangerous bacteria like *Staphylococcus aurea* is becoming an increasing problem worldwide, due to the combined overuse of both antibacterial agents in soaps and other personal-care products as well as overprescription of pharmaceutical antibiotics.

Do we really need this extra level of "clean"? Not according to Dr. Stuart Levy, director of the Center for Adaptation Genetics and Drug Resistance at the Tufts University School of Medicine, in Boston. "No current data demonstrate any health benefits from having antibacterial-containing cleansers in a healthy household," he says.

Besides building resistance, Dr. Levy adds, the antibacterial craze has another potential consequence. Studies show that people who have been raised in a more sterile environment actually experience *more* allergies, asthma, and eczema than those allowed to live with germs. Ironically, excessive hygiene may interfere with the normal maturation of the immune system by eliminating opportunities for the immune system to "exercise itself" against germs using the body's natural defense mechanisms.

Antibacterials take their toll on the natural environment as well. Minuscule amounts of triclosan, like the levels being found in many of America's streams and rivers, can upset thyroid function in frogs, for instance.

Professor Caren Helbing is researching that phenomenon on frogs at the University of British Columbia in Vancouver, Canada. Her studies show that not only does the chemical structure of triclosan closely resemble thyroid hormone, but also that triclosan is capable of intensifying the impact of the thyroid hormone. In the case of frogs, triclosan exposure leads to weight loss, accelerated limb development, and uncontrolled cell growth in certain parts of the brain.

What's bad for frogs, Professor Helbing fears, is probably bad for people, too.

A tadpole needs normal thyroid hormone in order to change into a healthy frog. People need thyroid hormone "especially during early development around the birth period" to develop healthy organs, notes Professor Helbing. "Throughout life in adolescence and in adulthood the brain is very dependent on proper levels of thyroid hormone. So even though there are some obvious differences between frogs and people, the fundamental biology is very, very similar," she says.

"I would certainly think twice about whether you need and want triclosan in the products you're using," Professor Helbing advises.

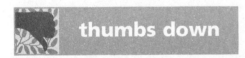

thumbs down

Are the drugs you take giving the fish in the lake conniptions?

If you're pouring them down the drain or flushing them down the toilet, they could be. Studies by the U.S. Geological Survey and the Environmental Protection Agency have found fish, frogs, and other aquatic animals with both male and female sex organs, freaks of nature they attribute to the growing amounts of pharmaceuticals showing up in rivers, lakes, and streams.

The pharmaceuticals include narcotics, birth control drugs, antidepressants, and other controlled substances that most wastewater treatment plants aren't equipped

Buy products made from fewer ingredients overall

Compare the contents of Aubrey Organics J.A.Y. Desert Herb Shampoo to L'Oréal Vive Nutri-Moisture Shampoo.

Aubrey Organics contains: coconut oil soap, olive oil castile, desert herb complex (organic jojoba oil, organic aloe vera, and yucca root extract), water, and citrus seed extract with vitamins A, C, and E as preservatives.

L'Oréal Vive contains: water, sodium laureth sulfate, coco betaine, dimethicone, cetyl alcohol, hydroxystearyl cetyl ether, cocamide MIPA, sodium cetearyl sulfate, fragrance, polyquaternium-10, carbomer, sodium methylparaben, DMDM hydantoin, propylene glycol, phenoxyethanol, 2-oleamido-1, 3-octadecanediol, methylparaben, butylparaben, ethylparaben, isobutylparaben, propylparaben.

The more ingredients a product contains, the more your chemical exposures add up. Remember the Green Purse Principle to buy products made from the fewest ingredients as a way to minimize health and environmental risk.

to remove. One study found nine male smallmouth bass in the Potomac River near Washington, D.C., carrying female eggs inside their sex organs.

What to do with pharmaceuticals you no longer need?

- Toss them in the trash, not down the toilet.
- Contact Earth Keepers, 906-228-6095, a grassroots group that organized a highly successful program in Michigan to collect old drugs to keep them out of the water.
- Follow the example of Milwaukee-based Capital Returns Inc., which in 2006 incinerated 6.5 million pounds of pills and other pharmaceuticals sent from pharmacies and drug manufacturers around the country. The "fuel" generated enough energy to power more than 220 homes for a year.

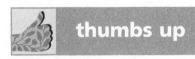

Less Is More

The fewer ingredients you expose yourself to, the better. The following companies offer cosmetics that consist of simple, unadulterated minerals:

Everyday Minerals (www.everydayminerals.com). These American-made products contain no pthalates or parabens.
Alima Cosmetics (www.alimacosmetics.com). You can recycle the jars for a free eye shadow.
Monave (www.monave.com). The company offers a cosmetics color line particularly developed for African-American, Asian, and Latin complexions.

Whatever you buy, keep on the watch for "greenwashing." Remember that manufacturers can use words like "natural" and "hypoallergenic" to create marketing buzz without having to prove actual results. Ignore words like "nontoxic," "cruelty-free," "ecosafe," "dermatologist tested," and "nature's friend" unless the manufacturer substantiates the claim with third-party verification or a transparent explanation of the product's ingredients.

To see how your favorite brand or product measures up, visit the Environmental Working Group's Skin Deep Cosmetic Safety Data Base (www.cosmetics database.com).

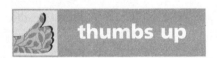

Straight Talk

Tom's of Maine gets a thumbs up for putting a clear statement on its label that lets you know exactly what's inside: "This product does not contain triclosan; saccharin; artificial sweeteners, preservatives, colors, or flavors; or animal ingredients. Tom's of Maine products are tested for safety without the use of animals."

Shop for Safer Products

Now that you're aware of key ingredients in cosmetics and personal-care products, take the next critical step. Shift your spending to safer goods. You'll send manufacturers an unmistakable message to clean up their act, and protect the planet and yourself.

One product to consider in this category is hair dye. We don't know much about the safety of hair dyes, especially during pregnancy. It's likely that when you apply hair dye, a small amount is absorbed into your system. However, in the few animal and human studies that have been done, no changes were seen in the developing baby. Some precautions you can take:

- Check the safety of the ingredients in your hair coloring against the Environmental Working Group's cosmetics database (www.cosmeticsdata base.com), where you can also find alternative, safer products.
- Buy hair-color products that meet the higher safety standards imposed by the European Union. Look for them at Whole Foods, food co-ops, and online.
- Don't start coloring hair until you really have to! Highlight rather than dye your entire head.
- Use color sticks (available at beauty-supply stores like Ulta and Sephora) to touch up gray spots at your temples or hairline to reduce the number of times in a year you dye your hair.
- Tell the men in your life to avoid any hair color products that contain lead, a neurotoxin.
- Know that the chemicals in darker hair dyes seem to be linked to more health problems than lighter colors. If you're going for a new you, lighten up.

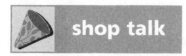

Don't see a product that meets your needs for safe ingredients? Ask the store manager to order it. Specify not just a product but the manufacturer, too, for example, Burt's Bees Herbal Treatment Shampoo, Honeybee Gardens Peel Off Nail Polish, or Alba Organic Facial Toner.

big green purse

make the shift

Buy Safer Products

Of the hundreds of cosmetic and personal-care manufacturers in the marketplace, the following are among the best at limiting the number of toxic ingredients they use.

Burt's Bees (www.burtsbees.com). Burt's includes a complete line of lip balms, glosses, sticks, and shimmers; face cleansers, toners, complexion bars, moisturizers, eye creams, and exfoliating scrubs; shampoos and conditioners; toothpaste and peppermint breath drops; eye makeup and face powder; various Baby Bee products and a growing list of men's grooming choices. Increasingly available in mainstream grocery stores, drugstores, and pharmacies.

Tom's of Maine (www.tomsofmaine.com). The company's ninety oral and body-care products include toothpaste, deodorant, mouthwash, soap, shaving cream, and dental floss. Sold at 40,000 retail outlets in the United States and around the world.

Ecco Bella (www.eccobella.com). Includes perfumes, bath and body products, cosmetics, and skin and hair-care products. Often available in organic and natural food stores and food co-ops.

Aubrey Organics (www.aubrey-organics.com). Products are made primarily with herbals, essential oils, and vitamins. Includes baby care, bath products, hair care and color, hand and body lotions, makeup, skin care, soaps, toiletries, sun protection, and hair and skin essentials for men. Often available in organic and natural food stores and food co-ops.

Pangea Organics (www.pangeaorganics.com). Pangea's soaps, shower gels, skin cleansers, toners, masks, and creams are made from organic, plant-based ingredients according to fair-trade principles. You won't find artificial-fragrance chemicals or petroleum derivatives in these products, either.

Honeybee Gardens (www.honeybeegardens.com). In addition to a variety of lipsticks, powders, eyeliner, eye shadow, hair spray, shampoo, and conditioner, Honeybee manufactures water-based nail polish, including one brand that can peel off without need of nail polish remover.

Terressentials (www.terressentials.com). Claims that every single ingredient they use in their products is 100 percent certified organic by the U.S. Department of Agriculture. Their line consists mostly of face and body cleansers, shampoos, body oils and creams, and baby products. Often available in organic and natural food stores and food co-ops.

Dr. Bronner (www.drbronner.com). A longstanding manufacturer of soaps, lotions, and lip balms. Available in organic and natural food stores and food co-ops, as well as online.

Vermont Soapworks (www.vermontsoap.com). Manufacturers of 100 percent certified organic bar soap, liquid soap, shower gel, and bath salts.

The Organic Make-up Company (www.organicmakeup.ca). Products include face cream, lip balm, hand lotion, cleansers, lipstick and lip gloss, foundation, makeup remover, eye shadow, blush, concealer, and mascara. Many products are organic: none use synthetic or petroleum-derived ingredients; genetically modified substances are held to a minimum. There's no animal testing, and the containers can be reused.

Miessence (www.miessenceproducts.com). Offers a line of certified organic products that includes skin conditioners, toners, cleansers, exfoliants, and masks; lip balms, creams, and shimmers; eye creams; powders, blushes, and concealers; shampoos; and mascara.

Especially for Men

Shaving Creams

Aubrey Organics Herbal Mint & Ginseng Shaving Cream (www.aubrey-organics .com/about/articles/shavingcream.cfm) and *Men's Stock Shave Systems* (www .aubrey-organics.com/spec_prods/mens_shave.cfm). Ingredients are free of triethanolamine (TEA) and diethanolamine (DEA) which, in combination, are suspected of being carcinogenic. Products contain no synthetic fragrances or parabens, and are cruelty free and consciously green in manufacturing. Available at health stores and online.

Tom's of Maine Natural Conditioning Shave Cream (www.tomsofmaine.com). Mint or calendula scent, cruelty-free vegetable ingredients. Widely available at pharmacies and grocery stores but also online.

Deodorants

Jason Naturally Fresh Stick Deodorant for Men (unscented) (http://Jason-natural .com/products/deodorants.php). Certified organic and formulated without alu-

Need to Contact Corporate Headquarters?

Urge your favorite drugstore to carry better brands: Free of phthalates, antibacterials, parabens, and other harmful chemicals.

Costco
P.O. Box 34331
Seattle, WA 98124
800-774-2678
www.costco.com

CVS Corporation
Corporate Headquarters
One CVS Drive
Woonsocket, RI 02895
888-607-4287
e-mail: customercare@cvs.com

Duane Reade Inc.
440 Ninth Avenue
New York, NY 10001
212-273-5700

Eckerd Pharmacy
50 Service Avenue
Warwick, RI 02886
1-800-ECKERDS (1-800-325-3737)
Fax: 401-825-3587

Target
1-800-440-0680

Longs Drug Stores Corporation
141 North Civic Drive
Walnut Creek, CA 94596
925-937-1170
1-800-TO-LONGS (1-800-865-6647)
www.longs.com and click on
   Customer Service

Rite Aid Corporation
Customer Support
P.O. Box 3165
Harrisburg, PA 17105
1-800-RITE-AID (1-800-748-3243)

Walgreens
200 Wilmot Road
Deerfield, IL 60015
847-914-2500

Wal-Mart Stores, Inc.
Attn: Customer Service
702 S.W. 8th Street
Bentonville, AR 72716
1-800-WAL-MART (1-800-925-6278)

minum chlorohydrate. Combines green tea extract, vitamin E, and cornstarch. May be purchased online and at major natural and health food stores.

Aubrey Organics Men's Stock Natural Dry Herbal Pine Deodorant (www.aubrey-organics.com/product1.cfm?product_id=408&cat=11). Cruelty-free vegan product made from natural grain alcohol, witch hazel, arnica flower extract, calamine, vitamin E, calendula oil, and pine needle oil. Available at health and natural food stores and online.

French Transit, Ltd. Crystal Body Deodorant Men's Stick (www.thecrystal.com/product.cfm/Id/2). These mineral salts form a topical layer on the skin and leave no residue. Contains no aluminum chlorohydrate or dyes. Fragrance free. May be purchased online from several retailers.

Hand and Body Lotion

Anthony Logistics for Men Glycerin Hand & Body Lotion (www.anthony.com/index.cfm/a/catalog.prodshow/vid/421/catid/212). All of Anthony Logistics grooming products are designed specifically for men and are based on natural ingredients. This lotion is created from sea kelp, shea butter, aloe vera, glycerin, chamomile, and vitamins A, B_5, C, and E. It is allergy tested and fragrance free. Available at Nordstrom, Bath & Body Works, and Sephora (online or at retail outlets).

WildWays Studio Hand Balm Just for Men (www.wildwaysstudio.com/herbals/man.html). Organic, sandalwood-scented hand and body lotion contains water, cold-pressed oils (hazelnut, coconut, avocado, wheat germ), shea butter, aloe vera, vitamin E, lemon verbena, beeswax, and sandalwood essential oil. Wildways Studio (www.wildwaysstudio.com).

Shampoo

Ahava Mineral Shampoo for Men (http://ahavaus.com/site/men.html). This Israeli company, which has a branch in America, utilizes the mineral salts of the Dead Sea to create a wide variety of cosmetic products. Oil free, alcohol free, hypoallergenic, and not tested on animals, the mineral compounds are mixed with gingko and ginseng. The shampoo is said to have anti-dandruff properties. It may be bought online at the Ahava's North American site, as well as at Bath & Body Works.

Gaia Made for Men Shampoo (www.gaiaskinnaturals.com/pages/default.cfm?

page_id=34414). Gaia uses natural extracts in combination with ingredients certified as organic in Australia. The shampoo is low-foaming, vegan, and cruelty free and made without soap, sulfates, mineral oils, petrochemicals, parabens, propylene glycol, or artificial fragrances. The scent is a blend of certified organic orange, certified organic chamomile, certified organic spearmint, and certified organic aloe vera. The shampoo may be purchased online in America through Tender Care International (www.gaiamensorganictoiletries .com/Shampoo .html).

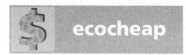

Some safer shampoos, lotions, conditioners, and makeup may be more expensive than the goods you normally use. How can you shift your spending but stay within your budget?

- **Cut back on the number of products you use overall.** I have shifted at least $15 a month from face toner, throwaway cleansing wipes, and facial masks to a simple organic-based face wash.
- **Use products less frequently, to last longer.** I take a makeup break every Saturday.
- **Shop on sale.** I buy two-for-one or buy one, get one half-price.
- **Prioritize your spending.** I shifted first to products like safer deodorant and makeup that stay on my skin; then as my budget allowed I focused on alternative soaps, shampoos, conditioners, and other products that rinse off.

Feeling Sexy?

I'm all for going "natural," but when it comes to sex, what's a girl to do? Rhythm and withdrawal are the only birth control methods that leave no trace behind . . . until they fail. Then their impact on the planet is a lasting one.

Other options?

Condoms do double duty: they prevent unwanted pregnancy and promote safe sex. However, millions of condoms are unwittingly flushed down the toilet every year, where they escape wastewater-treatment systems and end up in lakes, rivers, and streams, fouling waterways and sometimes choking wildlife.

- Latex condoms, which usually contain animal-based casein (a drawback for many vegetarians), are biodegradable and prevent HIV.
- Lambskin condoms, another vegan no-no, are too porous to prevent a sexually transmitted disease but will keep your genes in your jeans, so to speak.
- Glyde latex condoms, available from www.pristineplanet.com, and the Condomi brand, sold at www.britishcondoms.com, contain no animal products.
- Polyurethane condoms for men and women and female polyurethane sponges offer an alternative if you're allergic to latex, but the polyurethane will not decompose should the darn thing end up on a riverbank somewhere.

Regardless of what you choose, wrap it in tissue or toilet paper and toss it in the trash—not the toilet—after use. Then tie your trash bag closed before it goes to the landfill. No need for runaway rubbers to litter the terrain.

As for female contraceptives, the pill, the patch, and the Depo-Provera shot are popular but not especially eco. Because they're hormone-based, we end up urinating synthetic estrogen every day. These chemicals elude most water-treatment systems and sneak into our waterways, where they've been blamed for feminizing male fish and frogs and affecting the animals' fertility rates. Some choices to consider:

- If you're with a partner you trust and sexually transmitted diseases (STDs) are not a risk, ask your doctor about nonhormone-based alternatives like an IUD. (A diaphragm uses spermicide, which gets rinsed into the water, too.)
- If you're finished having children, talk to your partner about having a vasectomy or consider sterilization for yourself.
- And remember, don't douche. Douching will not prevent pregnancy or protect you from STDs. It will simply wash away healthy vaginal bacteria, a practice that could cause infections in the reproductive organs.

What's that, you say? You just want to have fun?

- Skip the jelly and vinyl sex toys that contain endocrine-disrupting phthalates and other chemicals, and aim for those made from silicone and even glass (if you don't mind the hard surface). Consider solar-powered vibrators; at the least, power your standard model with rechargeable batteries. You've got more options than you can probably imagine at www.blowfish.com.

- Sympathical formulas (www.sympathical.com) sells "personal lubricants" in three varieties: peach, raspberry, and unflavored. Chemical-, paraben-, glycerin-, and hormone-free, these organic products, claim the company, are also water-based and cruelty-free. How could they be anything but . . . stimulating?

Sunscreens

Skin cancer is on the rise. Every year, more than 800,000 Americans are affected by basal cell skin cancer alone. Exposure to the ultraviolet (UV) rays of the sun appears to be the biggest cause of skin cancer and a primary cause of lip cancer. UVA, which penetrates beyond the top layer of human skin, is the most abundant source of solar radiation, but UVB also contributes to this disease.

It turns out that, ironically, some popular sunscreens break down when exposed to sunlight. Others penetrate the skin and present significant health concerns. Choose the option that will best protect you from the sun. Blue Lizard Australian Suncream SPF 30/Baby, California Baby Water Resistant Hypo-Allergenic Sunscreen SPF 30-plus, and Aveeno Baby Continuous Protection Sunblock Lotion with SPF 45 all get top ratings for effectiveness in the sun and staying on in the water.

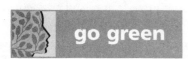

Protect Yourself from Skin Cancer

- **Avoid outdoor activities during midday.** The sun's rays are strongest between 10 A.M. and 4 P.M.
- **Cover up.** Wear a wide-brimmed hat, long-sleeved shirt, and long pants.
- **Protect your eyes.** Wear wraparound sunglasses that provide 100 percent UV ray protection.
- **Consider Solarweave® (www.sunprotectiveclothing.com).** This fabric is specially

manufactured to block more than 97.5 percent of all UVA and UVB radiation; available in bathing suit cover-ups, long-sleeved shirts, T-shirts, pants, and hats.

- **Try Coolibar (www.coolibar.com).** These tunics, blouses, hoodies, pants, and cover-ups include a hang tag that lists the ultraviolet protection factor (UPF) rating. Some clothes claim to block 98 percent UV.

- **Wear a broad-spectrum lotion.** Aim for at least SPF 15 to guard against both UVA and UVB rays. To find the most effective brands, check the sunscreen database at the Environmenal Working Group (www.ewg.org).

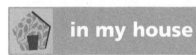

in my house

My family is particularly susceptible to skin cancer. My father's had it, my brother's had it, and I've had it—several times. Needless to say, I'm a borderline fanatic when it comes to wearing sunscreen. My daily face lotion contains SPF 15, and if I'm at the beach I always use a sunscreen of at least SPF 45. We all wear hats and sunglasses in the sun, and I wear long-sleeved cover-ups and pants. It's easy enough to use a little makeup if I feel I'm looking pale. I have to admit, it took a while to get over my desire for a "summer tan." But there's nothing like a few bouts of skin cancer to put vanity into perspective.

Send Companies a Message

Europe is far ahead of the United States in requiring manufacturers of cosmetics and personal-care products to avoid chemicals that could threaten the health or safety of people or the environment. Here in the United States, the Campaign for Safe Cosmetics, an alliance of consumer, environmental, and health organizations, is urging American industries to pledge that "all of the cosmetics and personal-care products made by our company anywhere in the world will meet the standards and deadlines set by the European Union . . . to be free of chemicals that are known or strongly suspected of causing cancer, mutation, or birth defects."

The pledge, called the Compact for Safe Cosmetics, commits cosmetic manufacturers to phase out 450 hazardous chemicals and replace them with safer, nontoxic alternatives. As of July 2007, eighty-seven organic and "natural products"

Message for Moms: What Are Your Daughters Doing?

There are lots of reasons you may not want your daughter to wear makeup. Until now, the health of your future grandchildren probably wasn't high on the list. But as increasing research shows, girls who apply cosmetics at an extremely early age may be putting themselves and their eventual offspring at risk. What can you do?

- Set a reasonable age for your daughter to begin to wear cosmetics.
- Set a good example by showing restraint yourself.
- Teach your daughter to read labels on the products she buys.
- Teach her where to shop.

companies had signed up. But the cosmetics giants, including L'Oréal, makers of Maybelline, Lancôme, and Redken; Clairol; and Revlon had not.

Contact your favorite cosmetic brands and urge them to sign the Compact for Safe Cosmetics. You can get more information at www.safecosmetics.org.

 shop talk

Urge Your Favorite Company to Sign the Compact for Safe Cosmetics

Almay
1-800-992-5629
www.almay.com/pg/help/contactus.aspx
  ?catid=0&catnm=ContactUs&subid=0
  &subnm=ContactUs

Avon
1345 Avenue of the Americas
New York, NY 10020
212-282-5000

Clairol
World Headquarters
1 Blanchley Road
Stamford, CT 06922
1-800-CLAIROL

Clinique
767 Fifth Avenue
New York, NY 10153
212-572-3800
www.clinique.com/customerservice/
cservice_clinique.tmpl#corp

Estée Lauder
Corporate Headquarters
767 Fifth Avenue
New York, NY 10153
212-572-4200

Lancôme
www2.lancome.com/_int/_en/services/
contact.aspx

L'Oréal
575 Fifth Avenue
New York, NY 10017
212-984-4000
www.loreal.com

Maybelline
1-800-944-0730
www.maybelline.com/contactus.aspx

Procter & Gamble
(Cover Girl, Crest, Clairol, Gillette
Complete Skin Care, Herbal Essence
Shampoo, Olay, Old Spice,
Secret Deodorant)
www.pg.com/en_US/products/all_
products/index.jhtml

Revlon
1-800-473-8566
www.revlon.com/Corporate/ContactUs.
aspx

Choose Less Packaging

Why cosmetics are packaged the way they are is a mystery to me.

Often, face powder will be boxed, but blush—a similar powder sold in a similar type of container—will be sold as is, with a simple adhesive seal secured over the opening. Lipstick tubes may be secured with a simple strip of tape; mascara tubes almost always come sheathed in plastic glued to cardboard.

Even the most evocative packages—the ones that use alluring faces and beckoning body parts to stoke your imagination—lose their appeal in the amount of time it takes to rip them open, retrieve their contents, and toss all that fancy wrapping into the trash bin and, ultimately, the landfill.

Companies that use point-of-purchase displays to educate shoppers about their products seem to get away with less-elaborate individual packages, reducing overall resource use. That's a good environmental strategy and one that should be rewarded, all other factors being equal and given the fact that a dollar of every eleven we spend on products goes for packaging we just throw away.

Look for the following low-impact packages when choosing your products:

- The least amount of packaging
- Cosmetics that are simply sealed, rather than boxed or encased in plastic
- Packages that are made from post-consumer materials, meaning the paper, plastic, and glass have been previously used, recycled, and remanufactured into the new packaging. Post-consumer materials are better for the environment because they reduce our use of virgin materials, energy, and water.
- Packaging, like cardboard and paper, that you can recycle. You cannot recycle most packaging made from plastic or polystyrene (such as Styrofoam).

 make the shift

Packaging

Yes	No
Cosmetics sealed with simple adhesive strip	Cosmetics encased in plastic, glued to cardboard backing
Packaging made from post-consumer recycled materials	Packaging made from PVC plastic
Packaging that can be recycled (e.g., paper, cardboard, glass containers, number 1 or 2 plastic)	Packaging that cannot be recycled (e.g., most cosmetic containers, number 3, 4, 5, 6, or 7 plastic)
Containers that can be refilled	Containers used once and discarded
In-store displays to explain product benefits	Elaborate packaging for each item to explain product benefits
Bulk-size to save energy and other resources	Bulk-size unavailable

Good Packaging Choices

Aveda. All Aveda's shampoo and conditioner bottles are made of 80 percent post-consumer recycled content, which the company claims is one of the highest levels in the industry. Aveda urges its customers to toss less trash by buying shampoo and conditioner in liter sizes, which use 40 percent less plastic and cost 30 percent less than the equivalent product in regular-size bottles.

Bath and Body Works. The company is phasing out PVC (polyvinyl chloride) plastic, a major source of dioxin, in its personal-care products, and switching to polyethylene terephthalate (PET, PETE), which can be recycled in most community recycling programs.

Johnson & Johnson. J&J is also phasing PVC out of most of its packaging, replacing it with PLA, a material whose building block is field corn and which the company says requires 65 percent less fossil fuel to manufacture than traditional plastics.

Burt's Bees. Rather than publish full catalogs that consume a lot of paper, Burt's Bees prints simple inserts to announce a new product and relies on in-store displays to advertise benefits. Some Burt's Bees products, like Cucumber and Chamomile, Lavender, and Grapefruit Complexion Mists, are packaged in aluminum containers that can be recycled curbside.

Tampons

If you're like most women, you'll use as many as 11,000 tampons during your lifetime. Add to that a couple of thousand pads and panty liners, and the ecological impact of your monthly cycle really starts to add up. Particularly egregious are the plastic applicators that come with some tampons. They can escape from any landfill—or wastebasket, for that matter—and plop down in a lake, river, playground, or just about anywhere else you'd rather not see them. The darn things are so indestructible even a car can run over them and not destroy them.

Conventional products may contain a mixture of rayon and cotton. Rayon has been implicated in toxic shock syndrome, particularly for superabsorbent tampons. Cotton is highly pesticide-intensive; 25 percent of pesticides used globally are devoted to growing cotton. To look as white as possible, conventional pads and tampons are usually bleached with chlorine, a process that can create dioxin, a known carcinogen.

Tampons, pads, and panty liners made from organic cotton are becoming increasingly available online and in the marketplace. If you're going to use conventional products, choose those sold in the simplest packaging.

Options:

O.b. tampons come in a small box with no applicator. They're compact and easy to use, and take up very little room in your purse.

Original-style *Tampax* are wrapped in paper and have a cardboard applicator that breaks down relatively quickly if they happen to get loose in the environment. They're preferable to the Pearl brand, which has an almost indestructible plastic applicator and is wrapped in coated paper.

Natracare and *Seventh Generation* chemical-free, nonchlorine-bleached biodegradable pads, panty liners, and tampons are available from natural food stores and food co-ops, as well as online at www.natracare.com and www.seventh generation.com.

The *DivaCup* (www.divacup.com) is worn internally like a birth control diaphragm. It may require emptying two to four times a day depending on your flow. This reusable option generates no trash, but is not quite as convenient as a tampon. Some women swear by it; others think it's, well, pretty messy. Take a look and decide for yourself.

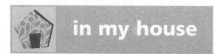

Sometimes what you try is all about convenience. Initially it was a little easier for me to come by Natracare products, so those are the ones I'm personally most familiar with. I've been satisfied with them, but I can only get them at the food co-op or Whole Foods. If I'm at the grocery store and I'm in a pinch, I'll buy O.b. or Tampax Original. Then I go see the store manager and ask him to order Natracare. He usually takes my information pretty quickly, since he doesn't really want to stand in the aisle very long talking to me about tampons. Someday, I expect to be pleasantly surprised to see the low-polluting, chlorine-free, eco-friendly tampons sitting right there on the shelf next to the indestructible plastic-coated options!

big green purse

What About Nanotechnology?

Nanoparticles are being engineered at the atomic and molecular level to enhance the consumer appeal of cosmetics and personal-care products. In some cases, nanomaterials enrich the color of a product; in others, they make the product easier to apply. With still others, they serve as "penetration enhancers," helping the product get below the surface of the skin to the blood vessels below.

Because these particles are essentially invisible—a nanometer measures a mere one billionth of a meter, compared to a molecule of DNA, at roughly 2.5 nm; a red blood cell at 7,000 nm; or a human hair cell, which is 80,000 nm wide—they can exist in your lipstick or body lotion and you would never know. Manufacturers are not required to inform you if they include nanomaterials in their ingredients.

Nanoparticles are being used in almost every personal-care product on the market, including deodorant, soap, toothpaste, shampoo, hair conditioner, sunscreen, antiwrinkle cream, moisturizer, foundation, face powder, lipstick, blush, eye shadow, nail polish, perfume, and aftershave lotion.

Despite such widespread and growing use, consumer groups, scientists, and environmentalists are concerned that the safety of nanotechnology has not been fully validated. Some scientific research has shown that certain types of nanoparticles can be toxic to human tissue and cell cultures. There is very little research on the impact that nanoparticles may have if they get loose in the environment. Activists worry that they could be like DDT or asbestos: once released into the air, water, or soil, they could have dire consequences that take decades or longer to sort out.

The nonprofit Friends of the Earth believes there should be a moratorium on the release of new products containing nanomaterials until adequate research demonstrates the health and environmental safety of this technology. Friends of the Earth also recommends that cosmetics and personal-care products that contain nanomaterials be withdrawn from the market until adequate safety studies have been conducted. At the very least, products containing nanomaterials should include that information on the label so consumers have the option of choosing an alternative.

The organization has compiled a database of cosmetics, personal-care products, and sunscreens that contain nanomaterials. The database, as well as the report "Nanomaterials, Sunscreens and Cosmetics: Small Ingredients, Big Risks," is available at www.foe.org.

The California Safe Cosmetics Act

The California Safe Cosmetics Act took effect in January 2007. The first legislation of its kind, it requires manufacturers to disclose product ingredients that cause cancer or birth defects. The law authorizes the state to investigate the health impacts of chemicals in cosmetics. The act also enables the state to regulate products in order to assure the safety of salon workers.

The bill, which was opposed by the Cosmetic, Toiletry and Fragrance Association, attempts to resolve the uncertainties created by the fact that the Food and Drug Administration does not review the ingredients in cosmetic and beauty-care products. Instead, the FDA relies on self-regulation by the industry's own Cosmetic Ingredient Review (CIR) panel.

One provision in the bill is designed specifically to protect the safety of nail-salon and cosmetology workers. Though these people come in contact with solvents, chemical solutions, and glues every day, little research has been conducted on the chronic health effects they face. Few appropriate educational materials exist to help workers and salon owners deal with these materials safely. During the course of the campaign to pass the California Safe Cosmetics Act, the California Healthy Nail Salons Collaborative was formed. It now advocates for greater workplace safety, protective policies, research, and community education.

Cosmetics Wrap-up

- **Give your body a break.** Use fewer or no cosmetics on the days you don't go to work.
- **Cut back.** Reduce the number of personal-care products you use overall by three.
- **Read labels.** Choose items that have the fewest, and safest, ingredients.
- **Limit or avoid purchase** of products that contain fragrance, phthalates, parabens, and triclosan or other antibacterial agents.
- **Prioritize your spending.** Shift first to products like safer deodorant and makeup that stay on your skin, and focusing on soaps, shampoos, conditioners, and other products that rinse off as your budget can afford it.
- **Ask local stores to carry more organic options.** Meanwhile, find brands online that you can trust.
- **Cut back on trash.** Choose products sold in the least amount of packaging.

And if you can do only one thing, create a line item in your budget for earth-friendly cosmetics and personal-care products. Shift at least 20 percent of the money you annually spend on shampoo, makeup, soaps, and lotions to safer, greener options. If you reduce the number of products you use overall, you can budget the money you save for the purchase of the sometimes higher-priced eco options.

big green purse

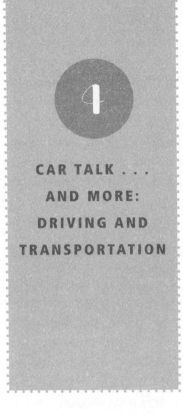

4

CAR TALK . . . AND MORE: DRIVING AND TRANSPORTATION

LET'S BE REAL.

As much as we dislike the environmental, health, and even national security consequences associated with driving our own cars, many of us still aren't ready to let go of our vehicles, or even change the way we drive. After all, we are *busy*. We have jobs to get to, families to attend to, religious obligations to meet, social appointments to keep, volunteer time to put in, community commitments to fit in, and, if a few precious seconds allow, "me" time to squeeze in so we don't go stark raving mad.

In other words, we have a lot of ground to cover, and covering it in our own car seems like the fastest, easiest, least stressful way, despite the impact we may have on the rest of the world. Do we really want to forgo the freedom our own four wheels affords—even if it means the planet will breathe a sigh of relief?

Often, the answer is no.

It's not that we wouldn't like to make the right choice. More often than not, we feel like we don't have much choice at all. Two-thirds of us living in rural areas have no access to mass transit right now. Those of us living in suburban and urban communities just can't see lugging all the kids and their gear on the bus. Given how many people (and pets, and backpacks, and other stuff) we have to cart around, and how many different places we need to be (often at the same time), it seems like the only way to do it all is by driving—even if we drive ourselves crazy in the process.

Then, there's the question of *what* we drive. We've all seen the ads calculated to make us feel secure and snug in a great big powerful car or SUV—you know, one that gets about fifteen miles for every gallon of climate-changing gas we pump into it. Don't we need to sacrifice fuel efficiency for family safety?

So sure, it would be terrific to drive less, and make a smaller impact when we do drive. But how do we manage that and still safely get where we need to go?

Good News

Hopefully, this chapter will help you answer these questions, and more. It starts by asking you to shift not just your money, but also your *mind*.

For the most part, we assume we have to drive everywhere we need to go. But all that driving complicates and stresses our lives, costs us a lot of money, pollutes the planet, and is even changing our climate. Thus, the most important shift you can make when it comes to transportation is to take stock of how much driving you do and figure out where you can cut back but still meet your transportation needs.

The list on page 81 should help you pinpoint opportunities to lighten your driving load. It's followed by dozens of ways you can conserve gas, share your ride, and explore alternative modes of transportation. You'll also find information on hybrids, diesels, and electric cars if you're in the market for a new vehicle, plus plenty of websites where you can get additional details.

Throughout this chapter, look for solid information on the environmental and health benefits you'll gain if you do cut back on driving or switch to a more fuel-efficient vehicle. The evidence is in. Cars are among the largest sources of air pollution, one of the biggest contributors to climate change, a major cause of water pollution, and a key factor behind asthma and even heart disease. Convenient or no, surely it's time we figured out how to meet our transportation needs without killing ourselves and the planet, too. Manufacturers will make the vehicles we demand. Women buy or influence the purchase of 59 percent of all vehicles. Let's throw the power of our purse behind the most fuel-efficient vehicles available.

How Much Do You Drive? It All Adds Up

Most of us, on average, drive about 11,500 miles a year. But it's not only the total number of miles that complicates our lives, it's also the number of trips we take that adds to the stress. Whether your work propels you outside the house or not, trips for family and personal business dominate women's transportation needs. That's a big distinction between men and women. About half of women's travel focuses on family and personal business, like grocery shopping and taking kids to school, doctor and dentist appointments, dance practice, music lessons, and after-school sports practice. The rate for men is significantly less.

How many of these trips do you make? Check all that apply.

__ Work (outside your home)

__ School

__ Doctor appointment

__ Dentist appointment

__ Sports practice (multiply for each child, and for number of times each child has practice during the week)

__ Sports game

__ Dance rehearsal

__ Dance performance

__ Art lesson

__ Music lesson

__ Religious class

__ Religious service

__ Regular weekly grocery shopping

__ Miscellaneous mall shopping

__ "In and out" shopping (to pick up milk, bread, eggs, etc.)

__ PTA meeting

__ Miscellaneous school activities

__ Exercise class for you

__ Community gathering

__ Volunteer work

__ Political activity

__ Social engagement for you

__ Play date for the kids

__ Caretaking for your parents

__ Social engagement for your family

__ Pets to the veterinarian

__ Pets to pet grooming

__ Pet store

__ Hardware store

__ Garden-supply center

__ Dry cleaner

__ Shoe repair

__ Family outing

__ Manicure/pedicure

__ Hair salon for you

__ Hair salon for kids

__ Video store

__ Restaurant

__ Carryout

__ Other?

We make most of these trips without giving them a second thought. We've gotten so used to the hectic pace of everyday life, we just hop in our car, step on the gas, and take off. But at what cost?

Let's take a quick look at the personal, environmental, and health impacts driving creates—and the benefits you'll gain from shifting your transportation dollars to more fuel-efficient options that offer the greatest opportunity to save gas, reduce climate change, and clean up the air.

Why Make the Shift to More Fuel-Efficient Transportation Options?

- Save time
- Save money
- Reduce climate change
- Save energy
- Protect water and wildlife
- Breathe easier
- Prevent heart disease
- Strengthen national security
- Improve your neighborhood

Save Time

If you're sixteen or older, you're probably spending at least an hour and a half behind the wheel every day, says *Consumer Reports*. In fact, it's taking 10 percent longer to cover commuting distances, given how much traffic there is. According to the most recent Texas Transportation Institute (TTI) report, congestion caused an average annual delay per traveler of forty-seven hours. In other words, you spent more than a work week of your life being late, just because you were sitting in traffic. Now, compare that to how much more efficiently you can use your time when you take mass transit and let someone else do the driving. Working at home could actually save you one to three hours a day, depending on the length of your commute. Even by grouping shopping expeditions so you can make one longer trip instead of several shorter ones, you can save yourself some time and hassle.

Save Money

Our dependency on oil is attached to a stupendous price tag, and it's a lot more than what we pay for a gallon of gasoline at the pump. California's Santa Cruz County Regional Transportation Commission has calculated that the hidden cost of the automobile to the average American taxpayer is $1.19 per mile, once the expense of building and maintaining roads, regulating and policing traffic, caring for accident victims, rectifying air pollution damage, and loss of land to paved roads is computed into the price. In other words, in addition to the three dollars per gallon it might cost you to drive twenty-five miles, you're being socked an additional $29.74 in real though behind-the-scenes charges generated specifically to maintain our car culture.

Meanwhile, every year, the average U.S. household spends more than a sixth of its budget buying, repairing, and fueling cars, more than on food and second only to housing; poor households spend twice that proportion.

You can save twenty to fifty dollars every month on gasoline by economizing on the trips you make and driving more fuel efficiently. A two-adult household that also relies on mass transit can save as much as $6,251 every year compared to an equivalent household with two cars and no access to mass transportation, once wear and tear on a second vehicle, insurance, fees, gasoline, tolls, and parking are taken into account.

Reduce Climate Change

The ten years between 1995 and 2005 marked the hottest decade on record, thanks in large part to the carbon dioxide emissions cars, light trucks, and sport-utility vehicles (SUVs) pumped into the atmosphere. Unless we go easy on the gas, the earth's average temperature will increase by as much as 10 degrees Fahrenheit during this century, bringing record heat waves, droughts, more frequent severe storms, rising sea levels, and the spread of tropical diseases like malaria.

If you drive an SUV, you spew up to 30 percent more air-polluting carbon monoxide and hydrocarbons than your neighbor in a sedan, and up to 75 percent more nitrogen oxide, one of the pollutants that cause acid rain. Pickup trucks get even worse mileage than either SUVs or cars, creating even greater problems. But whether you're driving the monster truck or a miserly hybrid, every gallon of gas you burn shoots twenty pounds of climate-changing carbon dioxide and five pounds of pure carbon into the atmosphere, which one analyst likened to throwing a five-pound bag of charcoal briquets out the window every twenty miles or so you drive. The good news is, for every additional mile you go on a gallon, you keep one ton of CO_2 out of the atmosphere in a year, writes *Vanity Fair* reporter Alex Shoumatoff. The less gas we burn, the better—knowledge that should be just as fundamental to us as the ABCs are to kindergartners.

Save Energy

Right now, our cars and light trucks depend on oil for 95 percent of their fuel. Common sense should tell us to diversify—especially since American vehicles consume more petroleum than American producers extract from our own reserves. Increasingly we're being put at the mercy of foreign oil sources, a situation that threatens our national security and weakens our economy. Even if we weren't, there's only so much oil in the ground. Using energy wisely now will help us bridge the gap as we transition to non-petroleum-based fuels and development of better systems that meet more of our transportation needs.

Protect Water and Wildlife

We all know oil and water don't mix. That's especially true when there's an oil spill. In the United States, an average of 8,100 oil spills, more than twenty-two a day, are reported annually. About half come from vessels like tankers or barges; the rest of the oil oozes out of pipelines, refining and storage facilities, and tanker trucks or train cars. Large spills, those of more than ten million gallons, occur at a rate of one to three a year worldwide. When they happen they're unforgettable—by nature as well as by those of us who witness it or watch it on TV. In 1989, the *Exxon Valdez* oil tanker dumped close to eleven million gallons of crude oil in Alaska's Prince William Sound, contaminating beaches and devastating hunting and fishing grounds in the largest oil spill in U.S. or Canadian history. *Valdez* oil coated thirteen hundred miles of pristine shoreline, killed hundreds of harbor seals, thousands of sea otters, and hundreds of thousands of marbled murrelets, harlequin ducks, and bald eagles, among other birds. Six years later, none of these species had recovered. Ten years later, only the bald eagle was on the road to recovery. Even today, almost two decades after the calamity struck, some species still haven't made up their losses.

big green purse

Petroleum fuels also leak from underground storage tanks, contaminating groundwater and streams. The U.S. Environmental Protection Agency has reported around two hundred confirmed releases each week since 2000. What the EPA catches far less frequently is the used motor oil car owners dump in their sewers or in the street, so much so that illicit disposal of used motor oil sends more petroleum into the water each year than even the largest tanker spill. Notes transportation activist and author Katie Alvord, just one gallon of oil can contaminate about a million gallons of water.

Breathe Easier

According to the EPA, cars, trucks, and other mobile sources account for almost a third of the total air pollution in the United States. In addition to the particulates they belch, these vehicles generate more than two-thirds of the carbon monoxide in the atmosphere, and a quarter of the hydrocarbons, another component of smog. Other pollutants emitted by cars and trucks include benzene, arsenic, formaldehyde, and lead, all of which could cause cancer. The EPA attributes the premature deaths of more than 64,000 Americans to air pollution each year.

Nitrogen oxides, another by-product of gasoline combustion, can also irritate the lungs, increase your chances of contracting respiratory disease, and even cause emphysema. In addition, nitrogen oxides contribute to acid rain by converting to nitric acid in the atmosphere, forming a compound so powerful, reports environmental analyst Jim Motavalli, it makes an average car's yearly NOx emissions high enough over time to dissolve a twenty-pound steel cannonball.

Prevent Heart Disease

Cars not only are one of the major contributors to air pollution. They also exacerbate heart disease. Women in particular face increased heart threats from dirty air simply due to our anatomy. Air pollution consists of minute particles of dirt, dust, soot, and grit, all of which come from burning fossil fuels. When we inhale this grime, the particulates lodge deep inside our lungs. If our lungs get inflamed, and our body has to work harder to breathe, we could have a heart attack or stroke. Women are more susceptible than men to air pollution and the heart problems it causes because our blood vessels are smaller than men's, among other reasons.

Scientists at the University of Washington made this discovery by analyzing data available through the Women's Health Initiative, a national research project that studied the health status of 65,893 women. Their study, published in *The New England Journal of Medicine* in February 2007, provides more reason for all of us to buy fuel-efficient cars; to drive the cars we have as efficiently as possible; and to use transportation alternatives when we can.

Strengthen National Security

If you're worried about national security, you should definitely drive "lite." Transportation in the United States relies heavily on oil, accounting for two-thirds of this country's petroleum use. Almost 60 percent of the oil we use right now is imported. Our dependence will only increase as we exhaust America's own reserves. Meanwhile, we're spending more than $100,000 a minute to purchase foreign oil and countless billions more defending our oil interests in the Middle East. Shifting those billions into creating a renewable energy economy here at home would help the United States build a viable energy future independent of unpredictable or hostile governments elsewhere in the world.

Improve Your Neighborhood

Worldwide, in the 1990s, the number of cars grew three times faster than the human population. In the United States, there are now more cars than licensed drivers, even more cars than adults.

With more cars come more roads, yet more roads do not necessarily improve our quality of life. In fact, the more roads we build, the more traffic and congestion increase, since additional roadways simply make it easier to accommodate spiraling traffic. The Surface Transportation Policy Project (STPP) found that cities that have spent billions for new roads have the same congestion levels as those that have not. Increasing road capacity can actually slow traffic, says the STPP; it may be better to place buildings and development more closely together to encourage walking and mass transit. One study comparing the narrow streets of Portsmouth, New Hampshire, to a conventional, low-density subdivision of the same size found that the subdivision and its wide roads generated three times the car trips. Economizing on trips, increasing mass transit, and supporting transit-oriented development are

Why Are We So Vulnerable?

The United States consumes 25 percent of all the oil produced in the world, yet we control just 2 to 3 percent of the world's oil reserves. We're on an energy seesaw, and most of the time we're stranded at the top, dangling our legs in distress.

Because of this imbalance, we rely too much on foreign oil, especially from regions in the world that are ridden with conflict and instability. Our dependence on oil from the Persian Gulf has almost tripled since the first gas lines in the 1970s. In 1974, the United States imported "just" one million barrels of oil a day from the Persian Gulf. Today, we import 2.5 million. As a result, our economy is vulnerable to extreme swings in the price and supply of oil.

We felt victimized after September 11. But we don't need acts of terrorism to put us at oil's mercy. Hurricanes Katrina and Rita knocked out 10 percent of the capacity of refineries based in Texas and Louisiana to convert oil into gasoline, sending gas prices skyrocketing and creating spot shortages in many parts of the country. As long as the United States remains dependent on petroleum—domestic or imported—the energy seesaw will never balance in our favor.

alternative approaches that will improve your neighborhood and lead to higher quality of life.

Mind Shift

Considering what driving costs in time, money, health, and environmental impact, the sooner we shift our mind-set away from a focus on driving our own cars, the better. The goal should be to meet our transportation needs, not necessarily to do all the driving ourselves. Take a minute to inventory the amount of driving you do day to day and week to week. Then ask yourself a few questions.

- **Where can you simplify?** Can you make fewer commitments, thereby reducing your time behind the wheel? Try alternating activities: volunteer at your church or other place of worship this year and on a community project next year. Freeing up your schedule will give you more leeway to create a "car-lite" transportation plan.
- **What about the kids?** Can you simplify your children's lives by having them alternate or drop activities so their lives aren't quite so transportation intensive, either?
- **Can you group errands and appointments in the same vicinity?** One longer trip is more efficient than several short trips; ask: "Do I really need to do that errand now, or can it wait until I go out for something else?"
- **Can you carpool?** If you have children, can you coordinate with other parents so you all drive less? Consider adult carpooling, too—for classes, social activities, school functions, and more.
- **Is online shopping an option?** Can delivery services take the place of the driving you would otherwise have to do?
- **Can you telecommute?** Is it feasible to work, volunteer, or perform some community service from home rather than drive to a location, at least part of the time?
- **Can you walk, bicycle, or take a bus or subway?** Can you cover shorter distances on foot or by bike? Will mass transit meet at least some of your transportation needs?

Once you identify ways to reduce the amount of driving you do, you may be surprised at how easy it is—and how much your quality of life improves. It might help if you set a goal that's reasonable given your circumstances. Can you reduce the amount of driving you do by 15 percent? Can you cut back the number of trips you make in a week by three? Team up with family, neighbors, and friends so that you work together to reduce driving and still get where you want to go.

Use Your Big Green Purse

Ideally, laws and regulations would continually improve automobile fuel efficiency while ensuring that America develops renewable, non-petroleum fuels as quickly as possible. In reality, quite the opposite has been true. Time and again, the federal government has sided with industry in opposing legislation that would require America's cars, trucks, and sport-utility vehicles to squeeze more miles out of every gallon of gas and transition to alternative sources of power.

For example, automakers are currently required to meet an average of only 27.5 mpg for cars and 22.2 mpg for SUVs and light trucks, a standard that has hardly changed since 1989. (Though the Bush Administration increased truck requirements slightly, as we went to press, a federal appeals court pronounced those requirements too weak and ordered the U.S. Transportation Department to toughen them.) In 2007, the U.S. Senate has finally passed an energy bill that would require cars, SUVs, and pickup trucks to achieve a 35 mpg fleet average by 2020. But this is at least five miles below the 40 mpg or higher that many environmental and public health advocates have long hoped could become the national standard. Automakers and their supporters on Capitol Hill also beat back a measure that would have required fleet vehicles to increase their average mpg by an additional 4 percent every year for ten years after 2020 until cars, trucks, and SUVs reached 52 mpg by 2030. Carmakers objected that such a goal was not feasible, even though a 2002 study by the National Academy of Sciences concluded that technological improvements should enable fuel economy to be increased by 50 percent without sacrificing safety, performance, or vehicle size.

Do fuel efficiency improvements make a difference? Increasing standards just to the 35 mpg proposed in the Senate would save more than two million barrels of oil per day by 2025—nearly the amount that the United States currently imports from the Persian Gulf. It would also reduce greenhouse gas emissions by 18 percent in the same period—the equivalent of taking sixty million cars off the road in one year.

The 35 mpg bill has not yet been passed by the House of Representatives or signed by the president. Whether it is or not, you don't have to wait until the law goes into effect to buy a vehicle that can achieve tremendous gas and climate-change savings. In fact, by using the power of your purse you can pull manufacturers in a greener direction precisely by spending your money on the greenest options that already exist:

- Mass transit
- Car-share membership
- Telecommuting
- Bicycling
- Walking
- A gas-sipper, not a gas-guzzler

Mass Transit

If you commute to work using mass transit rather than by driving alone, you could save two hundred gallons of gasoline per year, reduce the carbon dioxide and other air pollutants you pump into the atmosphere, and, at $3 per gallon, save $600.

Mass transit options include:

- **Electric railway and subway.** Electric rail is about six times as energy efficient as automobiles, with the added benefit that the electricity that runs rail can be generated by less-polluting sources that create far less smog. A six-car rail train can replace nine hundred cars that would otherwise clog sixty-eight city blocks at 15 mph, notes the Union of Concerned Scientists. Electric rail can use cleaner power, too. The light-rail system in Calgary, Canada, gets all the electricity used to power its trains from windmills.
- **City buses.** A growing number of cleaner transit vehicles is powered by compressed natural gas, which produces almost no air pollution. One full forty-foot bus helps keep fifty-eight cars off the road.
- **Long-distance trains and buses.** Amtrak train service and several national bus lines, including Greyhound and Trailways, provide energy-saving alternatives to both driving and flying.
- **Intracity rail.** Local rail lines connect suburban and rural cities and towns to metropolitan hubs, reducing traffic congestion, air pollution, and gas consumption.
- **Ferries.** Boats provide convenient shortcuts for commuters living in coastal communities.
- **Vanpools.** Dedicated minivans and small buses shuttle employees from central regional locations to company headquarters to reduce commuting stress, relieve traffic congestion, and minimize energy and air pollution costs associated with individual driving.

Use your transportation dollars to buy tickets for mass transit rather than pay for gasoline and parking.

- To determine what local mass transit options you have, do an Internet search for "mass transit in [city name]."
- To locate a convenient car pool, check http://carpoolconnect.com or www.erideshare.com.
- To participate in employer-provided vanpools, contact your company's human resources department.
- To book a train ticket, visit www.amtrak.com.
- To book a bus trip, log on to www.greyhound.com or www.trailways.com.

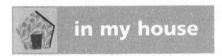

in my house

My family is lucky. We live in a suburb of Washington, D.C., one of the best metropolitan areas for mass transit in the country. We're only two blocks from the "Metro," so within five minutes we can walk to a subway that will whisk us to the cinema, performing arts complexes, museums, good restaurants, and the homes of friends.

For inconvenient destinations, we drive a hybrid car. It's been great in the city—easy to parallel park, with a great turning radius and maneuverability. Our hybrid is also peppy enough to wheel onto the Beltway with no worries. In addition, we have a Honda Odyssey minivan we're about to retire. We used the van for ten years when the kids were little to drive car pools, cart my son to Boy Scouts, and deliver my daughter to dance rehearsals. On its own, the vehicle wasn't very fuel efficient—it only got 26 mpg at the most—but it was effective at hauling six kids, the driver, and all their stuff. Now that our children are driving, we occasionally find ourselves in a transportation crunch. When the subway or our bicycles won't do, we call on Zipcar, a membership service that allows us to rent a car by the hour (see page 92).

The biggest challenge, regardless of the vehicle, is trying not to drive when we only have to go a few blocks. Engines generate the most air pollution running short distances when they're not yet operating efficiently. Still, sometimes it's irresistible to hop in the car and run up to the video store or over to 7-Eleven to get a gallon of milk, even though we could just as easily walk. Part of what we're trying to do in our own household is agree that we'll walk or bike to any location that's less than a mile. Teenagers just learning to drive don't particularly like this idea, but they'll get used to it.

Car-Share Membership

Car-sharing is becoming increasingly popular as more people want to give up their own car but still need wheels for various chores. Not having a car 24-7 reduces unnecessary trips (and the related air pollution and energy consumption they entail) while increasing biking, walking, and use of mass transit. At the same time, having access to a shared car still provides the opportunity to drive when it's necessary, even if that turns out to be only for an hour or two.

Car "sharing" differs from car "renting" in four ways:

1. *Billing.* You don't pay for an entire day if you only need the car for a short while.
2. *Convenience.* You manage your transaction over the Internet, including reservations, invoicing, and payment. It's fast and efficient.
3. *Location.* You can usually pick up your car in an easy-to-reach spot in your neighborhood or near a mass transit stop.
4. *Membership.* You pay a nominal annual membership fee ($40 to $50), which gives you access to a wide variety of cars—from energy-efficient hybrids to minivans to sedans.

What else is convenient about car sharing?

- You don't pay for fuel. Gas is on the company.
- You don't pay for extra insurance. The company covers that, too.
- Flat tire? Engine block cracks (whatever that means)? Call the company for a repair or a tow, free of charge.

In North America, two major companies offer car-sharing services:

- Zipcar (www. zipcar.com) operates in Boston, New York, San Francisco, Toronto, and Washington, D.C.
- Flex Car (www.flexcar.com) operates in Atlanta, Los Angeles, San Diego, San Francisco, Seattle, Portland, and Washington, D.C.

big green purse

Note: As we were going to press, Flex Car and Zipcar were planning to merge. Get the latest details on their websites. Local groups that offer similar services include:

- Austin—www.austincarshare.org
- Boulder—www.carshare.org
- Madison, Wisconsin—www.communitycar.com
- Minneapolis/St. Paul—www.hourcar.org
- Philadelphia—www.phillycarshare.org
- San Francisco—www.citycarshare.org

In Canada:

- Edmonton—www.web.net/~cce
- Ottawa—www.vrtucar.com
- Quebec City—www.communauto.com
- Vancouver—www.cooperativeauto.net
- Waterloo—www.peoplescar.org

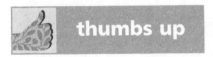

thumbs up

Eco-Friendly Car Services

Rentals. Increasingly, your fuel-efficient options at the rental desk include hybrids, diesels, and even biodiesels. Despite the efforts conventional car companies make to upgrade their customers to SUVs, stick with a model that is safe, fuel-efficient, and affordable. Alternatively, check out one of the companies listed below.

- **Bio-Beetle** (www.bio-beetle.com). The company, with operations in Los Angeles and on Maui, Hawaii, maintains a fleet of Volkswagen Beetles, Golfs, Jettas, and Passats, all running on 100 percent biodiesel fuel. The cars get between four hundred and eight hundred miles per tank, so refueling is usually not an issue on rentals of less than a week. Currently there are three fueling stations for 100 percent biodiesel (B99.9) in Los Angeles, and one on Maui.

- **EV Rental** (www.evrental.com). EV bills itself as "the nation's only environmental rental car company," and its exclusive line of hybrid vehicles bears it out. It operates exclusively in California and Arizona.
- **Alcatraz** (www.alcatraz.us). This San Francisco–based company rents two-seat electric cars for sightseeing in the Bay Area; the cars include a GPS audio tour guided by "hot spots" along three different routes.

Limo services. Want a chauffeur and some luxe but not the ozone usually associated with a limo? Try:

- **Eco-Limo** (www.eco-limo.com). Eco-Limo provides fuel-efficient, chauffeured ground transportation service in vehicles that include gas-electric, biodiesel, and compressed natural gas (cng) hybrids; available in Los Angeles, San Francisco, and Washington, D.C.
- **PlanetTran** (www.planettran.com). This hybrid shuttle service for New England and Northern California serves metropolitan airports and other destinations on call.
- **OzoCar** (www.ozocar). This hybrid service for New York City provides rides in a Toyota Prius or a Lexus RX 400h.

Alternative AAA. If you're looking for an eco-friendly auto service, check out:

- **Better World Club** (www.betterworldclub.com). The company offers emergency roadside assistance for cars and bikes, hotel and air bookings, eco-friendly travel options, and car insurance.

Telecommuting

Telecommuting works to the advantage of parents who prefer to be home when their kids arrive after school; baby boomers taking care of aging parents; and anyone looking to reduce travel stress, or simply save energy and money on gas. This option works best if your job involves research, writing, meetings with others you'd be "attending" by phone anyway, phone sales, and tasks that allow you to access your work computer from home. Check company policies to determine whether employees may telecommute one or more days a week, and whether you qualify to participate. If you do, shift the money you'd normally spend on gas, parking, and wear and tear on your car to a computer and other office equipment that will make working at home more pleasant and efficient. If you can't telecommute, suggest other options. Can you work a "flex time" schedule of four long days rather than five shorter ones? Can you task share with a coworker so that an employee is always on the job even if you're at home some of the time?

Bicycling

Use your bike to commute if your job is close by; to do errands; to socialize; to dine out; to take in a movie; to grocery shop; to relax and unwind. And if you're trying to stay in shape, remember: biking for transportation can take the place of other forms of exercise even while it reduces driving needs.

- You can learn about bike-to-work options at www.biketowork.com.
- Need tips on how to set up a bicycle commute? Check out the Bicycle Source, www.bicyclesource.com/you/commuting.
- Jennifer's Bicycle Commuting Suggestions (www.poplarware.com/personal/bicycle.html) can help you buy and outfit a bike you can use for work, shopping, and socializing.

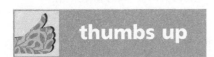
thumbs up

Electric Bikes and SUBs (Sport-Utility Bicycles)

Like the idea of biking but think all that pedaling will do you in? Consider an electric motorbike or bicycle. You'll reduce air pollution, relieve traffic congestion, and save money on gas and auto upkeep. Plus, says ElectricBikes.com, electric-powered bicycles pollute only one-tenth as much as driving a car the same distance.

The Enertia (www.enertiabike.com). This all-electric motorbike could reduce your carbon footprint by 92 percent. It requires no gas or oil, is nearly silent, has no exhaust, and doesn't get hot. The vehicle has a fifty-mile driving range at speeds of up to 60 mpg before its 110-volt battery needs a recharge. The standard model costs around twelve thousand dollars new.

eGo Cycle (www.gaiam.com). A simple turn of a key and a quick throttle twist en-

Meet . . .

Katie Alvord . . . This former librarian and freelance writer "divorced" her first car in 1992. In 1994, she moved to rural Upper Michigan, where she and her husband keep driving to a minimum. Instead, they've outfitted their bikes with snow tires for winter riding, haul groceries home in bike trailers, ski to social events, walk when it suits them, and rent bikes for getting around cities they visit. Read about her story in *Divorce Your Car! Ending the Love Affair with the Automobile.*

Janie Katz-Christie . . . An architect and mother of three, Janie invented her own oversize tricycle so she could cart all of her children to school at one time. The "Walk/Ride Days" she helps organize one day a month as part of the Green Streets Initiative in Cambridge, Massachusetts, encourage commuters to wear something green and bicycle, walk, or take the subway or train. "Just get out of your car," says Janie. "And have fun!" See more at www.gogreenstreets.org.

Karen Sagstetter . . . This editor at the National Gallery of Art in Washington, D.C., combines biking and busing to get to work from her home ten miles away in Glen Echo, Maryland. Going to work, she rides her bicycle along the C&O Canal and across the Mall to her Capitol Hill office. She takes the bus home, then catches the bus back to work the next day so she can ride her bicycle home again. "It's a great way to exercise," says Karen. Plus, she notes, "seeing great blue herons, beavers, turtles, deer, even a snowy owl once, combined with the camaraderie of Rollerbladers, joggers, and other bikers, is also part of the joy."

gage either of two electronically controlled operating modes ("Go Far" and "Go Fast"), letting you tailor your ride for either greater distance range or maximum speed. The standard model costs around fifteen hundred dollars new.

ScooterCommuter (www.scootercommuter.com). Electric scooters, standard electric bikes, and electric bikes with solar panels integrated into the wheels are among the nonpolluting transportation options offered by this innovator.

Schwinn (www.schwinnbike.com). The Continental, GSE, and Campus models all cover sixty miles on a four-hour battery charge.

Worksman (www.worksmancycles.com). Pedicabs, adult tricycles, "family chariots," and "Worksman Tough" are among the wheel combos this company retails.

BionX (www.bionx.ca). The BionX system can be installed on your own bicycle (road, mountain, tandem, folding, recumbent) by replacing the rear wheel with the BionX motor-wheel.

Want to load up your bike with groceries, your laptop, or even a kayak (yes, a kayak), but worry that you'll lose your balance when you pedal off?

Xtracycle (www.xtracycle.com). The FreeRadical kit available at Xtracycle.com converts your bike into a stable "sport-utility bicycle," complete with spacious saddlebags and a rear platform for a load or passenger.

Walking

Shift your spending to a new pair of shoes, and walk distances of at least a mile or less. To make shopping easier, use a light but sturdy backpack, a wagon, or a compact rolling cart (available in many grocery and hardware stores).

If you're wondering whether walking is a viable alternative to driving, just ask Edith McCrea, who has lived in Ithaca, New York; Chicago, Illinois; and Cambridge, Massachusetts, and never owned a car!

Says Edith of herself and her husband, Larry: "Our motives for remaining car-less include our distaste for driving and a desire to save money and avoid the other hassles associated with car ownership. Preserving the environment and getting a lot of exercise are added bonuses. We generally do not feel any particular need for other forms of exercise, and prefer actually going somewhere to, for example, using a treadmill.

"Chicago is a good city for public transportation. You can get pretty much anywhere on the bus and 'L' combined with walking, although you sometimes have to

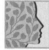

be patient—the buses tend to run behind schedule. It is also easy to find your way around, as it is mapped out on a grid, unlike the Boston area!

"I walked home from the hospital, which was in our neighborhood, after giving birth to both of our children, carrying my son in a Snugli and my daughter in a cloth sling.

"Our kids are used to walking everywhere. We used Baby Björns, backpack carriers, and strollers, in combination with public transit. We decided to put our son's stroller away before our second child was born rather than opt for one of those big double strollers. Taking a small child on foot requires a lot of patience; allow yourself a LOT of extra time to 'stop and smell the roses,' and rest!

"In Cambridge, when we felt both kids were too big for a stroller, we sometimes traveled the mile from our apartment to our kids' preschool using a little red wagon. We have become somewhat famous in the neighborhood for our use of this wagon. People often stop us . . . to say that they have seen us walking with our kids everywhere, and that they think it's great."

You can read more about Edith, and other people who choose walking and biking over their cars, at www.gogreenstreets.org.

For suggestions on earth-friendly shoes, don't miss Chapter 8.

go green

Top 10 Ways to Use Less Gas

1. **Drive less.** Walk, bicycle, use a scooter or moped, combine trips, and telecommute.
2. **Drive smart.** Avoid quick starts and stops, don't tailgate, and don't idle.
3. **Drive the speed limit.** Remember, every 5 mph you drive above 60 mph is like paying an additional ten cents per gallon for gas.
4. **Use cruise control on the highway.** You can improve fuel economy by 4 to 14 percent by driving at a steady speed.
5. **Drive a more fuel-efficient car.** Consider one of the new hybrids; at the very least, choose from among the EPA's "Fuel Economy Leaders" in the class vehicle you're considering.
6. **Keep your engine tuned up.** Improve gas mileage by an average of 4.1 percent by maintaining your vehicle in top condition.

7. **Carpool.** According to the Natural Resources Defense Council, thirty-two million gallons of gasoline would be saved each day if every car carried just one more passenger on its daily commute.

8. **Use mass transit and "Ride Share" programs.** Why buy gasoline at all?

9. **Keep tires properly inflated.** Improve gas mileage by around 3.3 percent by keeping your tires inflated to the proper pressure. Replace worn tires with the same make and model as the originals.

10. **Support higher fuel-efficiency standards and the development of alternative fuels.** Ultimately, our best hope for reducing the amount of gas we burn is to increase fuel efficiency while we transition to renewable and non-petroleum-based fuels. Endorse efforts to boost average fuel efficiency to at least 40 mpg. Support programs that promote research and development of alternatives to transportation systems based on oil.

A Gas-Sipper, Not a Gas-Guzzler

In 2004 the Good Housekeeping Institute and automotive research firm J. D. Power & Associates queried 40,000 women on what they most looked for in a vehicle. Researchers found that 82 percent of women find environmentally friendly vehicles "extremely" or "somewhat" important. Women value the low emissions that minimize pollution and slow global warming by reducing greenhouse gases, the survey showed. Women also appreciate the better gas mileage more fuel-efficient cars get.

While the survey showed that protecting the planet is a priority, safety was our greatest concern. Isn't it ironic then, that SUVs, which are among the most dangerous vehicles to drive as well as the most polluting, have been marketed so heavily to women? Dr. Jeffery Runge, head of the National Highway Traffic Safety Administration in 2003, reported that SUV drivers are especially vulnerable to fatal rollovers because the vehicles' high center of gravity makes them more likely to tip during sudden maneuvers. According to Dr. Runge, rollovers accounted for just 3 percent of all U.S. auto accidents in 2001 but caused nearly a third of all vehicle-occupant fatalities. An SUV occupant was more than three times as likely to die as a result of a rollover than an occupant of a passenger car.

When compared to minivans on the safety spectrum, SUVs lose hands down. Malcolm Gladwell, author of the best sellers *The Tipping Point* and *Blink*, notes, "If consumers really wanted something that was big and heavy and comforting, they ought to buy minivans, since minivans, with their unit-body construction, do much better in accidents than SUVs. (In a 35 mph crash test, for instance, the driver of a Cadillac Escalade—the GM counterpart to the Lincoln Navigator—has a 16 percent chance of a life-threatening head injury, a 20 percent chance of a life-threatening chest injury, and a 35 percent chance of a leg injury. The same numbers in a Ford Windstar minivan—a vehicle engineered from the ground up, as opposed to simply being bolted onto a pickup-truck frame—are, respectively, 2 percent, 4 percent, and 1 percent.)"

Gladwell also points out that a major disadvantage of SUVs is the clumsy handling that is an inevitable, and dangerous, consequence of their big size. "Are the best performers the biggest and heaviest vehicles on the road? Not at all," he points out. "Among the safest cars are the midsize imports, like the Toyota Camry and the Honda Accord [both of which are available in energy-saving hybrid models]. Or consider the extraordinary performance of some subcompacts, like the Volkswagen Jetta [another fuel saver]. Drivers of the tiny Jetta die at a rate of just forty-seven per million, which is in the same range as drivers of the five-thousand-pound Chevrolet Suburban and almost half that of popular SUV models like the Ford Explorer or the GMC Jimmy."

Acknowledges Gladwell, "In a head-on crash, an Explorer or a Suburban would crush a Jetta or a Camry." But, he says, "clearly, the drivers of Camrys and Jettas are finding a way to avoid head-on crashes with Explorers and Suburbans. The benefits of being nimble—of being in an automobile that's capable of staying out of trouble—are in many cases greater than the benefits of being big."

Given that women are buying or influencing the purchase of 59 percent of all cars (another Good Housekeeping Institute survey statistic), why not throw our purse power behind vehicles that provide more safety and the greater fuel efficiency we value?

Before you get a new car, consider:

1. Your needs
2. Fuel efficiency
3. Size and weight
4. Lease, buy, or rent?
5. Hybrids
6. Diesels
7. Alternatively fueled vehicles
8. Can you recycle your car?

Take stock of how many people or how much weight you most commonly transport before you head to the car lot. Are you single? Will you mostly be driving yourself? Do you still drive a car pool for your kids and their friends? Are you an entrepreneur who operates a business out of the backseat of your vehicle? Will you use your wheels primarily for commuting to work, for doing errands around town, or for traveling long distances? "Don't buy more car than you need," advises Jamie Kitman, New York bureau chief of *Automobile Magazine*.

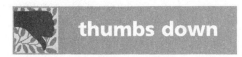

SUV Scam

I grew up in Michigan, before climate change was noticeable and nobody thought twice about plowing through snowfalls several feet deep. We didn't have SUVs. We had snow tires.

Today, women are being sold on sport-utility vehicles whether we need to drive in hazardous conditions or not (mostly, we don't). They're marketed to us as safe, reliable, and even fun. The record on SUVs tells a different story: when large SUVs hit cars head-on, according to a 1998 University of Michigan study, the occupants of the cars are five times more likely to die than if they'd been hit by another car.

SUVs are not any friendlier to the earth, either:

- Some SUVs attain only 13 or 14 mpg in the city compared to the 27.5 mpg a standard four-door car averages, giving new meaning to the term "gas-guzzler."
- Federal law actually permits SUVs to waste 33 percent more gasoline than passenger cars, spew out 30 percent more carbon monoxide and hydrocarbons, and emit 75 percent more nitrogen oxides.

At a time when every gallon of imported oil counts, asthma rates are rising, and climate change is the most serious environmental threat we face, surely we can find a better alternative to drive.

Consumer pressure has encouraged manufacturers to create a few fuel-efficient SUVs. If you still find yourself in the market for an SUV, the most fuel-efficient 2008 models are:

Ford Escape Hybrid—34 mpg city/30 mpg highway (Front-Wheel Drive)

Mercury Mariner Hybrid—34 city/30 highway (Front-Wheel Drive)

Lexus RX 400h—32 city/27 highway (Front-Wheel Drive)

Toyota Highlander Hybrid—32 city/27 highway

2. Fuel efficiency: Get the most efficient vehicle to meet your needs.

Once you've settled on the size and style vehicle you want, choose the most fuel-efficient option in that class by comparing mileage at www.fueleconomy.gov or the Edmunds "comparator tool" at www.edmunds.com/apps/nvc/edmunds/VehicleComparison. For example, if you want a family sedan, you can compare the Toyota Camry Hybrid, at 33 mpg city/ 34 mpg highway to the Chevy Malibu Hybrid at 24 mpg city/32 highway and determine which car offers the better choice.

You can also check the fuel economy label (see below) that's usually affixed to the window of every new car. Many vehicle models come in a range of engine sizes and trim lines, resulting in different fuel-economy values. When purchasing a vehicle, use the label to check the projected fuel economy for specific models you're considering. Similar ratings should be available for used cars; ask showroom dealers.

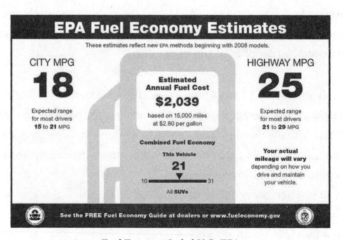

Fuel Economy Label U.S. EPA

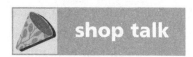
shop talk

When you go to buy or lease a new car, ask for some or all of the following performance-enhancing, fuel-saving technologies in the vehicle you choose.

WHAT TO LOOK FOR IN A NEW CAR	
Technology	*Average Efficiency Increase*
ENGINE TECHNOLOGIES	
Variable Valve Timing & Lift improve engine efficiency by optimizing the flow of fuel & air into the engine for various engine speeds.	5%
Cylinder Deactivation saves fuel by deactivating cylinders when they are not needed.	7.5%
Turbochargers & Superchargers increase engine power, allowing manufacturers to downsize engines without sacrificing performance or to increase performance without lowering fuel economy.	7.5%
Integrated Starter/Generator (ISG) Systems automatically turn the engine on/off when the vehicle is stopped to reduce fuel consumed during idling.	8%
Direct Fuel Injection (with turbocharging or supercharging) delivers higher performance with lower fuel consumption.	11–13%
TRANSMISSION TECHNOLOGIES	
Continuously Variable Transmissions (CVTs) have an infinite number of "gears," providing seamless acceleration and improved fuel economy.	6%
Automated Manual Transmissions (AMTs) combine the efficiency of manual transmissions with the convenience of automatics (gears shift automatically).	7%

Source: U.S. Dept. of Energy/U.S. Environmental Protection Agency

3. Size and weight: Pounds count.

Bigger cars use more gas, and cost more money to operate. An eight-passenger, fifty-five-hundred-pound Ford Expedition powered by a V-8 engine uses more fuel than an eight-passenger Honda Pilot with a V-6 engine that weighs less than forty-five hundred pounds. Unless you're towing a boat every weekend, do you really need an Expedition? Do you need any kind of SUV? Most people think of SUVs and light trucks generically as cars, and use them like cars; in reality, only about 14 percent of pickup buyers use them mainly as work trucks. On the excuse that they're work vehicles, SUVs and light trucks have been allowed to use more gasoline and emit more pollutants than regular cars, reducing air quality, accelerating global warming, and increasing our dependence on oil. But consider the difference this change makes for the driver who travels fifteen thousand miles in an average year. At 35 mpg, the compact burns about 428 gallons of fuel. At 15 mpg the SUV will consume about one thousand gallons of gas over fifteen thousand miles.

By the way, options like four-wheel drive and third-row seats increase the weight your vehicle carries, adding to its fuel consumption. If you don't need the extras, skip them. You'll be happy you did when you go to fill up your tank.

4. **Lease, buy, or rent? Owning a car doesn't always make sense.**
Given how quickly automotive technology is changing, next year's vehicles will undoubtedly be greener than this year's models. Rather than purchase a new car, consider leasing instead. You can benefit from the new technology, and be ready to transition to a more car-free lifestyle when it becomes more convenient to do so.

Another option: buy a gas sipper to meet your regular needs, then rent a larger vehicle when you want to pack in more vacation gear, work equipment, or home-improvement supplies.

 go green

Buying a New Car?

- Before you buy a new or used car, check with the U.S. EPA at www.fueleconomy.gov. Find the fuel economy leader in the class size you're interested in and choose the most fuel-efficient vehicles available.
- The federal government has also developed a Fuel Cost Calculator to help you anticipate annual fuel costs, as well as compare gas and money savings among vehicles. It makes clear how much gas and money you can save simply by driving

a more fuel-efficient vehicle. For example, a vehicle that gets 30 mpg will cost you $663 less to fuel each year than one that gets 20 mpg (assuming 15,000 miles of driving annually and a fuel cost of $2.65/gallon). Over a period of five years, the 30-mpg vehicle will save you $3,313. Visit www.fueleconomy.gov/feg/savemoney.shtml to download the calculator and look for ways to save money and gas.

- Check out Mothers for Clean and Safe Vehicles, a "gas roots" group of moms from diverse backgrounds and interests. But, says the group on its website www.dontbefueled.org, "one thing we have in common is definite opinions about vehicles and transportation. Our goal is to help people make educated and rational decisions by giving them access to lots of information about vehicles." At the site, you can sign a petition to major automakers and U.S. legislators asking that fuel efficiency and safety be made top priorities for every class vehicle, especially SUVs, pickup trucks, and minivans.

5. Hybrids: How they work.

Right now, existing technologies could quickly raise the average fuel economy of cars and light trucks to 40 mpg. But that's still not enough to help us conquer our dependence on oil. Over the long term, fuel cells and other alternatives will need to come to our rescue. These won't be ready for several years. Fuel efficiency and hybrid technology can fill the gap.

HOW DOES A HYBRID WORK?

Current hybrid vehicles simply combine a smaller gasoline engine with a battery-powered electric motor. In doing so, they can more than double the mileage of conventional cars. Hybrids burn little fuel as they slow down, and can come to a complete stop when waiting in traffic. You recharge their batteries every time you hit the brakes. You don't have to plug them into an electrical socket; they use the same gasoline other cars do, though less of it. The EPA website www.fueleconomy.gov/feg/hybrid_sbs.shtml compares the various hybrid cars, trucks, and SUVs currently on the market in terms of fuel efficiency and environmental impact.

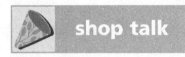

shop talk

Showroom Selections

Before you car shop, consider your choices. Every year, new vehicle models enter the marketplace offering more energy-efficiency options and environmental benefits. The list below gives you an idea of the top ten models available in 2007. Check www.biggreenpurse.com for updates on the most fuel-efficient, earth-friendly vehicles available this year.

	FUEL ECONOMY LEADERS: 2007 MODEL YEAR	
Rank	Manufacturer/Model	MPG city/highway
1	Toyota Prius (hybrid-electric)	60/51
2	Honda Civic Hybrid	49/51
3	Toyota Camry Hybrid	40/38
4	Ford Escape Hybrid FWD	36/31
5	Toyota Yaris (manual)	34/40
6	Toyota Yaris (automatic)	34/39
7	Honda Fit (manual)	33/38
8	Toyota Corolla (manual)	32/41
9	Hyundai Accent (manual)	32/35
	Kia Rio (manual)	32/35
10	Ford Escape Hybrid 4WD	32/29
	Mercury Mariner Hybrid 4WD	32/29

big green purse

Do One-Day Gas Boycotts Work?

You open your e-mail box and there it is—the call to boycott a single oil company on a particular day. Should you do it? Will it reduce the price of gas, increase oil supply, or minimize pollution?

The honest answer is, none of the above.

Often, boycotters simply top off their tanks a day in advance, or wait to fill them up until the day after the boycott. So while they may buy or use less gas on the appointed day, they're buying the same amount of gas overall.

The best way to bring the price of gas down, increase oil supply, and prevent pollution is to use less gas over time. Make it a habit to drive less, take the bus, carpool, walk, and bike. You'll have a much bigger impact than a one-day boycott because those activities actually leave more oil in the pipeline, ultimately increasing supply. In the long-term, you'll be fortifying your independence from petroleum, which is the best way to solve the problems created by burning gasoline.

thumbs down

Keep the Muscles for Opening a Jar of Spaghetti Sauce

A full hybrid like a Toyota Prius might get anywhere from 50 to 60 mpg. But so-called "muscle" hybrids only use hybrid technology to increase power and performance. They don't significantly increase the miles a vehicle wrings from a gallon of gas.

"Muscle" hybrids are usually more expensive than their gasoline-only counterparts and primarily benefit from the "hybrid" association in terms of the marketing pizzazz it provides.

The Chevrolet Tahoe is a perfect example of a "muscle" hybrid that reaps a marketing advantage from claiming to be a hybrid. The 2006 conventional Tahoe 2WD gets an estimated 17 mpg. GM is saying that its "dual mode" hybrid system will deliver approximately 25 percent better fuel economy. At only 21 mpg, that still doesn't pass muster as a highly fuel-efficient vehicle, even for an SUV.

Even if a car claims to be a "hybrid," check the fuel-economy label that comes with every vehicle. If it doesn't get at least 30 mpg, keep your money in your purse.

 thumbs up

News for Moms!

The Toyota Sienna Hybrid Minivan will be the first hybrid-powered minivan to hit the U.S. markets. Fuel economy should be in the high thirties to low forties, significantly above other standard minivans. The Sienna Hybrid will most likely have the same power train (the group of components that creates the vehicle's power, including the engine, transmission, and drive shaft) as the Highlander Hybrid SUV. The Sienna Hybrid will also sport an aerodynamic body design, insulated roof, and an "intuitive" humidity-sensing air-conditioning system, all meant to deliver better fuel efficiency while generating less pollution. The 1,500 watts of auxiliary power can be used to power appliances or laptops, or for emergency use. Check www.biggreen purse.com for availability.

 make the shift

Just Do the Math

Worried that a hybrid is out of your price range? Let's do the math. Depending on what model Camry you buy, a Prius Hybrid could be significantly cheaper. The middle-upper level Camry (SE), with a V-6 engine, bodyside molding, spoiler, mudguards, sunroof, leather seats, and a navigation system costs $32,319 ($24,815 is the MSRP; $32,319 with options).

How a Hybrid Saves Energy

- Regenerative braking captures energy normally lost during braking to charge the electric motor.
- High-strength, lightweight materials like aluminum reduce weight without compromising safety.
- Continuously variable transmission boosts fuel economy through better "gear ratios."
- Aerodynamic design improves fuel economy by reducing drag and wind resistance.
- Integrated starter/generator saves fuel by shutting down gas engine when idling in traffic.
- Hybrid engine combines small internal combustion engine with electric motor; variable valve control improves performance by controlling the mix of air and fuel more precisely.

Source: Sierra Club

A Prius (Touring Version—a step up from the basic) with a set of all-weather mats costs $26,682 ($23,070 is the MSRP; with options added it's $26,682).

Plus, in the case of the Prius, you have at least two additional advantages:

- **Save money on gasoline.** The EPA estimates you'll spend $908 a year on gas driving a Prius Hybrid, compared to $1745 driving the same distance in a standard Camry, a savings of $840 a year.

- **Take a tax credit.** Beginning January 1, 2006, you could take a tax credit ranging from four hundred to thirty-four hundred dollars if you bought a hybrid vehicle. The tax credit directly reduces the taxes you owe, as opposed to simply reducing taxable income. The tax credit varies, depending on which vehicle you buy. According to calculations by automotive website Edmunds.com, a Toyota Prius Hybrid generates an estimated $3,150 tax credit, while a Ford Escape Hybrid SUV generates $2,600 and the Honda Insight Hybrid tax credit is worth $1,950. The tax credit is set to expire in 2009, but for many hybrid models the incentive will end sooner, once a certain number of vehicles is sold. For more information, check with the IRS at www.irs.gov/newsroom/article/ 0,,id=161076,00.html and the EPA by visiting www.fueleconomy.gov/FEG/TAX_HYBRID.SHTML.

OTHER HYBRID PERKS

When I bought my hybrid sedan, I got a two-thousand-dollar federal tax credit as well as a two-thousand-dollar state tax credit from the state of Maryland. Nearby Virginia lets me drive in the HOV lane during rush hour, even if I'm alone. Local and state governments and private employers offer hybrid drivers a variety of similar incentives to choose highly fuel-efficient vehicles, including:

- **Customer discounts.** Travelers, the second-largest writer of auto and homeowners' insurance through independent agents, offers a 10 percent discount on auto insurance for hybrid owners. The Farmers Insurance Group of Companies makes an insurance discount available to customers who own a hybrid or alternative-fuel vehicle, including gas-electric hybrids, electric only, natural gas, ethanol, methanol, and propane. Hybrid-driving overnight guests at the Fairmont Hotel in San Jose, California, get free parking. The Argent Hotel in San Francisco cuts its rate for overnight parking in half—from forty-two dollars to twenty-one dollars—for hybrid drivers.
- **Cash back.** In February 2007, Bank of America announced that it is expanding its program to reimburse three thousand dollars to employees purchasing a new hybrid vehicle. Hyperion, a software company based in Santa Clara, California, offers its employees five thousand dollars if they purchase a hybrid. Google gives its full-time U.S.-based workers a five-thousand-dollar subsidy toward the purchase of a vehicle with an EPA fuel economy rating of 45 mpg or higher. Outdoor apparel company Timberland in New Hampshire put three thousand dollars toward hybrid purchases by any of its six thousand employees who have worked at least two years at the company. For more examples, visit the corporate incentives page of the Hybrid Cars website www.hybridcars.com/corporate-incentives.html.

HybridCenter.org maintains an updated list of state and federal incentives available to hybrid owners. See what additional benefits you can enjoy once you purchase a hybrid.

6. Diesels: New and improved.

Today, Volkswagen, Renault, Fiat, BMW, Jaguar, and Alfa Romeo are among the most popular diesel cars being sold . . . in Europe. Here in the United States, our choices have been limited. Formerly, even though a diesel engine got more miles to the gallon than a gasoline engine, because it generated more particulate matter, or soot, it was a lot worse for our air.

Starting in January 2007, all new diesel cars and trucks sold in the United States were required to reduce nitrous oxide (NOx), particulate matter, and other pollutants that cause smog. According to the EPA, once these standards take effect, diesels sold in America should be as clean as their gasoline counterparts. Due to their engine design, they'll still use less gas. At that point, if there's a diesel model that appeals to you over its gasoline counterpart, you can save more money and gas driving diesel.

If you already own a diesel, you don't need to trade it in for a new model if you want to be eco-friendly. You can drive it on biodiesel, a renewable fuel made from vegetable oil, with little or no modification to your car engine. Learn more at www.biodiesel.com; to locate biodiesel fuel, visit www.grassolean.com.

7. Alternative fuels: From ethanol to electricity.

ETHANOL

Should we eat corn—or drive with it?

Fuel derived from corn and other grains is called ethanol. It is the most widely used alternative transportation fuel in America. Thanks to General Motors, more than two million FlexFuel vehicles ply the roads today, cars, trucks, and SUVS that are able to operate either on gasoline or on a blend of 85 percent ethanol and 15 percent gasoline. By 2012, GM and other automobile manufacturers are aiming for half of their annual vehicle production to be E85 flexible fuel (or biodiesel) capable.

But is that what we want? Already, ethanol production is claiming the lion's share of America's corn crop. The U.S. Department of Agriculture projected that of the twenty million tons of grain grown in 2006, fourteen million tons would be used to produce fuel for cars, leaving only six million for food. We could have more ethanol, but a lot less corn to feed animals, so less meat, milk, and eggs.

Or maybe our groceries will just get more expensive. The Reuters news service reported that "U.S. popcorn prices have risen more than 40 percent since 2006 as soaring demand for feed corn to fuel the ethanol boom has spilled over into the favorite snack of American moviegoers." Reports the Canadian *National Post*, "Italians are grumbling because Canadian farmers are diverting wheat crops to biofuel production and not into making pasta. In Mexico, the rise in American corn prices has caused a spike in the tortilla prices that has the poor in that country on edge." In the United States, food prices were up 3.9 percent in April 2007 compared to a year earlier (the overall inflation rate in the same period: 2.6 percent). Over the past five years, food prices have risen 12.2 percent nationwide. Among the fastest-rising items, says the *Chicago Sun-Times*? Beef and eggs, two foods that are produced as a direct result of feeding cows and chickens corn.

Ironically, we may not be achieving the energy independence we want from the feed corn we're converting into agricultural oil. Since a gallon of ethanol contains less energy than a gallon of gasoline, flexible fuel vehicles typically get about 20 to 30 percent fewer miles per gallon when fueled with E85. So to use ethanol, you may end up paying more at the pump—along with those higher grocery bills.

Plus, when farmers grow grain, they use, literally, tons of fertilizer—fertilizer that runs off into streams and rivers and, ultimately, into the Gulf of Mexico, where a large "dead zone" is already being attributed to agricultural runoff. Scientists and environmentalists worry that growing more grain for fuel will spawn an even larger underwater region incapable of supporting the rich sea life that thrives in less toxic parts of the Gulf.

Fortunately, there are alternatives. The equivalent of the projected 3 percent gain in automotive fuel supplies from ethanol could be achieved several times over—and at a fraction of the cost—simply by raising auto fuel-efficiency standards by 20 percent, notes the Earth Policy Institute, a nonprofit Washington, D.C.-based research group. Investing in public transport could reduce overall dependence on cars with even greater impact on America's energy future. We could power our cars with electricity (see pages 113–114). We could also make fuel out of food that is being wasted. Researchers at the University of Arizona have determined that 40 to 50 percent of all food ready for harvest never gets eaten. Food is being discarded at farms and orchards, warehouses, retail outlets, dining rooms, and landfills. Nationwide, says Timothy Jones at the University of Arizona Bureau of Applied Research in Anthropology, household food waste alone adds up to $43 billion, a sizable amount that conceivably could be converted into transportation energy.

ELECTRIC VEHICLES

According to the Department of Energy, enough excess generating capacity exists at night in the United States to charge 180 million electric vehicles (EVs) without adding any new capacity. Though we don't yet have electric vehicles, several "plug-in" hybrids are in development by the major automobile manufacturers. General Motors may build as many as sixty thousand Volt electric cars their first year on the market, which could come as early as 2009 or 2010. Production at that level may allow GM to sell the plug-in Volt, designed to go forty miles on a single charge, for less than thirty thousand dollars.

When plug-ins do become available, make sure you take a look. At night, you'll plug them into a standard 110-volt outlet in your garage. Several hours later you'll be able to travel a distance of forty or fifty miles completely on electricity before needing to switch to gasoline.

The environmental benefits could be tremendous. If your car gets 20 mpg, you generate almost twenty-four pounds of carbon dioxide driving twenty miles, while burning one gallon of gasoline. By contrast, a twenty-mile-range plug-in hybrid might consume 5kW hours of electricity, emitting two-thirds less CO_2 than a gasoline-only car.

The cost-saving benefits could be significant, too. If you are getting 20 miles per gallon at $3 per gallon and you drive 30,000 miles, calculates the Grassroots Electric Vehicle Company, you will spend about $4,500 dollars for gas alone. If you average 30 miles a day in your electric vehicle at 60 cents per charge, traveling 30,000 miles will cost about $600. Though you may also have to change your electric battery after 30,000 miles, at a cost of around $1,800 dollars, you will still have spent only $2,400. Figure in that electric motors are not running when you are at traffic lights or in traffic jams so you are not spending energy when standing still. You will not have to change oil or spark plugs every 5,000 miles, and the electric motor can last ten times longer than a gas engine. After 150,000 miles, you will spend more than $22,500 in gas alone compared to less than $12,000 in electricity and batteries.

Meanwhile, some hybrid owners are also turning to electric scooters, golf carts, mopeds, and bicycles as fuel prices rise and people make independent decisions to use less oil.

You can check out the latest electric vehicle options at www.biggreen purse.com (search: electric vehicles).

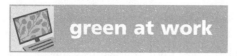

green at work

Save Gas on the Job

How can you encourage energy conservation where you work?

- Subsidize employees' use of mass transit. As part of their annual benefit, provide a mass transit allowance to discourage driving.
- Provide free or inexpensive vanpools so employees can leave their cars at home.
- Buy or lease vehicles that get at least 30 miles per gallon of gas.
- Choose fleet or company cars that feature advanced fuel-efficient component technologies, like continuously variable transmissions, variable valve timing, and cylinder deactivation.
- Track your fleet's fuel consumption, maintenance schedules, and performance to optimize fuel use.
- Permit employees to telecommute, alternate hours to avoid heavy traffic, and work fewer but longer days so they can stay home an extra day every two weeks.

For more ideas:

- Greener Fleets Fuel Economy Progress and Prospects (www.aceee.org/pubs/to24full.pdf)
- Clean Fleet Guide, U.S. Department of Energy, Energy Efficiency and Renewable Energy, www.eere.energy.gov/fleetguide/light-duty-vehicles.html

Because technology is changing so quickly, the models described in this chapter are only intended to give you an idea of what you might find on the car lot. If you decide to buy a new car, use the websites provided to track down the most recent information available on the vehicles you're considering. You can also check the cars page of the Big Green Purse website (www.biggreenpurse.com; search: transportation) for updates and additional Web links.

8. Can you recycle your car?

Manufacturing a car creates pollution you probably never thought about. Extracting and transporting the raw materials that go into components like the seats you sit on and the steering wheel you turn generates twenty-nine tons of solid waste and 1,207 million cubic yards of air emissions. In fact, while the majority of pollution is generated by driving, a third is incurred in car manufacture. Disposal of tires, lead-acid batteries, air conditioners, upholstery, and other materials adds to the trash pile, reports Katie Alvord in *Divorce Your Car.*

Manufacturers are taking notice by increasing the amount of recycled materials they weave into new-car production. Ford Motor Company has integrated recycled material into the cloth seating of the 2008 Escape. If it expanded the program, InterfaceFABRIC, the materials supplier, estimates that Ford could save at least sixty thousand gallons of water, 1.8 million pounds of carbon dioxide equivalents, and the equivalent of more than 7 million kilowatt hours of electricity annually.

Mazda and Toyta recycled used bumpers to make components for new ones. Cadillac's SRX uses 50 percent recycled tire rubber for its radiator side baffles, a process that in 2004 kept two thousand scrap tires out of landfills. Both Honda and Toyota recycle the battery packs in their hybrids to capture everything from the precious metals to the plastics and the wiring. Edmunds.com reports that Toyota even puts a phone number (for recycling information) on each battery and pays dealers two hundred dollars for each battery pack. Ten percent of the plastic in a new Mini Cooper consists of recycled material. In fact, according to Ward's Motor Vehicle Facts and Figures, at least 84 percent of an average car's material content gets recycled; automotive recycling ranks as the sixteenth-largest industry in the United States. Recycling those vehicles provides enough steel to make nearly thirteen million new cars, while also providing jobs for 46,000 people.

You can keep the cycle going:

- **Make sure to recycle your own motor oil.** If you change the oil yourself, take it and the oil filter to a recycling center. If you have it changed, double-check that the service center recycles all used oil.
- **Have your tires changed at a shop that recycles them.** Recycled rubber may become asphalt, playground material, athletic track, furniture, or apparel (like purses and jewelry).

- **Use your purse.** Buy playground equipment, personal accessories, tools, garden gear, and other consumer goods made from recycled rubber tires.

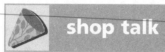

Encourage Car Companies to Make Eco-Friendly, Fuel-Efficient Vehicles

Despite their increasing use of recycled materials and the growing number of hybrids in their designs, auto manufacturers continue to oppose higher fuel-efficiency standards while encouraging consumers to buy gas-guzzlers like SUVs. You can send the industry a message in two ways: choose a highly fuel-efficient vehicle if you buy; and contact company CEOs directly to let them know you expect them to be more environmentally responsible. You can find a sample letter at www.biggreenpurse.com (search: car letter).

BMW
Tom Purves, Chairman and CEO of
BMW North America
BMW of North America, LLC
P.O. Box 1227
Westwood, NJ 07675-1227
www.bmwusa.com/contact/default

Chrysler
Robert Nardelli, Chairman and CEO
P.O. Box 21-8004
Auburn Hills, MI 48231-8004
www-5.chrysler.com/webselfservice/
chrysler/index.jsp

Daimler AG
Dr. Dieter Zetsche, Chairman of the
Board of Management
70546 Stuttgart, Germany
www.daimler.com

Fiat
Sergio Marchionne, CEO
www.fiat.com

Ford
Alan Mullalay, CEO
Ford Motor Company
Customer Relationship Center
P.O. Box 6248
Dearborn, MI 48126
www.fordvehicles.com/help/contact/

GM
G. Richard Wagoner Jr., Chairman
and CEO
General Motors Corporation
P.O. Box 33170
Detroit, MI 48232-5170
www.gm.com/gmcomjsp/contactus/

big green purse

Honda
Takeo Fukui, President and CEO
American Honda Motor Company, Inc.
Honda Automobile Customer Service
1919 Torrance Boulevard
Mail Stop: 500—2N—7D
Torrance, CA 90501-2746
www.automobiles.honda.com/info/
     customer_relations.asp

Hyundai
Finbarr O'Neill, CEO
Hyundai Motor America
P.O. Box 20850
Fountain Valley, CA 92728-0850
www.hyundaiusa.com/global/
     contactus/main.aspx

Nissan
Carlos Ghosn, President and CEO
Nissan Consumer Affairs
P.O. Box 685003
Franklin, TN 37068-5003
www.nissanusa.com/apps/contactus

PSA
Christian Streiff, Chairman,
     Managing Board
Corporate Communications
75, avenue de la Grande-Armée—
     75116 Paris—France
www.psa-peugeot-citroen.com/en/
     hp1.php

Renault
Carlos Ghosn, President and CEO
Customer Services, Renault UK Ltd.

The Rivers Office Park
Denham Way
Maple Cross
Rickmansworth
Hertfordshire WD3 9YS
United Kingdom
www.renault.co.uk/ContactDealer.aspx

Suzuki
Osamu Suzuki
American Suzuki Motor Corporation
Attention: Customer
     Relations Department
Automotive Division
P.O. Box 1100
Brea, CA 92822-1100
www.suzukiauto.com/owners/
     contact_us.php

Toyota
Toshiaki "Tag" Taguchi, President
     and CEO
Toyota Motor Sales, U.S.A., Inc.
19001 South Western Avenue
Dept. WC11
Torrance, CA 90501
www.toyota.com/about/contact/
     index.html

Volkswagen
Martin Winterkorn, CEO
North American Headquarters
3800 Hamlin Road
Auburn Hills, MI 48326
www.vw.com/customerservice/
     contactus/en/us/

Car Talk Wrap-Up

- **Use mass transit.** Consider the bus, subway, rail, car pool, vanpool, ferry, or shuttle to help meet your transportation needs.
- **Telecommute.** Work, shop, and volunteer from home.
- **Bicycle or walk.** Use your own energy to get to work, school, shopping, social engagements, community events, and to exercise.
- **Drive smart.** Pump up your tires, keep your engine tuned, and stick to the speed limit.
- **Buy a gas-sipper, not a gas-guzzler.** When it's time to buy a vehicle, purchase the most fuel-efficient model possible. Also consider alternatives like membership in car-sharing clubs, car rentals, and car-leasing programs.

And if you can do only one thing, make a mind shift. Rather than focus on driving your own car, identify other fuel-efficient ways to meet your transportation needs. Make driving "lite" a cornerstone of your view of a high-quality, environmentally healthy lifestyle.

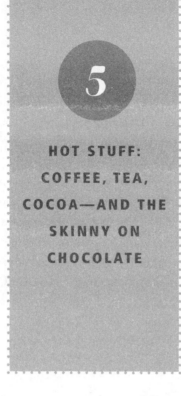

5

HOT STUFF: COFFEE, TEA, COCOA—AND THE SKINNY ON CHOCOLATE

COFFEE JUST USED TO WAKE YOU UP IN THE MORNING. NOW IT CAN HELP protect the songbirds in your backyard and enable the farmer who grew the beans to send his kids to school. As for that hot cup of cocoa or those delicious chocolate truffles you enjoy? They can help save the rain forests and maybe stop war. Even the tea you brew can preserve the environment while creating a better future for people living on three continents.

It all depends on what you choose to buy.

That's because most coffee, tea, and cocoa are grown on farms and plantations that don't give a second thought to protecting the planet. Workers are paid shameful wages for their labor, and children are often forced to work against their will. In the case of cocoa, sales in one country, Ivory Coast, are even being used to fund a war.

What you purchase at the supermarket or Starbucks, at the office or for the office party can help safeguard the Amazon and the wildlife that live there, plus keep kids learning how to spell coffee, not harvest it.

The Good News

~~If you're like me, you~~ probably had no idea how much difference your cup of coffee or pot of tea could make. This chapter not only provides background information on the environmental and social impacts of the conventional ways coffee, tea, and cocoa are grown, but also clarifies what the better alternatives are, explaining labels to look for so you can make meaningful choices when you shop.

In addition, the chapter lists a variety of companies and websites where you can find socially responsible, earth-friendly products (once you start looking on the Internet you'll find even more yourself). Hundreds of local shops and enterprising mail-order businesses are producing certifiably "eco" coffee, tea, cocoa, and chocolate. The more you shift your spending to the good stuff, the more it encourages other growers to change their practices, which is, of course, what using your big green purse is all about.

Coffee

Americans wield a lot of purse power when it comes to coffee because we drink so much of it. Nearly 52 percent of Americans over the age of eighteen, more than 100 million people, quaff four hundred million cups of coffee every day, making the United States the number-one coffee-consuming nation in the world. But we're not alone in our love for a jolt of java. Coffee is second only to oil as the most heavily traded legal commodity in the world.

The way coffee is farmed affects the environment in several key ways. Coffee is raised on estates in the rain forests that straddle the earth's equator. If coffee is grown in the shade, as it does naturally, that effect is more benign. Shady rain forest trees protect the coffee plants below them from rain and sun, help maintain soil quality, reduce the need for weeding, and naturally control bugs. Organic matter from the shade trees provides an ecological mulch that reduces the coffee plants' demand for chemical fertilizers, controls erosion, and builds the soil. Shade-grown coffee plants and the rain forests that nurture them also provide a place for migrating North American birds to winter over. Those warblers, thrushes, tanagers, Baltimore orioles, redstarts, and vireos that nibble at your bird feeder during the spring and fall? Chances are they perched on a coffee bush in Brazil or Colombia while you were shoveling snow.

Coffee grown in the sun has the opposite effect. Such java is raised on "technified" estates that raze rain forests to make way for coffee varieties that require heavy doses of pesticides and chemical fertilizers to thrive. While growing coffee in the sun increases yields, the payoff comes with a big environmental price tag. In Costa Rica, *The Green Guide* reports, the government recommends that sun coffee producers apply thirty kilograms of nitrogen per hectare per year, compared with shade coffee producers, who use little or none. In Colombia, with some 86 percent of coffee production technified, the country applies more than 400,000 metric tons of chemical fertilizers annually, at least when growers can afford them. Over the last decade, governments throughout the Western Hemisphere have attempted to prohibit use of a number of pesticides banned in the United States that are being applied to sun-grown coffee. Costa Rica, reports the Natural Resources Defense Council, continues to permit chlordane, a highly toxic insecticide that persists for years in the environment.

The toll on wildlife alone is enough to rattle your coffee cup: studies have found up to 97 percent fewer bird species on sun coffee farms than on shady ones, says Smithsonian's Migratory Bird Center. Compare that to eastern Chiapas, Mexico, where Smithsonian biologists discovered that traditionally managed shade coffee and cacao (chocolate) plantations support more than one hundred fifty species of birds, a number exceeded only in undisturbed tropical forest. In addition to your backyard songbirds, shade-grown coffee estates provide a haven for parrots, toucans, and macaws, as well as many species of insects, mammals, and reptiles. It's practically the difference between paradise and, to borrow Joni Mitchell's lyric, a parking lot.

Given their ecological impact, you might wonder why any grower would choose to raise coffee plants that prefer the sun. The reason has to do with yield. Sun coffee plants produce more beans than their shadier cousins. Since the 1970s, when sun coffee was introduced, almost half of cultivation in Latin America has abandoned the traditional shade method in favor of "full sun" techniques, reports *The Green Guide*. But producing more beans doesn't mean that farmers plant fewer plants. The most serious impact of coffee cultivation continues to be the conversion of natural forest areas to more and more coffee. Of the fifty countries in the world with the highest deforestation rates from 1990 to 1995, thirty-seven were coffee producers.

Producing more sun-coffee beans doesn't mean farmers earn more money, either. In fact, just the opposite is true. Farmers who raise their coffee in the shade may be paid as much as twice what their sun-growing colleagues earn . . . if they have a chance to garner the fairer wage. Global Exchange, a nonprofit organization that promotes fair wages for coffee farmers, calls most coffee farms "sweatshops in the fields" to describe the labor intensity of handpicking, preparing, and roasting coffee beans. The coffee market tends to fluctuate wildly; in bust cycles, when excess coffee beans flood the market, growers are often forced to sell their commodity below production costs, pushing coffee growers into debt. Coffee farmers may earn as little as fifty cents a pound for their product, even when a retailer is charging more than eleven dollars a pound for the same beans.

When you buy coffee that is grown organically in the shade by farmers who are paid a fair wage for their work, you dangle an economic carrot in front of conventional growers that can persuade them to convert to more eco-friendly production. You can make a difference by buying coffee that's been certified to protect the environment as well as workers. Several labels help make your choices clearer.

Fair Trade Certified, a label sponsored by TransFair USA, indicates that the coffee was grown by adults, not children, who were paid a premium for their beans, and that the farmers use the extra money to invest in health care, education, and other benefits for their families and communities. In addition to paying sometimes as much as twice the market price of conventionally grown coffee, importers who do business with Fair Trade Certified growers must also extend credit to them if they need it and provide technical assistance, support that helps them switch to organic farming. The Fair Trade Certified label limits eligibility to small-holder farms organized into cooperatives.

Certified Organic means the coffee has been grown free of harmful pesticides, fertilizers, and herbicides; meets USDA organic standards; protects farmworkers, wildlife, and waterways from toxic chemicals; and is generally grown in the shade.

Shade Grown indicates that the coffee was grown under the rain forest canopy. Sometimes the coffee box, bag, or can will simply use the words "shade grown." A more reliable shade-grown-certification label is managed by the Smithsonian Migratory Bird Center itself. It certifies coffee as "**Bird Friendly**"® if it is organically grown in the shade under conditions it deems ecologically sound for migratory birds. The Northwest Shade Coffee Campaign also certifies shade-grown coffee that protects habitat for migratory birds that winter in Latin America and the Caribbean.

Rainforest Alliance Certified is guaranteed to be shade grown using low or no pesticides; farmers are required to maintain the variety of animals and trees on the land that characterizes biodiversity. To gain Rainforest

Alliance certification, workers must also be treated in accordance with International Labor Organization standards that ensure fair treatment and good living conditions. Unlike Fair Trade Certified, the Rain Forest Alliance works with farms of all sizes, from the small family farms to larger estates.

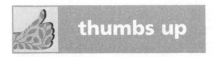

thumbs up

Triple-Certified Coffee, which is organic, shade grown, and fairly traded, is the preferable choice. The companies listed below meet these criteria and offer their coffee by mail order.

Adam's Organic Coffees, San Mateo, California, 800-439-5506, www.mothernature .com.

Allegro Coffee, Boulder, Colorado, www.allegrocoffee.com.

Alta Gracia (author Julia Alvarez's coffee farm), Dominican Republic, 802-453-2776, www.cafealtagracia.com.

Arbuckle Coffee Roasters, Tucson, Arizona, 800-533-8278, www.arbucklecoffee.com.

The Art of Coffee, La Jolla, California, 800-570-9010, www.theartofcoffee.com.

Avalon Organic Coffees, Albuquerque, New Mexico, 800-662-2575, www.avalon coffee.com.

Batdorf & Bronson Coffee Roasters, Olympia, Washington, 800-955-5282, www .batdorf.com.

Bisbee Coffee Company, Bisbee, Arizona, 800-215-2611, www.bisbeecoffee.com.

Boyd Coffee Company, Portland, Oregon, 800-545-4077, 800-223-8211, www .boyds.com.

Café Altura, Clean Foods, Inc., Santa Paula, California, 800-526-8328, www.cafe altura.com.

Café Bom Dia, Coral Gables, Florida, 888-470-8010, www.cafebomdia.com.

Café Canopy, FMZ International, San Diego, California, 858-449-4033, www.cafe canopy.com.

Café Mam, Royal Blue Organics, Eugene, Oregon, 888-CAFE-MAM, www.cafe mam.com.

Café Moto, San Diego, California, 800-818-3363, www.cafemoto.com.

Café Sombra, Miami, Florida, 305-591-9405, www.cafesombra.com.

Caffe Ibis, Logan, Utah, 888-740-4777, www.caffeibis.com.

Catskill Mountain Coffee, Kingston, New York, 888-SAY-JAVA, www.catskillmt coffee.com.

CoffeeAM.com, Woodstock, Georgia, 800-803-7774, www.coffeeam.com.

Coffee Bean & Tea Leaf, Camarillo, California, 800-TEA-LEAF, www.coffee bean.com.

Cooperative Trading, Fort Wayne, Indiana, 260-422-6821, www.friendsofthethird world.org.

Counter Culture Coffee, Durham, North Carolina, 888-238-5282, www.counter culturecoffee.com. Look for Sanctuary shade-grown label; some shade-grown is also organic.

Dean's Beans, New Salem, Massachusetts, 800-325-3008, www.deansbeans.com.

Elan Organic Coffee, San Diego, California, 619-235-0392, www.elanorganic.com.

Equal Exchange, West Bridgewater, Massachusetts, 774-776-7400, www.equal exchange.com.

Frontier Coffee, Norway, Iowa, 800-669-3275, www.frontiercoop.com.

Global Exchange Fair Trade Store, San Francisco, California, 800-505-4410, www.store .globalexchange.org.

The Good Coffee Company of Charleston, www.goodcoffeeonline.com; online re-tailer of Rainforest Alliance–certified coffees.

Green Mountain Coffee Roasters, Waterbury, Vermont, 888-879-4627, www.green mountaincoffee.com.

Grounds For Change, 800-796-6820, www.groundsforchange.com.

Higher Ground Roasters, Leeds, Alabama, 800-794-8575, www.higherground roasters.com.

Jim's Organic Coffee, West Wareham, Massachusetts, 800-999-9218, www.jims organiccoffee.com.

Kalani Organica, Seattle, Washington, 800-200-4377, www.kalanicoffee.com.

Larry's Beans, Raleigh, North Carolina, 919-828-1234, www.larrysbeans.com.

Montana Coffee Traders, Whitefish, Montana, 800-345-5282, www.coffeetraders .com.

Mount Hagen Organic Coffee, InterNatural Foods, Paramus, New Jersey, 973-338-1499, www.internaturalfoods.com; organic instant coffee.

Peace Coffee, Minneapolis, Minnesota, 888-324-7872, www.peacecoffee.com.

Pura Vida, Seattle, Washington, 877-469-1431, www.puravidacoffee.com.

Rocamojo, Los Angeles, California, 310-479-2151, www.rocamojo.com; certified organic soy coffee.

Starbucks Coffee, Seattle, Washington, 800-782-7282, www.starbucks.com.

big green purse

Swiss Water Decaffeinated Coffee Company, Burnaby, British Columbia, Canada, 800-667-6181; 604-420-4050, www.swisswater.com.

Taylor Maid, Sebastopol, California, 888-688-7272, www.taylormaidfarms.com.

Tesoros Del Sol Coffee, St. Louis, Missouri, 314-570-9659, www.tesdelsol.com.

Thanksgiving Coffee Co., Fort Bragg, California, 800-648-6491, www.thanksgiving coffee.com; wholesale. Look for Song Bird shade-grown line, www.songbird coffee.com.

Well-Bean Coffee Co., Webster, New York, 800-633-9850, www.wellbeancoffee.com; certified organic and fair-trade soy.

Who's NOT Selling Shade-Grown, Fair-Trade, Organic Coffee?

Most major commercial brands, like Taster's Choice (Nestlé), and Maxwell House, either don't sell shade-grown, fair-trade, organic coffee or only make it available on-line. For example, Folger's Signature Collection includes Mountain Moonlight Fair Trade Certified Coffee, but it is only available to U.S. residents by direct order via the phone or Internet. Send companies a letter. Urge them to become triple-certified as soon as possible, and to sell the "green" coffee they do produce in grocery stores and other retailers where it's easy to buy.

Folgers Millstone Coffee
Charles Pierce, President
4740 North Interstate Drive #3
Cincinnati, OH 45202
513-860-2146

Maxwell House Coffee, Inc.
Consumer Relations Group
Box 153FPD
Rye Brook, NY 10573
800-432-6333
www.maxwellhouse.com

Hills Bros. Coffee
Write to:
Massimo Zanetti Beverage USA
Donald McIntyre, CEO & President
1370 Progress Road
Suffolk, VA 23434
757-538-8083

Nestlé USA
Brad Alford, Chairman and CEO
800 North Brand Boulevard
Glendale, CA 91203
818-549-6000

big green purse

What About Decaf?

Often, chemical solvents are used to decaffeinate coffee. The most widely used are methylene chloride, a suspected carcinogen, and ethyl acetate, which may lead to skin problems. The ecoalternative? The Swiss Water Method soaks beans in water to remove caffeine; the supercritical carbon dioxide method soaks them in carbon dioxide. These are the only safe methods that can be used if the coffee is organic.

What If It's Either . . . Or?

Ideally, all coffee you'd buy would be "triple certified"—shade grown, organic, and fair trade.

In reality, not many coffee growers have been able to afford the cost of certifying their farms in all three categories. The number is increasing, and the more certified coffee you buy, the more you enable farmers to meet certification requirements.

If your primary concern is for treatment of workers, choose Fair Trade Certified.™ You'll probably still get a "two-fer." More than 80 percent of fair trade coffee sold in the United States is shade grown. Fair trade also encourages farmers to adopt other environmentally friendly practices. For example, many fair trade farmers compost coffee pulp rather than dump it into local waterways. Some cooperatives have invested in processing mills that greatly reduce resource use. Even nonorganic fair trade farms are required to use integrated pest-management systems that emphasize alternatives to toxic chemicals. Plus, farmers who participate in the Fair Trade Certified program usually terrace to reduce runoff, and reforest areas that may have been clear-cut.

Around six hundred U.S. companies now sell Fair Trade Certified products in nearly 40,000 retail locations nationwide, including supermarkets, club stores, cafés, restaurants, specialty food stores, college campuses, and faith-based organizations. Fair Trade Certified coffee is the fastest-growing segment of the $11 billion U.S. specialty coffee market, growing an average of nearly 80 percent every year since 1999. If you drink most of your coffee on the go, you might be happy to know that Starbucks is the largest purchaser, roaster, and distributor of Fair Trade Certified coffee in North America.

If you want to try to influence the largest coffee merchants specifically, choose Rain Forest Alliance certified. Rainforest Alliance works with the major coffee producers, as opposed to small farmer cooperatives. Though less profit may reach individual farmers, the RA program does aim to reduce pesticide use, protect the environment, and improve conditions for farmers on large coffee estates. Caribou Coffee has pledged that 50 percent of its coffees will come from Rainforest Alliance–certified farms.

If your primary concern is songbirds, choose Smithsonian's Bird Friendly Coffee or coffee that's been certified by the Northwest Shade Coffee Campaign (www.shadecoffee.org). These coffees will have been grown on farms that safeguard diversity in the rain forest, helping a multitude of birds thrive.

And honestly, if you don't have time to do anything but pick up a bag of coffee and throw it into your shopping cart, just look for the organic seal and carry on, remembering that if it's organic it was in all likelihood grown in the shade, which means it's bird-friendly and people-safe, too. Plus, organic coffee benefits from having the credibility of the U.S. Department of Agriculture standards behind it. (When you get the bag home, call the company's customer service number or visit its website, and encourage it to get Fair Trade Certified as soon as possible!)

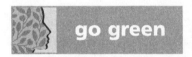

Reusable Coffee Filters

Grocery stores, coffee shops, and online outlets all sell a variety of reusable coffee filters for pots and cups so you can avoid the waste of throwing away single-use paper filters. Just query "reusable coffee filter" on your favorite search engine, or visit www.biggreenpurse.com (search: coffee filter) for links to some of the best filters on the market.

If you'd rather not buy a reusable filter just yet, at least choose nonbleached paper filters. You can compost the paper with the coffee grounds when you're finished making your brew.

What About the Coffeepot?

Consumers buy more automatic-drip coffeemakers than any other small kitchen appliance, so it's no wonder they use about $400 million worth of electricity just brewing coffee every year. To make an energy-efficient but still high-voltage cup of java, start with the pot:

- **French press (www.bodumusa.com).** Bodum Chambord's elegant but inexpensive model makes delicious coffee; the Columbia design contains the coffee in a thermal carafe to keep the beverage warm without the need for an electric hot plate.
- **Chemex manual drip coffeepots (www.ourcoffeebarn.com).** This hourglass-shaped flask can use recycled paper filters. Make as little as one cup of coffee, or as many as ten.
- **Chef's Choice electric French press plus (www.chefsresource.com/chef choicelf.html).** This technology combines the French press and an energy-saving electric kettle in one pot.
- **One-cup coffeemakers.** These efficient pots can brew coffee in less than a minute, eliminating the need to prepare a whole pot. Check the housewares section of Target, Wal-Mart, or your local department store.

When buying any new coffeemaker:

- **Consider how much you consume at any given time.** If you drink only one cup of coffee in the morning, and maybe one again in the evening, don't buy a machine that automatically brews eight or ten or twelve cups. You'll be wasting energy, water, coffee—and ultimately, money.
- **Get a carafe.** If you sip coffee sporadically through the morning or afternoon, rather than keep a pot warm on an electric hot plate, buy a good insulated carafe to keep the coffee hot.
- **If you buy an electric-drip appliance, choose one that shuts off automatically.**

And for those of you who like to grind your own beans, try:

- **Vermont Country Store coffee grinder** (www.vermontcountrystore.com). A metal grinder mounted on a compact wooden box, it lets you efficiently grind coffee beans from fine to coarse using no kilowatts but your own.

 shop talk

Take-out Tip

You might think the 12, 000 coffee shops on our streets, in the malls, and at the markets are overwhelming now, but that's nothing compared with what you'll find in 2010, when 50,000 coffee-serving cafes will be able to meet any need you have for a skim milk latte, caramel cappuccino, or double-double decaf. Many shops offer roasted shade-grown, Fair Trade Certified, organic beans for sale; they don't often have a pot of earth-friendly coffee brewing. Ask for a cup of the best ecobrand available whenever you order.

Where Can You Find Shade-Grown, Organic, Fair-Trade Coffee?

Coffee Shops

Dunkin' Donuts (espresso)
Green Mountain Coffee Roasters
McDonald's restaurants in the Northeast United States
Newman's Own Organics Blend
Peet's Coffee & Tea
Starbucks
Tully's
Dozens of independent coffeehouses

Supermarkets

Albertsons	Stop & Shop
Giant Eagle	Target
Kroger	Trader Joe's
Publix	Whole Foods
Safeway	Wild Oats

Club Stores

Costco, Sam's Clubs, Wal-Mart, and Target all offer organic and Fair Trade Certified coffees.

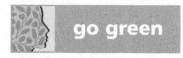

Use Your Own Mug

In 2005, Americans used and discarded 14.4 billion disposable paper cups for hot beverages, Green Mountain Coffee Roasters of Vermont calculated.

That's so many cups that if put end to end they would circle the earth fifty-five times. Based on anticipated growth of specialty coffees, reports Green Mountain, that number will grow to 23 billion by 2010—enough to circle the globe eighty-eight times.

Come on. It's one thing to pay two or three or even four dollars for a cup of coffee. It's another to throw cup after cup after cup away. If we do it every day, it amounts to almost twenty-five pounds of waste every year. The petrochemicals consumed in making the cups just one coffee drinker throws away could heat 8,300 homes for one year. Carting them to a landfill burns additional energy and each one takes about five hundred years to decompose.

What good does it do if you buy the "right" coffee (i.e., organic, shade-grown, Fair Trade Certified) if you drink it out of a paper or Styrofoam cup you just toss in the garbage?

Beat the disposable rap by using your own mug. Every coffee shop sells them. Some places even give you a little discount if you use your own cup instead of theirs—if they don't, ask for one. They'll get the message after a while.

And if you forget your mug and need a take-out cup, ask the shop if they're using the new ones made from recycled fibers that save trees. Do they make a difference? Starbucks' recycled paper cup protects about 78,000 trees a year.

Cocoa and Chocolate

Chocolatl—Aztec for "cocoa" and the source of our word "chocolate"—originated in the rain forests that once dominated Central and South America. Sweetened,

big green purse

solid chocolate was not invented until after cocoa was taken to Europe late in the sixteenth century.

Cocoa was so valuable in ancient Mesoamerica that the beans served as a form of regional currency, one that literally grew on trees. The coastal lands where cocoa grew best were highly valued by Indians and Spanish colonists alike. Along the Mosquito Coast of Honduras, cocoa seeds were used as money in village markets as late as the 1980s. In the state of Bahia and other cocoa-producing areas of Brazil, "cacao," the Portuguese term for cocoa, is still slang for money.

Debra Waterhouse, a registered dietitian and the author of the 1999 book *Why Women Need Chocolate*, thinks both culture and chemicals figure into women's love of this rich, dark confection. Chemicals in chocolate alter our body's mood-affecting chemicals, she says, including serotonin, endorphins, and phenylethylamine, which the body releases in response to romance. But culture is a factor, too. Delicious chocolate seems so decadent, we sometimes think it should be taboo.

Today, there are reasons beyond the sensual why chocolate could be considered taboo. The cocoa it's made from is grown primarily in the tropical rain forests of Africa and South America. And therein lies the problem. Like coffee, cocoa trees grow best in the shade of other trees. When very young, they require deep shade. As they mature, they require more filtered sunlight. Under the proper conditions, shade-grown cocoa trees can produce fruit for seventy-five to one hundred years or more.

But in the frenzy to meet the growing worldwide demand for cocoa and chocolate, cocoa growing is now responsible for 14 percent of the deforestation in the rain forests of West Africa and a large percentage of the deforestation in South America, reports *Sierra* magazine. Many cocoa farmers who work on large plantations live in horrible poverty, earning as little as thirty to one hundred dollars a year. Children labor as slaves on these plantations as well, applying pesticides and using machetes to clear forests. Even though Americans spend $13 billion a year on cocoa products, many small-scale family cocoa farmers earn a pittance, due to the local middlemen they must sell their harvest to and who take virtually all the profits for themselves.

There is an alternative. TransFair USA (www.transfairusa.org), the nonprofit organization that certifies coffee, also certifies fair trade chocolate and cocoa. In fact, you can buy Fair Trade Certified cocoa, chocolate bars, and chocolate chips in more than sixteen hundred retail locations around the United States, including food co-ops, and several Safeway, Tully's, and Whole Foods stores. Fair Trade certification ensures that cocoa farmers receive a fair price for their harvest. It creates direct trade links between farmer-owned cooperatives and buyers, and makes it easier for farmers to get access to affordable credit. Fair trade farms strictly prohibit slave labor, too.

On the environmental front, Fair Trade Certified cocoa is more likely to be grown on small organic farms that grow their cocoa trees in the shade so they don't have to chop down the forests or douse the plants in pesticides to repel bugs that thrive when the plants are grown on sun-loving plantations.

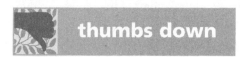

thumbs down

"Blood" Cocoa

Côte d'Ivoire in West Africa produces 40 percent of the world's cocoa. The majority is imported into the United States and Europe by Nestlé, Archer Daniels Midland, and Cargill for manufacture into chocolate and other cocoa products by such companies as M&M/Mars and Hershey's.

As the world's largest producer of cocoa, Côte d'Ivoire, or Ivory Coast, depends on the commodity to bolster its economy. On average, says the nonprofit human rights organization Global Witness, cocoa represents $1.4 billion, or 35 percent, of the total value of exports from the region.

This money does not come morally. Hundreds of thousands of children are enslaved on cocoa farms, reports the U.S. State Department. Since a military coup in 1999, Ivory Coast has been wrenched by political instability and, more recently, a civil war that both sides fund through cocoa sales. At least $118 million from the cocoa trade has been used to "fuel the conflict," according to reporting done by *The New York Times*. Apparently both the government, which rules the south, and the rebels, who control the north, benefit from cocoa profits. At one point, 30 percent of the government's military costs during one six-month period were provided by cocoa proceeds; roughly $30 million each year infuses the rebel side alone.

Global Witness is working to document the atrocities. The group recommends that any business trading in cocoa reveal where it buys its products and trace how its sales money is used. According to Fair Trade Certified, a 2002 report from the International Institute of Tropical Agriculture estimated that more than 284,000 children were enslaved in hazardous conditions in Ivory Coast and other African countries, where they worked on cocoa plantations applying pesticides and using machetes.

U.S. *chocolate* manufacturers refuse responsibility for the situation since they do not own the actual *cocoa* farms. But chocolate is made from cocoa, and Hershey's and M&M/Mars together control two-thirds of the $13 billion U.S. chocolate market. The premier chocolate companies in this country—and the consumers of that chocolate, like you and me—help perpetuate the horrendous working conditions for children in Ivory Coast if we don't use our purses to make a difference.

Contact the companies listed below. Urge them to use organic, Fair Trade Certified cocoa in the chocolate they make.

Archer Daniels Midland Company
4666 Faries Parkway
Decatur, IL 62526
800-637-5843
www.admworld.com

Cargill, Inc.
Warren R. Staley, Chairman and CEO
Gregory R. Page, President and Chief
   Operating Officer
P.O. Box 9300
Minneapolis, MN 55440-9300
800-CARGILL (227-4455)
www.cargill.com

Cocoa Specific Contact Info:
Patricia A. Woertz, President and CEO
12500 West Carmen Avenue
Milwaukee, WI 53225
414-358-5700 or 800-558-9958

The Hershey Company
Richard H. Lenny, Chairman of the
   Board, President, and CEO
P.O. Box 810
100 Crystal A Drive

Hershey, PA 17033
800-468-1714
www.hersheys.com

M&M/Mars Inc.
Paul Michaels, President
6885 Elm Street
McLean, VA 22101
800-627-7852
E-mail: consumer.affairs@mmmars.com
      and askmms@mmmars.com

Nestlé CEO Contact Info:
Peter Brabeck-Letmathe
Chairman and CEO
800 North Brand Boulevard
Glendale, CA 91203
818-549-6000
www.nestle.com

Nestlé® USA
Consumer Services Center
P. O. Box 2178
Wilkes-Barre, PA 18703
800-851-0512

make the shift

Kid-Safe Cocoa

Online, at natural food stores and food co-ops, and increasingly at neighborhood grocery stores, you can choose organic, fair trade cocoa and chocolates:

- Dagoba (www.dagobachocolate.com/)
- Divine Milk Chocolate (www.agreatergift.org/Kitchen/ChocolateFood/Divine/MilkLrgBars.aspx)
- Endangered Species Organic Chocolate (www.chocolatebar.com/shop/pc/viewCat_h.asp?idCategory=3)
- Equal Exchange (www.equalexchange.com)
- Green & Black's (www. greenandblacks.com/uk)
- Theo (www.theochocolate.com)

At the mall, Sam's Club, or a drugstore like CVS or Walgreens, look for these organic options:

- Russell Stover assorted organic chocolates, organic pecan delights, organic coconut-covered chocolates
- Dove Organic Chocolates dark chocolate, citrus spice, milk chocolate

The downside? Neither company appears to use suppliers whose ingredients come from fair trade sources. Contact them at the numbers below and urge them to source their cocoa from estates that don't use children as slave laborers:

Russell Stover: 800-777-4028

Dove: 800-551-0704

A Final Thought

In 2006, fair trade–registered cooperatives produced approximately two hundred million pounds of cocoa. Unfortunately, lack of consumer appreciation for the benefits of this eco-friendly and socially important product led to minimal consumer demand: less than thirteen million pounds of Fair Trade Certified cocoa were actually sold; the remaining 187 million pounds had to be unloaded on the conventional market at a financial loss.

Our purses only have power when we show we're willing to use them. If we create demand for products that are better for people and the planet, let's make sure we buy them.

Tea

After water, tea is the second-most-consumed beverage in the world. Virtually every country in the world serves it one way or another. In 2003, Americans alone consumed more than fifty billion servings of tea, 85 percent of which was iced.

Hundreds of different teas line grocery store shelves. Herbal "teas" are not true teas at all, but rather mixtures of dried herbs and/or flowers. Actual tea is derived primarily from the *Camellia sinensis* plant. Regional climatic and soil conditions, handling, plucking, and processing, plus the plant's variety determine the specific type of tea—white, green, black, oolong—the leaf will become. Different products like mint Jasmine, Lady Grey, or English Breakfast result from the ingenuity of packagers who blend different teas, add flavors and seasonings, and otherwise enhance the tiny leaf that unfurls in boiling water.

While it is packaged in dozens of countries, *Camellia sinensis* is grown primarily in China, Japan, India, Sri Lanka, and Taiwan. Unlike coffee and cocoa, the evergreen *Camellia* shrub thrives in the full sun that shines in subtropical and highland tropical climes. But like those plants, tea needs to be raised ecologically and according to fair trade practices in order to be a green purse priority.

The most destructive environmental aspect of tea production involves cultivation of the plant itself. *Camellia sinensis* is usually planted in steep, remote areas on terrain that tends to host a high—and vulnerable—concentration of animals and plants. Converting rugged natural landscapes to tea production takes an eco toll. Not only does it endanger species; due to the slope of the land, considerable soil can be lost to erosion before tea plantations are fully established. Since all tea must be dried with hot air after it is picked, and wood is the common source of heat, deforestation in regions that grow tea is common.

On conventional tea estates, health security for the workers is very low. Oxfam, a British nonprofit agency working to end poverty worldwide, reports that pesticides are often sprayed by untrained casual daily wage workers, sometimes even by children and adolescents, who are illiterate and cannot read the warnings on the containers. Many tea farmers douse their plants fifteen to twenty times each year, depending on pest infestations. Most of the chemicals they use (such as Aldrin 20E, Carbofuran 30, Endosulfan 35 EC, Malathion 50 EC, Tetradifon 8 EC, and Calixin 80 EC) are listed as hazardous and toxic; a number of them are banned in Western countries. Despite the dangers of toxic exposure, workers frequently go barefoot and wear only shorts rather than protective safety gear like masks, gloves, rubber boots, and aprons. The chemicals also endanger wildlife. *The Times of India* reported that at least ten leopards and five elephants died between 1999 and 2001 due to pesticides that leaked from "tea gardens" in West Bengal.

Growing tea organically offers many benefits.

- It improves the fertility of the soil by adding compost, natural organic matter, and plants rather than herbicides and pesticides.
- It protects all kinds of creatures. The Soil Association, an international organization that promotes organic cultivation practices, notes that a typical organic field hosts five times as many wild plants, 57 percent more animal species, and 44 percent more birds than a conventionally cultivated farm.
- It's safer for the workers in the fields.

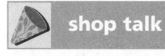

shop talk

Contact the Companies

Contact the major U.S. tea companies and urge them to expand their line into fair trade, organic offerings.

Bigelow Tea Company
R.C. Bigelow
201 Black Rock Turnpike
Fairfield, CT 06825
888-244-3569
www.bigelowtea.com

Salada/Red Rose
Redco Foods, Inc.
One Hansen Island
Little Falls, NY 13365
315-823-1300
www.redcofoods.com/contactus.asp

Note: Bigelow offers certified organic green and decaffeinated green tea along with its conventional teas. Now, encourage it to adopt fair-trade standards.

Should you give up the tea bag?

Most tea bags are filled with finely ground tea leaves that the industry refers to as "dust." Prepackaged months in advance, tea bags can sometimes be quite stale even before they reach the store shelf. Thus, the inferior leaves found in tea bags create a strong, harsh drink that is a far cry from what the true flavor of the tea should be. In buying loose leaves, you avoid both the tea bag and the extra foil package it may be wrapped in. A tea stick, ball, or strainer lets you brew your own full-bodied beverage, then use the brewed leaves for compost or side dressing in the garden. If you do use tea bags, compost them with the rest of your kitchen scraps or yard waste.

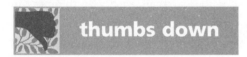

Tea Forté

You've probably seen the chic, pale green Tea Forté boxes the same places I have: specialty gift shops, tourist traps, and knickknack boutiques. In my region, they're sold in stores with names like "Artsy Fartsy" and "La De Da" (I'm not kidding). What's the problem? Wait till you see all the packaging you need to go through just to get a cup of tea. Shrink-wrap surrounds a tin box that contains finely designed paper pyramids that encase silken bags that finally contain the tea. Wouldn't a simple (and nonwasteful) tea ball work just as well?!!

What About Decaf?

For a tea to be legally labeled "decaffeinated" in the United States, 98 percent of the caffeine must be removed. The main decaffeination processes use one of three solvents: carbon dioxide, methylene chloride, or ethyl acetate. Carbon dioxide appears to have no environmental or health side effects. Both methylene chloride and ethyl acetate are powerful chemical compounds that have been linked to human health problems and hazardous waste disposal. Organic tea is more likely to have been decaffeinated using harmless carbon dioxide.

If you brew loose tea, you have the option of decaffeinating it yourself. Caffeine is highly water soluble; nearly 80 percent of the total caffeine content of the tea leaves will be extracted within the first thirty seconds of steeping. Simply pour boiling water over the tea leaves, steep for half a minute, then empty this water off, and pour fresh boiling water over the rinsed leaves to brew for the prescribed time.

 make the shift

Fair Trade Teas

The practice of paying people a fair wage while protecting children and adults from unfair labor is starting to gain more than a toehold in the tea industry. Tea is one of the fastest-growing fair trade categories, with more than seventy North American companies and a wider variety of brands offering certified specialty tea and herb products, including loose-leaf, bagged teas; ready-to-drink bottled teas and chai blends; kombucha bottled teas; and tea-based foods like mints, ice cream, and nutritional bars. Given the abundance of fair trade tea now available—online, at such retailers as Whole Foods and Trader Joe's, from food co-ops, in chain restaurants like Panera, at coffee shops like Starbucks and Caribou Coffee, and in neighborhood cafes—you could practically drink a different cup every day. Look for any of the following organic, fair trade teas online or at local retailers. If you don't see what you want on store shelves, ask for it.

- Alter Eco (www.altereco-usa.com/main.php). Cey lonchai, Darjeeling black, Green Dew, and other exotic choices.
- The Art of Tea (www.artoftea.com). Teas, fusions, gifts, and teaware.
- Assam Tea Company (www.tfactor.us). Breakfast teas grown biodynamically.
- China Mist (www.chinamist.com). Iced teas, hot teas, and herbal teas.

- Choice Organic Teas (www.choiceorganicteas.com). White, green, black, oolong, chai, and herbal teas.
- Davidson's Tea (www.davidsonstea.com). Holiday, children's, honey, red, green, white, classic, and dessert teas.
- Eco Teas (www.ecoteas.com). Organic and fair trade yerba maté, gourds, and straws called bombillas.
- New World Tea (www.newworldteac.com). In addition to a wide variety of teas, a wonderful assortment of teapots, tea cups, tea tumblers, and other "teaware."
- Numi Tea (www.numitea.com). Teas and "teasans," flowering teas, plus glass teapots and bamboo accessories.
- Quintessential Tea (www.qleaftea.com). Black and green teas, plus rooibos red and Earl Green, a cross between Earl Grey and green tea. Loose tea is sold in re- fillable tins that offer a discount when you refill.
- The Republic of Tea (www.republicoftea.com). Wide variety of teas and teapots; teas now being sold at Panera cafes.
- Upton Tea (www.uptontea.com). More than 420 varieties to choose from, listed on a website that provides informative details about tea.

Looking for Lipton? Here's the Scoop

Starting in 2007, Unilever, the world's largest tea company and maker of the Lipton brand, began to purchase all of its tea from growers who met environmen- tal and worker standards set by the nonprofit Rainforest Alliance. Unilever's program affects tea estates in Kenya, Tanzania, Malawi, Indonesia, India, Argen- tina, and Sri Lanka. Lipton, the world's best-selling tea, and PG Tips, the No. 1 tea in the United Kingdom, are the first brands to seek certification under Unilever's initiative. The company aims to certify all Lipton Yellow Label and PG Tips tea bags sold in Western Europe by 2010 and all Lipton tea bags sold glob- ally by 2015.

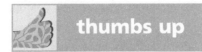

thumbs up

Celestial Seasonings

Celestial Seasonings uses as little packaging as possible to market its teas.

- The company's unique pillow tea bag requires no strings, tags, staples, individual overwrapping, or foil envelopes, keeping more than fifteen hundred tons of waste out of landfills each year.
- Tea bag papers are blended from chlorine-free natural fibers.
- Filled bags are packaged in cardboard boxes made from 100 percent recycled paperboard, which itself derives from at least 35 percent post-consumer waste.
- The boxes include resealable interior liners to keep the tea fresh.
- You can recycle the liners and box, and compost the bags.

Paying attention, Tea Forté?

Grow Your Own Tea

Many herbal teas are made from plants you may already be growing in your own garden. Mint, chamomile, lemongrass, rose hips, and bee balm are among the most common. To make your own tea, add one tablespoon of fresh leaves or one teaspoon of dried leaves to a hot (not boiling) cup of water (add more leaves if you're making a pot of tea). Steep, then add honey, lemon, cinnamon, and other natural ingredients if you want richer flavor.

big green purse

What's It Going to Cost You?

The price of Fair Trade Certified coffee, cocoa, chocolate, and tea runs about the same as other gourmet or specialty coffees and chocolates. They are, however, more expensive than mass-produced, lower-quality products. You can make the certified goods affordable the same way you shop for other items that you think are out of your price range:

* Wait for sales.
* Buy at Trader Joe's or similar stores that offer discounts.
* Forgo a purchase that's a waste of money (like bottled water) so you have more money to spend on fair trade coffee, tea, or chocolate that actually makes a difference to the planet as well as to people.

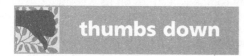

Tea in a Box

What were those people at Pacific Natural Foods thinking? Their latest offering is brewed tea . . . sold in a box. And it's not just any box, either. It's a 64-ounce, "shelf stable" box that can barely be recycled, since it's made from the same waxy material juice boxes are made from. All you can do is use up the ingredients inside—which, when you get down to it, are basically nothing more than tea you could easily brew yourself at home—and throw the box away.

The company calls its boxed tea "exciting." Somehow, the thrill of spending five dollars for a big box of flavored water I eventually have to send to a landfill is completely lost on me. And honestly, it doesn't matter if Pacific Natural's product is organic, fair trade, and otherwise "politically correct." This is a convenience food at an inconvenient time (i.e., with a global warming impact) that will only add to the trash you have to cart out to the curb or the dump every week. Want tea? Skip the box. Get a bag, or a tea ball, and brew your own.

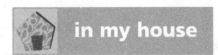

in my house

For years, my favorite tea was Good Earth Original caffeine-free sweet & spicy herbal tea. I loved its slightly sweet, slightly cinnamony taste; the fact that I could drink it right before I went to sleep and wouldn't stay awake all night was an extra plus. I also loved drinking a tea that seemed so eco-friendly. When I looked at the persuasive natural drawing on the box and thought of that appealing brand, it never occurred to me to question whether the product lived up to its name . . . good for the earth.

Once I finally took a closer look at the box, and read the ingredients in the tea itself, I had the sinking feeling that I'd been duped. My favorite Good Earth tea may be original, but it turned out not to be organic. It's not Fair Trade Certified either. And it contains artificial flavors, which the company justifies on its website as necessary to meet consumer demand.

It was a real lesson to me in how important it was to actually read the label on the box.

By the way, in 2007 Good Earth started offering an organic version of the tea. Unfortunately, it's not Fair Trade Certified and it still contains artificial flavors. Now I know—and can make (sadly) an alternative choice.

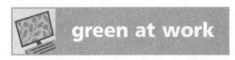

green at work

Green Coffee and Tea Service

Through Starbucks (www.starbucks.com/business/ocslist.asp) and Green Mountain Coffee (www.greenmountaincoffee.com/cstm_ocs.aspx) your company can order eco-friendly coffee and tea at work. Contact their services for more information.

Local coffee grinders sometimes supply businesses with their special shade-grown, organic, and fair trade blends as well. Ask around: you'll find them. While you're at it, replace the standard-issue orange pekoe tea with organic, fair trade varieties you can buy right off the shelf at the local Whole Foods, the food co-op or natural food store, and, increasingly, at any number of grocery stores.

big green purse

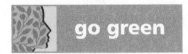 **go green**

How to Boil Water

Many government agencies and green groups advocate using a small electric kettle to boil water, claiming it's more energy efficient to use an electric heating element than a range top or microwave oven. I hesitate to follow suit. Already, fourteen million new coffeemakers are bought each year, suggesting that at least that many are being thrown away. If we start buying electric teapots, will we be perpetuating the resource-intense cycle of "buy, toss, and replace," especially noting that most electric teapots only carry a two-year warranty?

I've used the same kettle for at least fifteen years. Sure, it's lost its luster over time. But it's never failed to boil water. And there are several ways I maximize its energy efficiency:

- Use lukewarm rather than cold water to start.
- Boil only the amount of water needed.
- Use the heating element on the range that fits the kettle, to avoid overheating.
- Listen for the whistle; turn the kettle off as soon as the water boils.

If you do buy an electric kettle, choose a model that offers:

- an automatic shutoff mechanism
- a heat-resistant handle
- the option to heat only as much water as you want, rather than a full pot
- the heating element protected from the water to avoid mineral buildup that you'll otherwise have to clean regularly

Both the English Tea Store (www.englishteastore.com/kettles.html) and Target (www.target.com)—search: electric kettle—sell a wide variety of electric and traditional kettles in black, white, and stainless steel.

HOT STUFF: COFFEE, TEA, COCOA—AND THE SKINNY ON CHOCOLATE

Coffee, Tea, Cocoa, and Chocolate Wrap-up

- **Use your own mug.** Fill your own mug or thermos at the take-out counter.
- **Try reusable filters.** Brew coffee using filters that are reusable or made from recycled paper.
- **Use an energy-saving pot** that makes only as much coffee or tea as you need.
- **Keep extra coffee warm in an insulated carafe,** not on an electric hot plate.
- **Brew loose tea** in a tea stick, ball, or strainer.

And if you can do only one thing, make the shift to organic, Fair Trade Certified, shade-grown coffee, cocoa, and chocolate and organic fair trade tea. You'll help conserve the rain forest, save songbirds, and give the people who make your treats a chance to be treated fairly, too.

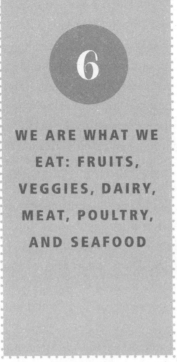

6

WE ARE WHAT WE EAT: FRUITS, VEGGIES, DAIRY, MEAT, POULTRY, AND SEAFOOD

WHAT ARE YOU MAKING FOR DINNER TONIGHT?

It used to be so easy to answer that question. You could shop for ingredients you thought were both delicious and safe, then decide on the meal once you got home: chicken or steak? Potatoes or pasta? Broccoli or beans?

These days, the more we learn about food's impact on the environment as well as our health, the more complicated grocery shopping gets. Should you buy organically grown produce or stick to conventional? Free-range or feedlot beef? Humanely raised or factory-farmed pork? No-hormone or "regular" milk?

The decision can be a weighty one. Convincing evidence now exists that pesticides, herbicides, and the industrial systems that produce most of the fruit, vegetables, dairy products, meat, fish, and poultry we eat are wrecking our world. They're also threatening our health and the well-being of those we count on to grow our food.

That said, women I've spoken with say their resolve to eat a more natural diet often "crumbles" by the time they wheel their shopping cart to the produce aisle. Buying organic fruits and vegetables can cost anywhere from 5 to 30 percent more, while organic meat can double the usual price. A mother of three in my neighborhood who regularly feeds not only her own kids but their friends, too, says she just doesn't think it's "worth it" to buy organic, especially given all the other demands on her family's budget. Even if they want to spend the money, some women don't have the choice. Only 3 percent of food is organic, and while most grocery stores carry some pesticide-free produce and dairy, almost 25 percent carry none at all.

What has made the journey from farm gate to kitchen plate so worrisome? And why pay the organic premium when other food is not only cheaper but also much more available?

The problem starts with modern agriculture itself. "Farming" may still conjure warm and fuzzy feelings, but the way food is raised today actually resembles practices you'd more likely find in a factory than on the quaint farm the song "Old MacDonald" brings to mind. There are 6.6 billion people on the planet, and they—we—all want to eat at least a few times a day. Mass-producing food is viewed, at least by agribusiness, as the most efficient way to meet demand, despite the environmental impacts industrial agriculture has on people and the planet:

- Agricultural chemicals and animal wastes leach into ground and surface water, threatening birds, fish, and beneficial insects like bees and ladybugs.
- A "dead zone" as big as the state of New Jersey spreads through the Gulf of Mexico every year as millions of tons of pesticides and fertilizers applied to Midwest farms are carried into the Gulf via the Mississippi River. U.S. coastal ecosystems are receiving 100 to 400 percent more nitrogen than natural systems should normally experience.
- The 50,000 cattle that reside in large feedlots at a given time produce as much manure as a city of several million people.
- Fattening up those cattle is none too easy on the earth, either. "It takes about seven pounds of corn [for a cow] to gain one pound of weight," reports Dr. Michael Jacobson in *Six Arguments for a Greener Diet*. "Over two hundred million acres of land are devoted to producing grains, oilseeds, pasture and hay for livestock. Cultivation of those crops requires 181 million pounds of pesticides, 22 billion pounds of fertilizer, and 17 trillion gallons of irrigation water per year. The fertilizer and pesticides pollute the air, water, and soil, while irrigation depletes natural aquifers built up over millennia."
- But growing fruits and vegetables can take their toll, too. A National Cancer Institute researcher who matched pesticide data and medical records in ten

California agricultural counties reported that pregnant women living within nine miles of farms where pesticides are sprayed may face increased risk of losing an unborn baby to birth defects.

• The EPA estimates that three hundred thousand farm workers suffer acute pesticide poisoning each year.

It's not as if we can turn to seafood for an alternative. The Environmental Protection Agency cautions everyone, but especially pregnant women and children, against eating tuna, due to contamination from mercury that precipitates out of air pollution generated by industrial smokestacks. But even if they're safe, many fish are becoming scarce. Nearly a third of the world's oceans and seas are "overfished," meaning that more fish are being caught than are reproducing. Fish in trouble include cod, haddock, sea bass, hake, red snapper, orange roughy, and grouper, among several other species.

The Good News

Given this grim gastronomical overview, you may feel as though you have no choice but to munch on organic nuts and berries for the rest of your life.

In fact, our options for safer, healthier, more abundant food are increasing with every trip to the grocery store, thanks almost entirely to consumer demand. This chapter lets you know what choices you have and how to make the most of them. It starts by encouraging you to eat less meat. There's just no getting around it. If we all cut more beef, chicken, and pork out of our diets, the environment would be cleaner, and we'd be healthier. How much you cut back is up to you. Hopefully, you'll get some guidance from these pages. The chapter also explains what organic is, why it's worth the extra dimes and sometimes dollars it costs, and how you can afford it. Fruit and vegetables receive a lot of attention here, but so do dairy products. If wine is more to your liking than milk, you'll find tips on how and where to buy it organically, too. And because life is such a rush these days, the chapter sneaks in (electronic) directions to locales where you can eat organically on the run.

If, indeed, we are what we eat, we've got every reason in the world to choose the safest, most delicious foods available. Let's get cookin'!

Use Your Big Green Purse

Because women have already been buying organic apples and oranges, hormone-free milk, and free-range chickens, we have many other choices as well. The more we shift our budget to organic and sustainably raised foods, the more choices we'll continue to have and the cheaper those choices will become.

- Eat less meat
- Choose sustainable seafood
- Buy organic
- Buy local
- BYOB

Eat Less Meat

Beef, Poultry, and Pork

More pasture is used to raise cattle than all other domesticated animals and crops combined. The United Nations Food and Agriculture project reported in 2006 that livestock now use 30 percent of the earth's entire land surface, either for permanent pasture or to produce feed for livestock. What else does that mean for the planet?

- **Deforestation.** According to World Wildlife Fund estimates, every year an area of the world's rain forests larger than New York State is destroyed to create grazing land. In Latin America, says the United Nations, some 70 percent of former forests in the Amazon have been cut down in favor of cows.
- **Manure.** Animal feeding operations also make you want to hold your nose. About 1.4 billion metric tons of solid manure are produced by U.S. farm animals each year—130 times the quantity produced by people. That amounts to 100,000 *metric tons of manure per minute*. This figure includes pigs and chickens as well as cattle, but cattle are the single largest source.
- **Global warming.** Dr. Michael Jacobson of the Center for Science in the Public Interest (CSPI) calculates that livestock manure (mostly cattle), plus the manure lagoons on factory farms (mostly hog), promote about as much global warming as the carbon dioxide generated by thirty-three million automobiles.

- **Health concerns.** Many consumers worry about pesticide residues on fruits and vegetables. "Fat-soluble pesticides in animal products actually pose the bigger risk," says CSPI's Dr. Jacobson. That's because livestock devour pesticide-tainted feed grains and stockpile chemical residues in their fat. While linking an infection or cancer to the steak you had for dinner is impossible, it still makes sense to reduce your pesticide exposure by purchasing beef produced organically or on farms that use integrated pest management and by eating less meat, poultry, dairy, and egg products overall.

- **Water pollution.** Two-thirds of the beef cattle raised in the United States are fattened up using hormones like steroids, testosterone, and progesterone. When these hormones are excreted, they can pollute surface and ground water, and affect the ability of frogs and fish to reproduce. If the lagoons break, animal manure can contaminate rivers and other waterways with stinky, slimy waste.

Chicken is often touted as a healthier, more eco-friendly alternative to meat and pork. Indeed, the British medical journal *The Lancet* in September 2007 encouraged consumers to switch from meat to chicken or fish not only to improve nutrition but also to reduce climate change. A cow, which has two stomachs, belches and poops far more than the significantly smaller, single-stomached chicken. When you eat less meat, you reduce the amount of manure your diet generates, curtailing some of the methane that contributes to climate change.

Still, poultry is nothing to cluck about:

- Like cattle, dairy cows, and hogs, chickens can be raised in "factory farm" environments that house hundreds of thousands of animals in inhumane conditions.
- Chicken wastes pollute the air with ammonia and the water with nitrogen.
- Along with hogs and ducks, chickens serve as repositories for flu viruses; public health officials are constantly on the lookout for "bird flu" and other epidemics that can spread like wildfire through the huge poultry sheds where chickens are raised.

Feeding antibiotics to farm animals sounds another alarm for many, including those in the medical community. "The reason to buy meat without antibiotics is not because the antibiotics in the meat are transferred to the person, but because of how the antibiotics increase the number of antibiotic-resistant bacteria," Dr. Stuart Levy, director of the Center of Adaptation Genetics and Drug Resistance at Tufts University Medical School, told *The New York Times*. The World Health Organization (WHO) has observed that antibiotics used to fatten livestock and poultry enable microbes to develop defenses against the drugs, scale the food chain, and assault human immune systems. The WHO encourages farmers to abandon antibiotics as a way to promote growth if similar antimicrobials are also used to treat people.

thumbs down

Antibiotics in Meat? Not a Good Idea

- Farm animals in the United States are fed or injected with 24.6 million pounds of antibiotics a year. The Union of Concerned Scientists notes that about 70 percent of all antibiotics made in the United States is used to fatten up livestock.
- Three studies published in the October 18, 2001, issue of *The New England Journal of Medicine* verified that antibiotic-resistant bacteria are widespread in American commercial meats and poultry and can be found in consumers' intestines. The studies indicate that routine use of antibiotics to enhance growth in farm animals can stimulate drug-resistant bacteria, which may endanger people who undercook their meat or consume food or water contaminated by animal droppings.
- The American Medical Association (AMA) has adopted a resolution opposing the use of antimicrobials at nontherapeutic levels in agriculture, or as pesticides or growth promoters. The AMA has urged that such practices be ended or phased out.

In addition to hormones and antibiotics, conventional meat producers routinely process their products using chemical additives and preservatives like phosphates and sodium nitrites. That makes them pinker, but not necessarily healthier. Sodium nitrites may react with amino acids to form carcinogenic nitrosamines; various studies have found a link between high processed-meat consumption and colon cancer, possibly attributable to preservatives like sodium nitrite.

Finally, you may be among the millions of consumers who are concerned about animal welfare. Hogs are raised in concentrated animal feed operations (CAFOs). Inside small pens about twenty-four inches wide, the hog's bedding is a metal grate that allows wastes to accumulate below. Most sows living in these conditions suffer joint damage, weak legs, impaired mobility, and urinary tract infections that require antibiotic treatment. Piglets are routinely castrated and have their teeth clipped, ears notched, and tails cut off, usually without anesthesia. Laying hens and dairy cows don't exist in much better conditions. The entire system is cruel and inhumane.

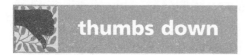

thumbs down

A Little Progesterone with Your Steak?

Feeding hormones to livestock has become standard practice in American stockyards and dairy barns. As many as two-thirds of American cattle raised for slaughter are injected with hormones to make them grow faster. America's dairy cows are fed the genetically engineered hormone rBGH to increase milk production. Both the USDA and FDA claim that these hormones are safe, but concern is growing that hormone residues in meat and milk may harm human health and the environment. The European Union's Scientific Committee on Veterinary Measures Relating to Public Health has questioned whether hormone residues in the meat of "growth enhanced" animals can disrupt *human* hormone balance, cause developmental problems, interfere with the reproductive system, and lead to the development of breast, prostate, and/or colon cancer.

Children, pregnant women, and the unborn are thought to be most susceptible. Hormone residues in beef have been implicated in the early onset of puberty in girls, which could put them at greater risk of developing breast and other forms of cancer. The European Union has banned meat imports from the United States because the meat comes from cattle raised on growth hormones.
Source: Sustainable Table

The Organic Alternative

After this rundown, is it any wonder so many shoppers are clamoring for organic meat?

Organic livestock are raised according to U.S. Department of Agriculture standards that require the following:

- **Organic feed.** Animals must be fed 100 percent certified organic feed or grass grown without toxic and persistent pesticides or fertilizers that harm the environment.
- **No animal by-products.** Animals may not be fed body parts of other animals, a practice linked to mad cow disease.
- **Humane treatment.** Livestock should be treated humanely, with access to the outdoors and uncrowded living conditions.
- **No antibiotics or hormones.** The use of antibiotics and hormones is strictly forbidden.
- **Preventive health practices.** Natural health practices are used to prevent disease. An animal treated with antibiotics will not continue to be certified organic.
- **Natural processing methods.** No synthetic chemicals, artificial preservatives, or harmful additives such as sodium nitrite may be used in processing the meat into sausage, patties, or other meat products.

go green

- **Eat less meat.** You can save 1.4 tons of greenhouse gases every year just from eating half as much meat. Start by replacing at least one meat meal a week with a vegetarian option. Try meat alternatives like tofu and veggie burgers. Get ideas from books on vegetarian cooking.
- **Buy local.** Check your farmers' market, food co-op, and natural food store for chicken, beef, and pork that's raised, packaged, and sold within two hundred miles of your kitchen. Advantages? You'll be dealing with farmers whose smaller operations allow the animals to graze freely and without the need for antibiotics or hormones. At www.localharvest.org you can connect with nearby farmers' markets, direct-sell farmers, and natural foods retailers that sell organic, hormone-free, and antibiotic-free meat.
- **Check the grocery store.** Coleman Natural Meats (www.colemannatural.com) and Laura's Lean Beef (www.laurasleanbeef.com) both sell hormone-free beef nationwide. Organic Prairie is more common in western states (http://organic valley.coop).
- **Order online.** The following companies are not USDA-certified organic, as some of them find it difficult to obtain organic feed for their animals; nevertheless,

they do not treat their animals with hormones or antibiotics, and they raise them in pastures.

- Blackwing Chicken (www.blackwingchicken.com)
- Diamond Organics Chicken and Turkey (www.diamondorganics.com)
- Grande Premium Meats (www.elkusa.com)
- Hollin Farm Natural Angus Beef (http://hollinfarms.com)
- Lobel's Free Range and Organic Poultry (www.lobels.com)
- Niman Ranch (www.nimanranch.com)
- Ranch Foods Direct (www.ranchfoodsdirectshop.com)

What Is the Difference Between "Organic," "Natural," and "Grass-fed" Meat?

- **Certified organic** farms must follow strict standards set by the USDA's National Organic Program, and are inspected by an independent third party each year for compliance. These standards prohibit the use of antibiotics, synthetic hormones, and pesticides.
- **"Natural"** meats may be minimally processed and free of preservatives and additives, but since no standards determine what qualifies as natural, you have no guarantee that hormones or antibiotics weren't used at some point unless the producer offers third-party verification.
- **"Grass-fed"** could mean the animals grazed for a day in a pasture, or most of its life. Again, without a standard to adhere to, it's difficult to judge.

Visit ranchers' websites to learn more about their operations and look for third-party verification of their marketing claims. Your biggest challenge will be finding organic pork. As of August 2004, the nation's largest organic hog farmer cooperative included only eight farmers—out of 80,010 hog farmers in the United States. During 2001, fewer than 3,500 hogs were certified organic in sixteen states—out of almost 185 million. Clearly, there's plenty of opportunity for hog farmers as well as cattle ranchers to convert more of their livestock operations to organic, a process that can take two years per cow in the case of beef. Your purchase now can make a difference by demonstrating, through your spending shifts, that the market will exist for the organic producer when he's ready for the market.

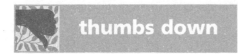

Empty Marketing Promises

Some marketing claims sound good, but don't mean a thing.

Hormone free. That's a favorite boast by supporters of free-range poultry products, but the truth is that growth hormones are banned from use for all poultry. Even conventionally raised chickens are free of added hormones.

Organic versus free-range. Organically raised hens are not given hormones, antibiotics, or pesticides. Their feed is 100 percent certified organic; it's never treated with synthetic fertilizers or pesticides. Organic farmers preserve the soil and protect the environment from degradation. Furthermore, farmers must follow strict rules about how the chickens are treated. Organic farmers allow chickens access to the outdoors rather than confine them in cages. These practices create healthier chickens and premium-quality eggs.

Producers of free-range chicken need follow no regulations or standards that hold them accountable for responsible production. They may or may not use antibiotics, hormones, and nonorganic feeds, depending on their preference.

Given the choice between organic and free-range, choose organic.

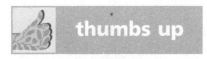

Certified Humane

If you're concerned about the way chickens, cows, pigs, and sheep are treated, look for the Certified Humane Raised & Handled label when you shop. The label, affixed to meat, poultry, egg, and dairy products, provides independent verification that livestock and poultry have had access to clean and sufficient food and water; a safe environment; protection from foul weather; and space to move naturally. The standards were created by animal scientists and veterinarians under the auspices of groups like the American Society for the Prevention of Cruelty to Animals (ASPCA) and the Humane Society of the United States (HSUS).

About Eggs: Brown or White?

There is no nutritional difference between caged and cage-free chicken or eggs. Some consumers believe that chickens allowed to roam free lay tastier eggs; you'll have to judge for yourself. Certainly, it is more humane to allow the animals to move about freely rather than confine them in a torturous pen.

As for the color of an egg's shell, it has to do neither with nutritional value nor with whether the bird was raised "free range" or confined. Rather, egg color simply reflects the hen's breed. It is more important to choose an egg based on how the chicken itself was raised than by the egg's color.

Become a Vegetarian?

Whether your primary concern is animal welfare, the impact food animals have on the environment, a healthy diet, or all of the above, you might consider becoming a vegetarian. See the Vegetarian Society's "Common Questions About Vegetarianism" at www.vegsoc.org/info/goingveg.html to determine whether a meat-free regime would work for you.

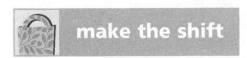

Start with Breakfast

Some women who join the Big Green Purse "One in a Million" campaign focus on shifting their spending to individual purchases. Mary Hunt, a marketing consultant in Orange, California, homed in on an entire meal: breakfast. She swapped her regular cereal for organic raisin bran, her regular milk for organic soy milk, and her fruit for organic fruit whenever it's available. "I love being reminded first thing in the morning that I can use my purse to make a difference," she says. "It affects the purchasing decisions I make about other products as I go through the day. Now, if there's a greener option, I'll choose it even if it's somewhat more expensive than the alternative."

Choose Sustainable Seafood

My grandfather was a cod fisherman in Nova Scotia. My father, his reluctant helper, spent many cold, bracing mornings in their small dory plying the icy North Atlantic waters where they fished. Dad was only a boy at the time, but he still remembers the thousands of cod they used to haul into their boat. There were so many fish, my father recalls, it was more a question of what to leave in the sea than what to sell to the merchants waiting for the catch on shore.

Those days are long gone. Today, more than 75 percent of the world's fisheries are either overfished or fished to capacity. And often, what remains, like tuna and swordfish, is too contaminated to eat with much frequency.

As hard as it is to believe, the oceans don't contain an infinite supply of fish. In fact, fish are being caught at such rapid rates that many of them face extinction. According to the Monterey Bay Aquarium, "between 1950 and 1994, ocean fishermen increased their catch 400 percent by doubling the number of boats and using more effective fishing gear." The aquarium says that catching more fish will drive some species to extinction. At the very least, they'll become so scarce it won't be worth it for commercial fishermen to go after them anymore. Then the fisheries themselves will collapse and a lot of people will lose their jobs.

This has already happened where my father and grandfather fished, in the North Atlantic waters of the United States and Canada. In 1992, reports the World Resources Institute, some 30,000 Canadians were suddenly without work when once-plentiful stocks of cod off the coast of Newfoundland disappeared.

The American Fisheries Society has identified a few geographic "hot spots" where several additional species face particular risk today. These include Florida's Indian River Lagoon, Keys, and Florida Bay; Puget Sound; and the northern Gulf of Mexico. Specific fish under siege include the Atlantic sturgeon and numerous varieties of rockfish. Scientists recommend creating marine preserves that would protect fish from hooks, trawlers, and nets.

How to Shop for Seafood

The Monterey Bay Aquarium's regional Seafood Watch guides contain the latest information on sustainable seafood choices available in different parts of the United States. "Best Choices" are abundant, well managed, and fished or farmed in environmentally friendly ways, like Pacific halibut on the West Coast or stone crabs in the Southeast. Seafood to "Avoid" is overfished or fished or farmed in ways that harm other marine life or the environment, like Chilean sea bass or red snapper, two species that are endangered nationwide. You can view the guides online or download a pocket-size version at www.mbayaq.org.

If it's too much trouble to keep track of the guides, shop for seafood sold under the Marine Stewardship Council (MSC) label, which certifies that those fish and shellfish come from sustainable sources. Creating a market for MSC seafood also helps discourage destructive overfishing.

STORES SELLING MSC-LABELED SEAFOOD

Costco (Kirkland brand)
Norm Thompson
Safeway
Sam's Club
Taku Store (order online at www .takustore.com)
Target (Archer Farms brand)
Wal-Mart
Whole Foods

Is Fish Farming the Solution?

Throughout the last decade, as concerns about eating beef have increased, American fish consumption has risen 29 percent. Fish offer a good source of heart-healthy, cancer-fighting omega-3 fatty acids. Plus, fish are generally lower in calories than meat. But with wild fish populations on the decline, the fishing industry is turning to fish farming to meet consumer demand. Unfortunately, fish farming can cause its own set of problems. "Enclosing thousands of fish in pens close to the shoreline is equivalent to cramming chickens and pigs into warehouses. The same results are achieved: drugged fish eating dubious-quality feed, then producing tons of feces," reports Luddene Perry, author of *A Field Guide to Buying Organic*.

WANT TO EAT FARMED FISH? THE MONTERREY BAY AQUARIUM SUGGESTS:	
Best Choices:	*Avoid:*
Barramundi, Catfish, Arctic char, Clams, Mussels, Oysters, Bay scallops, Striped bass, Sturgeon, Tilapia, Rainbow trout	Salmon (Atlantic, Norwegian, or other farmed salmon), Shrimp, Tilapia farmed in China or Taiwan

Farmed hybrid fish frequently escape from their cages, interbreed with native populations, and spread diseases like sea lice. Plus, fish farming can consume more fish than it generates. Producing one pound of farm-raised salmon or shrimp requires two to three pounds of wild fish for feed.

Are Fish Safe to Eat?

The omega-3 benefits aside, some fish are contaminated with heavy metals like mercury and lead, industrial chemicals including PCBs, and such pesticides as DDT and dieldrin. These contaminants enter the water in several ways: from factory discharges, runoff from farms and lawns, and air pollution that falls into lakes, rivers, streams, and the sea from power plant cooling towers and automobile emissions. Fish can absorb these toxins in their skin, organs, and fatty tissue.

Over time, contaminants can build up in your body. Mothers who eat contaminated fish before becoming pregnant may have children who are slower to develop and learn. Developing fetuses are exposed to toxins that pass through the placenta. Women beyond their childbearing years and men face fewer health risks from contaminants than children do.

You've probably heard the most about mercury in canned tuna. Both the Environmental Protection Agency and Environmental Defense recommend that adults and children limit consumption of canned white albacore tuna because of the mercury it contains.

Canned light tuna usually consists of skipjack, a smaller species with approximately one-third the mercury levels of albacore. Therefore, Environmental Defense recommends that only young children (ages zero through six) limit consumption. However, recent news reports suggest that some canned light tuna actually contains yellowfin, a species similar in size and mercury content to albacore. These foods may be labeled "gourmet" or "tonno," and their consumption should be restricted by adults as well as children. Overall, it's best to exercise caution in how much tuna you (and especially your children) consume.

Fish that are low in contaminants include wild salmon from Alaska (fresh, frozen, and canned), Atlantic mackerel and herring, sardines, sablefish, anchovies, farmed oysters, and tilapia.

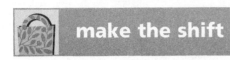

make the shift

Sustainable Seafood Strategies

- Look for seafood sold under the Marine Stewardship Council label.
- Substitute wild Alaskan salmon for farmed salmon. (Atlantic salmon in United States stores and restaurants is always farmed.)
- If you live in New England and want to serve cod, opt for hook-caught instead of trawl-caught Atlantic cod. If you live on the West Coast, sablefish/black cod is a good replacement.
- Farmed striped bass can be used as a substitute for Pacific rockfish, grouper, snapper, orange roughy, and Patagonian toothfish (often called Chilean sea bass).
- Tilapia farmed in the United States (rather than China) is another tasty alternative.
- Try Mary Lu Seafoods (www.maryluseafoods.com). This West Coast albacore tuna is sustainably harvested and canned in its own juice; it claims to contain less mercury than other tuna brands.
- EcoFish (www.ecofish.com) sells fish from ecologically sound sources. Try shrimp, mahimahi, wild Alaskan salmon, and canned and fresh-frozen delicacies.

You can also benefit from fish-oil supplements, though capsules should be made from purified oil that is free of environmental contaminants. According to an Environmental Defense (ED) survey on the safest supplements, some of your best choices include:

* CVS brand	* Kirkland brand (Costco)	* Nutra Sea
* Health Pride	* Nature's Valley	* Omega3, 6, 9

You can get the complete list at ED's Ocean's Alive website, www.oceans alive.org.

Going out to dinner? Steer clear of the large predators, especially shark, tuna, Chilean sea bass, and swordfish. Big fish play a critical role in marine ecosystems; they also concentrate the most toxins. Select smaller wild fish from well-managed fisheries, or U.S.-farmed catfish or tilapia instead.

WE ARE WHAT WE EAT: FRUITS, VEGGIES, DAIRY, MEAT, POULTRY, AND SEAFOOD

Buy Organic

Via local grocery stores, superstores like Wal-Mart and Sam's Club, farmers' markets, community-supported agriculture (CSA), and the Internet, most of us can shop and eat organically. Though only a small percentage of the entire food supply qualifies, enough fruits, vegetables, meat, chicken, dairy, oil, and spices abound sans pesticides, herbicides, and added hormones to enable you to prepare almost any recipe. Organic food sales are growing 15 to 21 percent each year, reports *Forbes*, faster than any other segment of the food industry, so your options are only destined to increase.

What Does "Organic" Mean?

Organic refers to the way agricultural products—food and fiber—are grown and processed, explains the Organic Trade Association (OTA).

- **Good for the soil.** Organic food production is "based on a system of farming that maintains and replenishes soil fertility without the use of toxic fertilizers and pesticides that persist in the environment for decades or even generations."
- **Minimal processing.** Plus, says the OTA, "Organic foods are minimally processed without artificial ingredients, preservatives, or irradiation to maintain the integrity of the food."
- **Organic standards.** "Certified Organic" means the item has been grown according to strict government standards that have been verified by independent state or private organizations. These independent certifiers inspect farm fields and processing facilities, periodically test soil and water, and examine the detailed records that growers and handlers keep to ensure that the standards are being met.
- **Smart farming.** "Prevention" is the organic farmer's watchword when it comes to fighting diseases, weeds, and damaging insects. Organic producers also cultivate species that are well suited to the climate. If pest populations get out of balance, growers will deploy insect predators, traps, and barriers or strategies to disrupt mating habits. Permission may be granted by the certifier to apply plant-based botanical or other nonpersistent pest controls that break down quickly if all else fails.

Organically grown crops also require less fossil fuel than conventional crops. The fifteen-year "Farming Systems Trial" conducted by the Rodale Institute in Pennsylvania showed that organic agriculture can reduce greenhouse gas emissions by effectively locking more carbon into the soil rather than releasing it into the atmosphere, as happens in conventional agriculture. Because it relies more on human labor than machines while forgoing petroleum-based pesticides and fertilizers, organic farming consumes 50 percent less energy overall than conventional agricultural methods.

There is even some proof that organic food may be more nutritious. Research presented at England's Soil Association's annual conference in January 2005 showed that milk from cows raised organically had 75 percent higher levels of beta-carotene and 50 percent higher levels of vitamin E, and was two to three times richer in the antioxidants lutein and zeaxanthin. Organic fruits and vegetables averaged 33 percent more antioxidants than conventionally grown produce in thirteen out of fifteen studies, according to research conducted by Dr. Charles Benbrook of the Organic Center.

How Can You Tell If Food Is Organic?

"100 percent organic." Food must contain only organically produced ingredients according to standards set by the U.S. Department of Agriculture; may carry the *USDA Organic* seal.

"Organic." Food must be at least 95 percent organic by weight (excluding water and salt); may display the *USDA Organic* seal.

"Made with organic ingredients." Processed products that contain **at least 70 percent organic ingredients** may not use the "USDA Organic" seal but use the phrase "made with organic ingredients" and list up to three organic ingredients or food groups on the principal display panel. For example, soup made with at least 70 percent organic ingredients may be labeled either "made with organic peas, potatoes, and carrots," or "made with organic vegetables." The "USDA Organic" seal may not be used anywhere on the package.

Less than 70 percent organic ingredients. May not use the term "organic" on the main label; may identify specific organic ingredients on the product label.

USDA organic regulations:

- prohibit the use of irradiation, sewage sludge, or genetically modified organisms in organic production;
- prohibit antibiotics in organic meat and poultry; and
- require 100 percent organic feed for organic livestock.

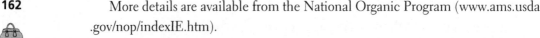

More details are available from the National Organic Program (www.ams.usda .gov/nop/indexIE.htm).

Beware Greenwashing

The word "organic" must reflect the federal standards governing its use. Other terms that appear on food labels may sound equally appealing yet could be meaningless.

Natural. "Natural" is a ubiquitous marketing claim, especially on processed foods. But what it means depends on how it's used. An apple off the tree or a carrot right out of the ground is clearly natural and there's no harm in saying so. But what if natural food is processed for convenience or packaging ease? In all likelihood, it will be combined with a variety of ingredients, some natural, some not. Your best bet? Read the label. Avoid artificial ingredients or added colors, and look for explanations that clarify how the food was made.

Who Does It Right?

Nature's Path Organic 8 Whole Grains Cereal ingredients list:

Organic whole wheat bran	Organic whole oat flour	Organic buckwheat flour
Organic whole wheat meal	Organic whole millet	Organic barley flour
Organic rolled oats	Organic oat bran	Organic barley malt extract
Organic evaporated cane juice	Organic brown rice flour	Organic sprouted whole rye kernels
	Organic yellow corn flour	
	Organic molasses	
	Organic quinoa	

No Detected Residues. This phrase implies that lab testing has been conducted to ensure that any toxic chemicals applied to produce have degraded and are therefore harmless. The problem with this label is that it doesn't ensure that no pesticides or herbicides were applied in the first place. Further, only those chemicals that the farmer asked to be tested for residues were evaluated. "No Detected Residues" is not a blanket seal of approval for any and all chemicals that might be found on a particular crop. This is essentially a meaningless claim.

Other Food Label Lingo

In addition to "organic," you may see these descriptions of ecogrowing practices on the labels of food you buy.

Biodynamic. Biodynamic agriculture is supposed to incorporate organic growing principles into a holistic farming approach that recycles nutrients, rotates crops, and builds and maintains the soil. Biodynamic farmers also attempt to tap "cosmic rhythms" (the phases of the sun and moon) to maximize soil and plant development and to keep the farm vital. "Biodynamic" is not a federally defined classification; there are no guarantees it represents what it implies. However, Consumers Union analysts say that "biodynamic" as certified by the Demeter Association (www.demeter-usa.org) is "highly meaningful." If a company's biodymanic claim is backed up by Demeter, you may have confidence in it.

Sustainable. "Sustainable" agriculture promotes farming that protects and perpetuates the natural environment. But like "biodynamic" and "traditional," no federal standards give the word any on-the-ground teeth. The Oregon-based Food Alliance (www.foodalliance.org) operates a comprehensive third-party certification program in North America for "sustainably" produced food. Food Alliance–certified distinguishes foods produced by farmers and ranchers who provide safe and fair working conditions; promote healthy and humane treatment of animals; raise animals without added hormones and antibiotics; grow crops without genetically modified organisms; reduce the use of pesticides; conserve soil and water resources; and preserve and protect wildlife habitat. Food Alliance–approved foods can be bought throughout the Midwest and Pacific Northwest.

Fair Trade. A limited amount of imported food is being certified as "fair trade." The label ensures that farmers are being treated fairly and paid a decent wage for their work. Look for the Fair Trade Certification label on coffee, bananas, cocoa, dried fruit, fresh fruit and vegetables, honey, juices, nuts and oil, seeds, rice, spices, sugar, tea, and wine. To learn more about fair trade, see Chapter 5.

Wonder if a product or marketing claim is as "eco" as it claims to be? Check it out, at www.eco-labels.org.

Why Does Organic Food Cost More?

About the price issue: no denying it, most of the time, organic food is more expensive than food grown with chemicals. Here's why:

- **The federal government favors conventional crops.** The federal Farm Bill financially subsidizes massive industrial agricultural operations and their pesticide-intensive practices; it provides comparatively little support to organic farmers, or to farmers who want to transition to organic, a process that takes at least three years. The subsidies to the pesticide-plied crops make them artificially low-cost—but more affordable nonetheless.

- **Organic farms are more labor intensive.** In organic agriculture, people do the work that keeps soil healthy and plants pest free. Conventional farms rely on inexpensive chemicals to bring their food to market, while ignoring the long-term costs society pays for health care and environmental cleanup as these chemicals accumulate in our bodies, on the land, and in the water.
- **Demand exceeds supply.** People are clamoring for more and more organic food. As supply increases, prices will decrease.

You can make a difference over the long-term by encouraging your elected officials to favor laws and regulations that will help family farmers compete in the marketplace. In the short term, pick some entry points—milk, fruit, salad greens, or meat—and shift ten dollars a week of money you already spend on these foods to their organic alternatives. Remember, your dollars will make a difference. The more you buy, the cheaper organic food will eventually get.

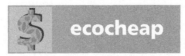

How to Afford Organics

You can minimize or avoid paying premium prices for organic food by following these smart shopping strategies:

- **Comparison shop.** Check prices among grocery stores to find the lowest costs. In my neighborhood, Trader Joe's is usually less expensive than my grocery store, which charges less than my local food co-op. And the food co-op sells fresh produce more cheaply than Whole Foods Market (though dairy and packaged goods are more expensive at the co-op).
- **Buy the store brand.** Due to consumer demand, my local supermarket is carrying its own, more-affordable organic brand, which I choose over the name brand whenever I have the option.
- **Buy in season.** It's usually cheaper to buy foods that are grown in season, rather than imports that travel across the country or from another hemisphere no matter what time of year it is.

Why Buy Organic?

1. **Keep chemicals out of the air, water, soil, and our bodies.** With only 0.5 percent of crop and pasture land organic, 99.5 percent of farm acres in the United States are at risk of exposure to noxious agricultural chemicals, according to the USDA. Organic agriculture reduces the toxic load on our natural systems as well as our human ones.

2. **Reduce if not eliminate off-farm pollution.** In addition to polluting farmland and adversely affecting farmworkers, industrial agriculture wreaks havoc on the environment downstream. Pesticide drift in the air pollutes nonfarm communities with odorless and invisible poisons. Synthetic fertilizer that runs off into rivers and streams is the main culprit behind the dead zones in delicate ocean environments like the Gulf of Mexico.

3. **Protect future generations.** Even before a mother first nurses her newborn, the baby's toxic risk from pesticides has begun. Studies show that infants are exposed to hundreds of harmful chemicals in utero—chemicals whose safety was determined based on adult tolerance levels, not on children's. According to the National Academy of Sciences, "Neurologic and behavioral effects may result from low-level exposure to pesticides." Numerous studies show that pesticides can alter the nervous system, increase the risk of cancer, heighten learning disabilities, and decrease fertility later in life.

4. **Protect farmworkers.** Farmworkers on conventional farms are exposed to inordinately high levels of pesticides, herbicides, and fertilizers that put them at risk for cancer, respiratory disease, and many other illnesses.

5. **Build healthy soil for better food.** Feeding the soil with organic matter instead of ammonia and other synthetic fertilizers increases nutrients in produce. Plus, higher levels of vitamins and minerals infuse

organic food, according to the 2005 study, "Elevating antioxidant levels in food through organic farming and food processing," by The Organic Center State of Science Review.

6. **Consider the yum factor.** It makes sense that strawberries taste yummier when raised in harmony with nature, but researchers at Washington State University proved this in lab taste trials where the organic berries were consistently judged to be sweeter.

7. **Support family farmers.** Organic family farms bring healthy food directly to our communities while protecting local landscapes from sprawl and overdevelopment.

8. **Avoid "FrankenFoods."** Cloned food, GMOs (genetically modified organisms), rBGH (recombinant bovine growth hormone). As recently as 1996, genetically modified food would not be served for supper; today an astounding 30 percent of our cropland is planted in GMOs. Organic is the only de facto seal of protection against these and other modern, lab-produced additions to our food basket.

9. **Save energy.** Organic agriculture uses, on average, about 30 percent less energy than conventional agriculture, helping to limit climate change and reduce our dependence on petroleum.

10. **Promote biodiversity.** Visit an organic farm and you'll notice something: a buzz of animal, bird, and insect activity. These organic oases are thriving, diverse habitats, especially when compared with the sterile landscape common to industrial agriculture.

Adapted from "Top 10 Reasons to Support Organic in the 21st Century," www.organic.org

- **Support CSAs.** Buy a share in community-supported agriculture, choosing a local organic farm that supplies you with a weekly shopping bag or two of seasonal fruits and vegetables. Check with Local Harvest (www.localharvest.org) for the CSA nearest you.
- **Buy in bulk.** Many grocery stores and food co-ops let you bag your own organic dry goods at more favorable prices than if you bought them prepackaged.

big green purse

- **Shop sales.** You may be able to find coupons at All Organic Links (http://frugal living.about.com/gi/dynamic/offsite.htm?zi=1/XJ&sdn=frugalliving&zu=http%3A %2F%2Fwww.allorganiclinks.com%2F). Many food co-ops and grocery stores discount organic food in their weekly, in-store shopping papers. Also, check the containers the food comes in for printed coupons on the can, box, or bag.
- **Shift money within your shopping budget.** Can you replace items like bottled water or paper towels with reusable options, and put the saved money toward organic food?
- **Grow your own.** Talk about cheap! All it will cost you is the price of the seeds, water, and compost (unless you make your own), and some work with the shovel and hoe. See Chapter 9 to get started.

Looking for the closest organic retailer? Check out www.eatwellguide.org.

Organics in Your Shopping Cart

Organic foods are available fresh. You can also buy a wide variety of prepared organic foods, including pasta, prepared sauces, frozen juices, frozen meals, milk, ice cream and frozen novelties, cereals, meat, poultry, breads, soups, chocolate, cookies, beer, wine, and vodka. Given all the choices, where should you start?

According to scientists at the Environmental Working Group (EWG), eating the twelve most contaminated fruits and vegetables exposes consumers to about twenty pesticides a day on average. Consuming the twelve least contaminated foods reduces pesticide exposure to about two pesticides a day. To be honest, we don't know what impact multiple exposures to pesticides will have on healthy adults. However, the U.S. Environmental Protection Agency believes that infants and children may be especially sensitive to pesticide-related health risks because kids' internal organs are still developing and maturing. Plus, in relation to their body weight, infants and children eat and drink more than adults, possibly increasing their chemical exposure.

Some fruits and vegetables are more likely than others to retain pesticides after they are harvested. Given that organic foods can be more expensive than those grown using pesticides, the EWG and other organizations say consumers who want to economize and still shop organically should focus their shopping dollars on the following produce first.

make the shift

Organic Produce Purchase Priorities

These fruits and vegetables consistently show the highest levels of pesticide residues. They would be the first place to spend shopping dollars on organic produce.

- Apples
- Carrots
- Celery
- Cherries
- Cucumbers
- Grapes (domestic and imported)
- Green beans
- Hot peppers
- Lettuce
- Nectarines
- Oranges
- Peaches
- Pears
- Plums
- Potatoes
- Raspberries
- Spinach
- Strawberries
- Sweet bell peppers

The following foods consistently show the lowest levels of pesticide residues. If you need to economize, don't worry as much about buying these foods organically.

- Asparagus
- Avocados
- Bananas
- Blueberries
- Broccoli
- Cabbage
- Cantaloupe
- Cauliflower
- Eggplant
- Grapefruit
- Honeydew melon
- Kiwi
- Lemon
- Mangoes
- Mushrooms
- Onions
- Papaya
- Pineapples
- Sweet corn (frozen)
- Sweet peas (frozen)
- Sweet potatoes
- Tangerines
- Tomatoes
- Watermelon
- Winter squash

For full details and a copy of the EWG's wallet-size advisory guide to take shopping with you, see www.foodnews.org/walletguide.php.

What If You Can't Buy Organic?

- **Still eat produce.** The health evidence overwhelmingly supports consuming more fruits and vegetables, especially compared to meat and processed foods, even if some pesticide residue remains. And growing fruits and vegetables is eas-

big green purse

ier on the environment than producing meat. Life is one big continuum anyway. Eat more veggies today, eat more organic veggies tomorrow.

- **Wash produce in clean running water.** There's no need to use detergent, soap, or fancy vegetable washes. Scrub produce that has a thicker skin (like potatoes and cucumbers) with a vegetable brush if you want to eat the peels. Otherwise, you can pare apples, pears, cucumbers, and potatoes, the four peelable foods on the "high" side of the pesticide spectrum.
- **Use the EWG list** to choose fruits and veggies that are consistently less contaminated.
- **Vary your diet.** By consuming different produce items you limit your exposure to any one kind of pesticide.
- **Grow your own.** Even if you don't have time to start veggies from seed, you can buy seedlings at the local garden store or farmers' market, or get patio planters for a kitchen garden of lettuce, spinach, and cherry tomatoes.

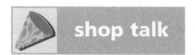 **shop talk**

Ask for Organic

No organic choice in your grocery store? Take a minute to ask the people stocking the produce bins when you can expect more-healthful fare. They won't know—but they'll be prompted to find the department manager so you can ask the question directly. That person may want to pass the buck up to the district manager for the store, the person who orders food from the regional warehouse. That's okay. Tell the department manager you'll check in with him or her next time you're shopping to find out what the store's organic timetable is. Then get the department manager's name. Encourage a few of your friends to ask that same manager for organics when they shop, too. It shouldn't take too long for your demand to increase supply. But be careful what you wish for: once the products show up, make sure you buy them. No sense going to all that trouble if you don't put your money where your mouth is.

What About the Spinach Scare?

Many consumers were frightened and confused in 2006 when bagged, raw spinach contaminated with E. coli sickened hundreds of people and killed three. How E. coli entered the bagged spinach hasn't been definitively determined, but it's possible that feral pigs or cattle left their contaminated droppings directly on the California field where the spinach was grown. In addition, a cattle feedlot located upstream from the field may have polluted irrigation water.

Most health professionals believe that because spinach and other salad vegetables are so nutritious, their benefits far outweigh the unlikely risk that they will transmit foodborne illness. Still, you can take precautions to protect yourself and your family.

- Wash your hands, cutting boards, knives, and other utensils after handling raw meat.
- Keep salad vegetables away from raw meat.
- Noting that E. coli can flourish in deteriorating salad greens, refrigerate spinach and lettuce. The U.S. Centers for Disease Control and Prevention (CDC) recommends storing all fresh produce at a temperature of 40 degrees Fahrenheit or below. Refrigerate all precut or peeled produce to maintain both quality and safety, says the CDC.
- Cook fresh spinach at 160 degrees Fahrenheit for 15 seconds to kill any E. coli present.
- Buy fresh greens from local markets where you trust farmers to grow your spinach and lettuce on land that will not be contaminated by animal waste.
- Grow your own. Spinach and lettuce are among the simplest foods to raise in your backyard or on your patio.

Full Disclosure

Is organic food 100 percent pesticide free? Not necessarily. Some organic crops may be inadvertently exposed to agricultural chemicals that have built up in rain and groundwater over the last fifty years. Organic fields are also victimized by pesticide-laden drift from wind, rain, and runoff from farms that use toxic chemicals today, according to the Organic Trade Association. But pesticide residue on organic food will be substantially lower than it will be on conventionally grown food. Buying organic food is about making better choices—not necessarily "perfect" choices. Besides, supporting organic agriculture is not only an attempt to protect ourselves today. It is truly an investment in the food we'll be eating tomorrow.

Buying organic milk is one of the easiest purchases you can make to improve the food you're offering your kids, especially if you're buying from family dairies that raise their cows in pastures. Here's why:

Health benefits. Organic milk provides 50 percent more vitamin E than conventionally produced milk and 75 percent more beta-carotene, which the body converts into vitamin A. It is also two to three times higher in antioxidants, according to the Danish Institute of Agricultural Research. Local organic dairies that allow their cows to graze on grass produce healthier milk than "mega" dairies that feed their cows organic grain in confined feedlots.

No hormones. Genetically engineered "bovine growth hormone" (known as rBGH or rBST) is injected into nonorganic cows to increase milk production, a procedure that can lead to infections requiring treatment with antibiotics. Milk from these cows often contains residues of these chemicals. The U.S. Food & Drug Administration has said that using rBGH poses no health risks. Consumer and health groups argue that we should not burden our bodies with synthetic hormones and unnecessary antibiotics.

Today, certified organic dairy products include:

- butter
- buttermilk
- cheeses and spreads
- cottage cheese
- cream

- half-and-half
- ice cream
- milk
- powdered milk and cheese
- yogurt

Organic dairy products are also used as ingredients in a diverse array of organic products, such as frozen and convenience foods, chocolate bars, and baby food.

Look for milk, cheese, and other dairy products that are produced locally by farmers who do not use hormones and antibiotics. Plug your zip code into the map at www.foodroutes.org/localfood to locate an organic dairy farmer nearby.

In your grocery store or food co-op, shop for brands like these:

- **Natural by Nature grass-fed organic milk** is 100 percent certified organic and produced without rBGH. It's available in large natural food stores and local food co-ops.

- **Green Valley Dairy** makes cheese from organic milk produced from cows that graze on grass all year long.
- **Organic Valley** sells eggs laid by chickens fed an organic diet.

The increasing demand for organic milk has put a strain on the industry nationally. Some "organic" operations have gotten as large as their conventional counterparts, raising thousands of cows on inadequate pasture and otherwise violating federal organic standards. The nonprofit Cornucopia Institute's Organic Integrity Project acts as a "corporate watchdog" to assure that "no compromises to the credibility of organic farming methods and the food it produces are made in the pursuit of profit." The Institute monitors organic farming practices and publicizes industry efforts to weaken organic standards. You can get more information at www.cornucopia.org.

 thumbs down

Organic Fish

There's no such thing as "organic" fish as far as the U.S. Department of Agriculture standards are concerned. Here's what Marion Nestle, public health professor at New York University and author of *What to Eat,* says on the subject: "The basis of organic food production is control over growing conditions. But big fish eat smaller fish and migrate thousands of miles over rivers and oceans. If they end up full of methylmercury and PCBs, how can they possibly be considered organic? Fish farming also seems anything but organic. Farm-raised fish are treated with pesticides to prevent lice, and they eat pellets containing artificial colors, parts of fish and other animals, and binders and thickeners made from soybeans that could be genetically modified. How . . . could any farmed fish be labeled 'organic'?" Ignore marketing campaigns that try to sell you organic fish.

 in my house

We drink at least three gallons of milk a week at our house, so we decided a long time ago that we'd buy organic. We're lucky because we live in the Chesapeake Bay region, where a couple of good local dairies provide a delicious alternative to industrial milk products. The downside of organic milk is that it's so darn expensive. I justify it in a lot of ways. Mostly, I figure if I can spend ten dollars to rent a couple of movies every week, I can spend an extra five or ten bucks on healthy milk for my family. I buy my eggs at the farmers' market—they're usually gathered the same morning I buy them, and the taste is worth the extra money they cost. Most of my cheese comes from the supermarket, and while it's functional, it's not very tasty. It does seem like the closer you can trace food back to the earth, the more delicious it is.

Wine, Beer, and Spirits

When it comes to drinks with dinner or a beer to go with the game, eco-options abound.

Wine

- "USDA-certified organic" means that the wine was produced without herbicides and pesticides and with no added sulfites, preservatives that help wine maintain its color and taste but that can cause serious allergic reactions and headaches in susceptible people. (Sulfites occur naturally, so no wine is sulfite free.)
- "Made from organically grown grapes" means grapes were grown without pesticides or chemicals; some sulfites may have been added as a preservative.
- "Sustainable" may indicate the vineyard practices pesticide-free viticulture, using sheep to suppress weeds and owls to kill rodents. However, "sustainable" is not as meaningful as "organic" unless it is backed up by independent third-party certification.
- "Biodynamic" practices rely on viticulture techniques that build healthy soil and keep the vineyard in tune with the cycles of the sun, moon, and planets. When certified by the Demeter Association, it's safe to assume the vineyard met standards for biodynamic production. Learn more about biodynamic wine at www.demeter-usa.org/.

WINES TO LOOK FOR

Benziger (biodynamic—California)
Ca'del Solo (biodynamic—California)
Cullen (organic—Western Australia)
Emiliana (organic—Chile)
Four Gates (organic, kosher—California)

Frey Vineyards (organic—California)
Frog's Leap (organic—California)
Grgich Hills (biodynamic—California)
Santa Julia (organic—Argentina)
Sobon Estate (organic—California)
Yarden Chardonnay (organic, kosher—Golan Heights)

See many more options at http://trade-organic-wine.com.

Beer

Organic beer is made the same way any beer is made, but under USDA standards at least 95 percent of its ingredients—usually barley and hops—must be grown without pesticides. Some organic beers to look for:

Butte Creek Brewing Co. (Chico, California)
Peak Organic Brewing Co. (Burlington, Massachusetts)
Stone Mill Pale Ale (Anheuser-Busch via Crooked Creek Brewing Co.)
Wild Hop Lager (Anheuser-Busch via Green Valley Brewing Co.)
Wolaver's Organic Ale (Middlebury, Vermont)

Spirits

If wines or beers aren't your drinks of choice, organic or not, the following spirits may be more appealing:

Square One Organic Vodka (Marin County, California)
Sunshine Vodka (Stowe, Vermont)
Vodka 14 (Thornton, Colorado)

Dining Out?

Whether you're looking for a fine dining experience or eating on the run, it's getting easier to find organic and unprocessed food on the menu.

Fast Food

- **Burgerville** (www.burgerville.com). Found throughout the Northwest, Burgerville features fresh local ingredients and serves seasonal specialties like huckleberry milk shakes and strawberry shortcake.

- **Chipotle** (www.chipotle.com). In addition to the vegetarian offerings, the meat (chicken, beef, pork) is produced without hormones; the company has made sustainable farming a key tenet of its operations.
- **Evos** (www.evos.com). This Florida-based chain uses hormone- and antibiotic-free beef in its burgers and spins salads from organic field greens.
- **O'Naturals** (www.onaturals.com). A new but growing franchise offering sandwiches, salads, noodles, soups, pizza, and "thirst quenchers."
- **Organic and natural foods grocery stores.** Try salad, soup, and entrée bars.

One thing about takeout that's true whether the food is organic or not: it generates a lot of trash if it's wrapped in plastic and paper. Minimize the garbage you throw away by skipping extra napkins. And if you're taking the food home, leave the plastic forks and knives at the restaurant.

Fine Dining

"Green" restaurants are sprouting in many cities, as chefs respond to consumer demand for locally grown and organic cuisine. Your best bet is to do an Internet search of "eco-friendly restaurant" plus the name of your city and give the establishment a try. You can also check out the Green Restaurant Association, a nonprofit that encourages its members to serve organic and locally grown food, save energy and water, and reduce use of paper products. Check the database for the nearest certified "green" restaurant at www.dinegreen.com.

Wherever you dine, don't forget to ask your waiter what organic entrées the restaurant is serving—especially if you don't see any listed on the menu. The message will make it back to the chef loud and clear.

Cooking on the Grill?

Check the Big Green Purse website (www.bigggreenpurse.com; search:Teflon pans) for the latest updates on the Teflon cookware controversy. You can also find reviews of the newest vegetarian and organic cookbooks on our blog www.biggreenpurse.com /blog.

Energy-efficient cooking tips are listed in the Appliances section of Chapter 11. If you do a lot of grilling, consider these ways to green it up:

Most grills use either natural gas, propane, charcoal, or electricity. Of these options, charcoal emits more carbon monoxide, particulate matter, and soot than any of the others. That means it also contributes more to ground-level ozone, or smog.

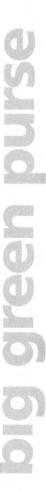

Alternatives?

Use lump charcoal instead of briquettes. Briquettes may contain coal dust and other additives. Lump charcoal actually comes from a tree, and you can find brands from sustainably managed forests certified by the Rainforest Alliance's SmartWood program.

Trade in your lighter fluid. This toxic petroleum distillate produces volatile organic compounds (VOCs) that create smog. No sense ruining your skewers or burgers with an air-quality alert, is there?

Try a chimney charcoal starter. Tuck crumpled newspaper into the bottom of the canister, load charcoal on top, and light with a match. You'll be able to pour hot coals onto the fire grate in about fifteen minutes.

Go solar. A solar stove cooks more slowly and won't get you the grilled flavor you enjoy off the barbie. But it can't be beat for a clean-cooking cookout.

Where to Buy

Chimney charcoal starter. It averages fifteen dollars online. You'll find several options at www.nextag.com/charcoal-chimney-starter/search-html.

Solar oven. The "sport solar oven" (http://pathtofreedom.com/peddlerswagon/ homestead/ecogoods/solaroven/sunoven-sport.shtml) costs one hundred fifty dollars, but you'll never buy charcoal or other cooking fuel again.

Gas grill. Log on to www.grillsearch.com/ for a list of dozens of grill choices by brand. Start with the page, "What to look for?" Don't buy a larger appliance than you need or you'll end up wasting energy and money.

Grilling or broiling meats at extremely high temperatures can form carcinogenic hydrocarbons if fat from the meat, fish, or poultry drips onto hot coals and shoots back onto your food. Have a healthier cookout by choosing lean meats; trimming the fat; and marinating in citrus juices, olive oils, and herbs. Be safer yet, and grill vegetable kebabs or skewers of pineapple, melon, and other fruit.

Buy Local

Buying food that's locally grown is among the most effective ways you can spend your money to get the world you want. First, buying local benefits the environment by reducing the amount of oil needed to transport food long distances. On average, most supermarket foods travel about fifteen hundred miles to get to your plate.

big green purse

Locally grown food averages around fifty-seven miles. An analysis done for the state of Iowa determined that growing 10 percent of the state's food elsewhere and transporting it back to market would burn four to seventeen times more fuel than growing food within Iowa itself. The same conventional system would generate five to seventeen times more climate-changing carbon dioxide than an Iowa-based system, while consuming 280 to 360 thousand gallons more fuel. Buying local eases our dependence on petroleum, helps clean up the air, and reduces the global warming that's associated with transportation.

Second, supporting nearby farmers strengthens the economy in your own backyard. Next time you make dinner, really take a look at your plate.If you're like most cooks, your meal will contain ingredients from five countries other than the United States. Those food purchases do not bolster the livelihoods of American farmers. Buying local does. A recent study by the Maine Organic Farms and Gardeners Association estimates that by encouraging Maine residents to spend just ten dollars a week on local food, $100 million would be invested back into farmers' pockets and the Maine economy each growing season. The same investment could be made in every state in the country if residents opted to buy local.

Third, because it is freshly picked and not overprocessed or packaged, locally grown food tastes better. You can also often find greater variety, including heirloom fruits and vegetables that chain stores never stock.

Fourth, locally grown food offers more quality control. In the wake of the lead paint scandal that forced the recall of millions of China-made toys, you might wonder whether food imported from abroad is any safer. Locally grown food, whether organic or conventional, provides reassurances that U.S. pesticide standards, which are usually higher than in Asia and Latin and Central America, are being met.

Finally, buying local helps save open space. More than one million acres of farmland are lost each year in the United States to residential and commercial development. Supporting local farmers helps them stay on their land and thrive economically while safeguarding beautiful landscapes.

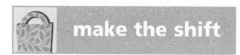

make the shift

big green purse

Want to Buy Local? Here's How

Shop at farmers' markets. You can buy fresh locally grown food at any one of the 3,100 farmers' markets in the United States. To find one in your state, start with the Department of Agriculture's list at www.ams.usda.gov/farmersmarkets/ map.htm.

Join a CSA. Community-supported agriculture (CSA) allows a group of "shareholders" to pledge in advance to cover the anticipated costs of the farm operation and the farmer's salary by paying a lump sum. In return, shareholders receive, usually on a weekly basis, a portion of the farm's bounty throughout the growing season. Growers earn better prices for their crops, gain some financial security, and are relieved of much of the burden of marketing. Consumers get a direct connection to the farm, very fresh food, and the satisfaction of helping promote sustainable agriculture. To find a CSA near you, go to http://newfarm.org/farmlocator/index.php ?type=cons&tab=consumer_seeking_farmer#consumer.

Ask your grocery store to carry more. Many grocery stores would carry more locally grown produce if they believed demand existed. Ask stock clerks and department managers to stock produce grown by neighborhood and regional farmers.

Pick your own. Check out your options at www.pickyourown.org.

Grow your own. If you don't have a backyard or a porch, take advantage of community gardens that provide a plot of land and a cohort of like-minded souls. Get started at www.communitygarden.org.

Find good food near you. Want fresh, locally grown food, but don't know where to find it? The Local Harvest community level map at www.foodroutes.org/local food/ makes it easy to locate sustainable farmers, farmers' markets, and Community-Supported Agriculture (CSA) projects in your area.

Organic versus Local

Ideally, you'll be able to find food that is both locally grown and organic. How do you choose when that's not possible?

Local growers strengthen your own economy, often use less energy transporting their produce from the farm gate to your kitchen plate, and probably apply fewer chemicals to preserve your food during transport. Organic produce may be available in the supermarket—but it might come from New Zealand, Latin America, or the other side of the country, racking up huge energy costs and losing a lot of flavor in the process.

Personally, I try to have it all.

- Whenever possible, I buy locally grown organic fruits and vegetables.
- If I shop seasonally, I'm more likely to meet my food-shopping goals.
- I buy fruits and vegetables that can't be cleaned adequately (like raspberries or cherries) organically, even if they come from afar.
- I do the best I can as often as I can, and try not to stress over it. Since it's impossible for me to meet all my food needs either buying local or organically, I buy as much as I can of both.

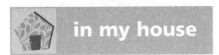

in my house

I have the good fortune of living three blocks from a farmers' market that's open year-round. The best time to shop there is midsummer to early fall, when the harvests start coming in and the food is so fresh it still shimmers with the morning dew. But regardless of the season, the stands overflow with delicious fruits and vegetables, freshly baked breads and pastries, homemade jams and cheeses, and organic eggs and pasta. If I can't get to the farmers' market, I make a point of asking for locally grown produce at my backups, the nearby supermarket and the neighborhood food co-op. Even though the supermarket is a big chain store, it's started carrying a lot more locally grown fruits and vegetables when they're in season. Besides, the supermarket is the only place I can get the exotic foods my kids love but that I can't buy locally: treats like kiwis, clementines, and chocolate, a rain forest goody that seems about as far away from my mid-Atlantic household as the moon. Is it inconvenient to have to shop at more than one place? Sometimes. But I usually have to get food more than once a week anyway. I make one trip to the farmers' market, one to the grocery store, and one to the food co-op. It evens out.

Buying local may require some getting used to, because it means that you're purchasing what's available on a seasonal basis. So no fresh tomatoes in January, at least not from the farmers' market. Try getting started in the summer, when there's a lot to choose from and delicious local produce is abundant and affordable.

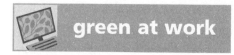
green at work

The Buy-Local Challenge

To encourage employees to eat locally, Vanguard Communications, a woman-owned company based in Washington, D.C. (which I cofounded years ago, by the way), challenges its employees, clients, friends, and acquaintances to buy food grown within a 250-mile radius of their current location. During the monthlong challenge, campaign participants can do as little as cook one meal using nothing but locally grown ingredients. Alternatively, they can commit to purchasing all their fruits, vegetables, dairy, and meat from local producers. The point is to learn about food and its role in the local economy. To ramp up the fun factor, the company sponsors cookoffs, posts recipes, maintains a blog, and buys snacks for the office from local food stocks. Get more details at www.vancomm.com.

BYOB

Sometimes, don't you feel like the biggest choice you make at the grocery store is when the cashier asks, Paper or plastic? And after all these years, you still don't know the answer. Frustrating, isn't it?

You know you're supposed to have your own reusable bag. But half the time, you're on your way home from work or from the kids' after-care; you simply don't have time to grab your own bags. The rest of the time, you're just happy you got out of the house with your grocery list. You don't even think about your own bags until you're parking the car and zooming toward the shopping cart in the hopes of whipping through the store as quickly as possible.

What can you do to avoid becoming a very stressed bag lady?

1. **Keep a couple of ChicoBags in your purse.** These small lightweight woven nylon bags (www.chicobag.com) fold up to the size of a small change purse; they unzip to a full-size shopping bag, with handles that fit over the plastic bag stands at the checkout counter. When you unpack your groceries at home, fold the bag up and pop it back in your purse.

2. **On your next few trips to the grocery store get one more durable bag;** they're usually sold right at the checkout counter. Depending on how much grocery

Slow Down!

Maybe we'd be more aware of the impact food was having on the environment and our lives if we spent a little more time cooking it. As inspired by the "Slow Food" movement, I'd like to suggest the following ways to slow down so we can savor the foods that make life's experiences worth living.

- Shop at farmers' markets, where you can browse the stalls, sample the goods, and talk to the people who grow, pick, and sell your food.
- Invite friends, neighbors, and family over for dinner; make it potluck so that everyone enjoys cooking together and sharing the essence of their kitchen.
- Cook with your kids at least once a week, taking the time to teach your child what you know and relearn how a child tastes what the earth grows.
- Chop it yourself; reacquaint yourself with the tools and techniques that turn your raw ingredients into a delicious meal.
- Start a kitchen garden, growing lettuces, herbs, tomatoes, and other vegetables you can easily toss in a salad, soup, or stew.
- Reestablish the dinner hour as a sacred time to reconnect with yourself and your family.

shopping you do, you'll ultimately need around six bags. When you get home and unpack your groceries, rather than put the bags back under the cupboard or in the pantry closet, walk right back out to the car and put the bags in your trunk (or pay one of the kids fifty cents to do it for you). If you live in an apartment and use a cart to transport your groceries, fold up the bags and slide them into the cart before you stow it until your next shopping trip.

3. **When you make your shopping list, write "Take bags" on the very top.** Make it a habit.

Back at the checkout counter, if you have to choose between plastic or paper, choose plastic—but make sure you recycle it.

Plastic Bags/Paper Bags

PLASTIC BAGS

Litter: In 2002 in Washington State alone, nearly 5,000 tons of plastic bags went to Seattle's landfills.

Wildlife impact: About one hundred thousand whales, seals, turtles, and other marine animals are killed by plastic bags each year worldwide, reports environmental watchdog Planet Ark.

Oil waste: It takes 430,000 gallons of oil to manufacture 100 million bags. Each year, Americans throw away some 100 billion polyethylene plastic bags. That's like throwing away almost 430 million gallons of oil every year.

Low recycling rates: only 1 percent of plastic bags are being recycled.

PAPER BAGS

Deforestation: Most paper comes from tree pulp, so the impact of paper bag production on forests is huge. In 1999, 14 million trees were cut to produce the ten billion paper bags used by Americans that year alone.

Global warming: Paper bag production delivers a global warming double whammy: when forests are cut down, we lose their ability to absorb carbon dioxide, plus making bags produces greenhouse gases.

Air and water pollution: Paper sacks generate 70 percent more air and fifty times more water pollutants than plastic bags.

Recycling rates: Twenty percent of paper bags are being recycled.

As you can see, neither option is an ecowinner, which is why several cities are considering banning plastic and paper bags. If you have to make a choice, plastic is slightly better than paper. Plastic bags require less energy to produce and generate less solid waste than paper bags. They also create less air and water pollution than paper sacks. And it takes 91 percent less energy to recycle a pound of plastic than it takes to recycle a pound of paper. According to research conducted in 2000, only 1 percent of plastic bags were recycled compared to 20 percent of paper bags, but

big green purse

most grocery stores now allow you to return plastic bags at convenient, in-store recycling bins.

Bottom line: Use your own reusable bag when you can, don't take a bag for single items, reuse bags as much as possible, and recycle when you're done.

And for bags at home? Try Bio-Bags (www.biogroupusa.com). They're 100 percent biodegradable, 100 percent compostable bags that fit into your kitchen or compost pail.

We Are What We Eat Wrap-up

- **Eat less meat.** Make one meat meal a week a vegetarian meal instead, or serve meat as a side dish instead of a main course.
- **Shift to sustainable seafood.** Select small fish like trout instead of big ones like tuna, shark, and Chilean sea bass. Choose safe-farmed tilapia and catfish over more problematic Atlantic salmon.
- **Buy organic.** To stretch your budget, purchase the foods where pesticides most likely persist: peaches, apples, sweet bell peppers, celery, necterines, cherries, berries, lettuce, domestic and imported grapes, pears, spinach, potatoes, carrots, green beans, hot peppers, cucumbers, plums, and oranges.
- **Create a line item in your food budget for organic cuisine.** Start with what you can afford, say, ten dollars a week of your total grocery purchases earmarked for organic foods. Or swap out a meal on a regular basis, for example, replacing your primary breakfast ingredients with organic alternatives.
- **Buy local.** Choose food grown within two hundred miles of where you live. Find it at farmers' markets or ask for it at restaurants, grocery stores, food co-ops, and online.
- **Bring your own bag.** When you forget, ask for the bag you can reuse and recycle the most.

And if you can do only one thing, eat less meat. You'll protect air and water, help reduce climate change, and contribute to a healthier, more humane world.

big green purse

7

CLEAN AND GREEN: CLEANSERS, SCRUBS, POLISHES, AND FRESHENERS

WHEN'S THE LAST TIME YOU READ A HEADLINE LIKE "HOUSEWIFE DROPS dead from dirty kitchen counters" or "Woman succumbs to fingerprints on wall"?

Probably never, right? Yet from all the marketing hype cleanser manufacturers throw at us you'd think that if we didn't keep our homes as spick-and-span as a hospital, we wouldn't live to tell the tale.

Ironically, the opposite is closer to the truth. It's the cleansers themselves that are harming us. The number of people becoming ill from lyes, soaps, detergents, solvents, polishes, scrubs, cleansers, and degreasers is on the rise. In 2005 (the most recent year for which statistics are available) the American Association of Poison Control Centers reported 218,000 calls involving cleaning products nationwide— a nearly 10 percent increase in just five years. Of those exposed, 121,498 were children under the age of six. Why are we cleaning up if it makes us sick?

Women and children are particularly at risk:

Women do most of the housework. Despite womens' advances in professions outside the home, on average we still do more than 70 percent of the housework. Stay-at-home moms may suffer even greater exposure to potentially hazardous cleaning chemicals, as they probably do more housecleaning and spend more time inside the home, where the chemicals persist and often contribute to high levels of indoor air pollution. In homes where aerosol sprays and air fresheners were used frequently, researchers at England's Bristol University found, mothers suffered from 25 percent more headaches and 19 percent more depression, while infants under six months of age experienced 30 percent more ear infections and a 22 percent higher incidence of diarrhea.

People who clean for a living are also at risk. The 3.4 million women and men who work in the cleaning industry need to be on the alert as well. Men make up nearly two-thirds of janitors and building cleaners, while women—often of color—comprise nearly 90 percent of maids and housekeepers. One San Francisco study found that 99 percent of hotel room cleaners were female. The "professional" cleaning products they tend to use can pack an even stronger punch than those used domestically. Occupational exposure to glycol ethers, common ingredients in chemical products, can reduce sperm counts in men. Pregnant women exposed to glycol ethers at work were significantly more likely to give birth to children with neural tube defects, cleft palates, and other disorders.

Children are disproportionately affected, not only in the womb and at home but at school, too. Because their internal organs and immune systems are not yet fully developed, kids are more vulnerable than grown-ups to cleansers, soaps, and other scrubs, most of which were developed with adult bodies in mind. Certain compounds may interfere with the development of young neurological, endocrine, and immune systems. At the same time, babies' and children's exposure to chemicals is more intense because they breathe more often and more deeply than adults and consume more food and water per pound of body weight. Toddlers crawl on the floor and frequently put their hands in their mouths, conveying chemicals from floor and carpet finishes, waxes, shampoos, and stain repellents directly into their bodies. Children are also at greater risk from accidental poisoning by cleaning products. Some kids might be confused by cleansers that smell like lemonade or resemble food.

Both children and adults face health hazards due to cleaning chemicals. As asthma rates increase for children and adults, household cleansers seem increasingly culpable. The EPA estimates that twenty million people in the United States, including 6.1 million children, suffer from this debilitating respiratory ailment, requiring more than fourteen million outpatient clinic visits and nearly two million emergency room visits each year. The National Center for Health Statistics reported that the incidence of asthma among preschool-aged children rose by 160 percent between 1980 and 1994, accounting for fourteen million missed school days each year and $3.2 million in treatment expenses. The most common serious chronic childhood disease, asthma is the third-ranking cause of hospitalization for children under age fifteen. In a groundbreaking report on the impact of cleaning products on women and children, the nonprofit research organization Women's Voices for the Earth identified several chemicals present in some household and industrial cleaning products that trigger asthma or aggravate existing respiratory ailments, including monoethanolamine, ammonium quaternary compounds, tall oil rosin, and chlorhexidine.

Cleaning products also degrade the environment. Detergents don't just disappear down the drain; soaps don't simply swirl down the sink. Though they're treated with other wastewater at municipal treatment plants, they're still discharged into lakes, rivers, and streams. Most of their ingredients break down into harmless substances at the treatment plant or soon thereafter, but others persist, threatening water quality, fish, and other wildlife. In 2000, the EPA found high levels of the carcinogen dioxin, a chlorine by-product, in San Francisco Bay. The source? Municipal gray water that had not been purged of chemical residue from laundry bleach. A May 2002 study by the U.S. Geological Survey (USGS) found detergent residue in 69 percent of the streams it tested. The residue included chemicals that have been shown to mimic the hormone estrogen. Scientists worry these estrogenic chemicals may be harming the reproduction and survival of salmon, trout, frogs, and other aquatic wildlife.

Industry's drive to create new (unnecessary?) product lines has seen the introduction of cleaning products infused with fragrances and antibacterial agents, even though the risks outweigh the benefits in both cases. Fragrances usually consist of phthalates, chemicals known to exacerbate asthma, trigger other respiratory ailments, cause headaches and general anxiety, and upset the ecological balance when they pass from our drains to our waterways. And the overuse of antibacterial agents, doctors fear, is breeding populations of "supergerms" against which we will have less and less immunity the more we use the very products intended to combat them.

Another irony: Cleaning products leave behind a mess that needs cleaning up. Think of the mounds of empty or semiempty cleaning bottles, cans, boxes, and bags you throw away every month just to keep your home spick-and-span. If a product is bottled in high-density polyethylene (HDPE, #2) or polyethylene terephthalate (PET, #1), the container may be accepted at a community recycling center. However, products bottled in polyvinyl chloride (PVC, #3) aren't so desirable. Made from cancer-causing chemicals like vinyl chloride, PVC devolves into the by-product dioxin when it is manufactured and incinerated. Most sanitation departments do not accept PVC for recycling; less than 1 percent of all PVC is recycled each year, not even denting the seven billion pounds from all sources (toys, household goods, and vinyl products, as well as cleaning products) that are discarded annually.

Finally, even if most cleansers were safe to use, you could question their source. Many laundry detergents, fabric softeners, and stain removers are petroleum-based. Thus, they contribute to the depletion of a nonrenewable resource and increase U.S. dependence on foreign oil.

The Good News

Now, I'm not advocating we stop cleaning our houses. No one wants to be able to write her name in an inch-thick coating of dust on the coffee table, or trip over Fido's accumulated furballs as they bounce across the floor. We want to prepare food in a clean kitchen, take baths in a ring-free tub, and enjoy a good night's sleep on freshly laundered sheets. We all have to wash our clothes. And if we didn't do the dishes, we probably would get sick.

What I am suggesting is that we need to live in our homes, not sterilize them. Just as important, we shouldn't upset nature's sink in order to clean our own.

Fortunately, we can exchange almost every cleaning product in our cupboards for a few earth-friendly items and a handful of ingredients that will go easier on our homes, our bodies, the environment, and our pocketbooks. This chapter shows you where to start.

You'll find suggestions for cutting back on the products you already use and tips for choosing the safest conventional options among the cleansers you still need to buy. The chapter's label-reading insights will help you shift your spending to the greenest cleaners available; there are dozens of new ecologically friendly scrubs, soaps, detergents, and polishes in stores and online, any of them worth putting to the test in your living room, kitchen, or bath. I've also included recipes for several cleansers you can easily mix yourself from simple ingredients you may already have at hand. The "In My House" sections share some of the challenges I've faced in greening the cleaning in my own home, as well as a few solutions that might work for you, too.

Everyone talks these days about simplifying—there's even a magazine devoted to the concept. But simplifying is not always so easy. Cleaning products offer one area where it is.

How Much Do You Use?

Whether your home is a palace or a studio apartment, you've probably been convinced you need a different cleaning product for every surface that's in it. Take a look at the list below. How many of these cleansers are taking up space in your bathroom or kitchen cupboard?

___ After-shower scum spray
___ Air freshener
___ Bleach
___ Brass, copper polish
___ Carpet shampoo
___ Clothes washing detergent
___ Counter and cupboard cleaner
___ Dishwasher detergent

___ Dishwashing liquid
___ Drain cleaner
___ Fabric softener
___ Floor cleaner
___ Furniture polish
___ Furniture shampoo
___ Jewelry polish
___ Mildew cleaner
___ Mothballs
___ Oven cleaner
___ Shoe polish

___ Silverware polish
___ Spot remover
___ Stain repellent
___ Swimming pool chemicals
___ Tub and tile cleaner
___ Wall cleaner
___ Window/glass cleaner
___ Wood cleaner

Your cleaning problems are limited in variety—dirt, grease, baked-on dirt and grease, mold and limescale in the bathroom, perhaps some tarnish or rust, and the occasional stain—yet companies use an almost unlimited number of questionable combinations to sell you more products than you need. Not only does this cost you more money, but also the more products you bring into your home, the more you expose yourself and the environment to unnecessary and undesirable chemicals.

Use Your Big Green Purse

If you decide to switch to greener cleaning products, you'll find plenty to choose from. The U.S. market for natural household cleansers has grown to $100 million

Common Ingredients in Conventional Household Cleaning Products

CHEMICAL	EFFECT
Ammonia	Fatal when swallowed; respiratory irritant
Ammonium hydroxide	Corrosive, irritant
Bleach	Potentially fatal if ingested; highly caustic
Chlorine	Respiratory and skin irritant
Ethyl glycol	Damages nerves
Formaldehyde	Highly toxic; known carcinogen
Hydrochloric acid	Corrosive; eye and skin irritant
Hydrochloric bleach	Eye, skin, and respiratory tract irritant
Lye	Severe damage to stomach and esophagus if swallowed
Naphtha	Suspected carcinogen and reproductive toxin
Nitrobenzene	Poisonous; carcinogenic
Perchloroethylene	Eyes, nose, throat, and skin irritant; possible carcinogen
Petroleum distillates	Highly flammable; suspected carcinogen
Phenol	Extremely dangerous; suspected carcinogen; fatal if swallowed
Propylene glycol	Immunogen; main ingredient in antifreeze
Sodium hypochlorite	Potentially fatal; highly caustic

CHEMICAL	EFFECT
Sodium lauryl sulfate	Carcinogen, toxin, skin irritant
Sodium tripolyphosphate	Irritant
Trichloroethane	Damages liver and kidneys

annually according to natural goods retailer Seventh Generation, and new options seem to pop up online or on the shelf with every trip to the market. But shifting your spending to greener cleaners will make a difference beyond your healthier household. Even though these options have been increasing by 18 to 25 percent a year for the last five years, ecocleaners still represent just 1 percent of the total household cleansers market. When you switch to greener products, you'll help pull the entire industry in a healthier, safer direction.

You'll also be doing in the marketplace what government has failed to do in the regulatory arena. Federal regulation of cleaning products is woefully inadequate. The U.S. Environmental Protection Agency is supposed to regulate chemicals that pose an "unreasonable" risk to human health and/or the environment. However, a report by the Government Accountability Office found that neither existing chemicals nor new ones are adequately assessed for any threat they pose. The U.S. Consumer Product Safety Commission is responsible for overseeing the safety of household cleaning products. But given how many products there are and how understaffed the CPSC is, the agency gets involved primarily in recalling merchandise once a problem surfaces. The CPSC does not require that individual chemicals be tested for safety.

While chemical companies must list storage instructions, first-aid information, and precautionary advice on their products' labels, they are not required to reveal individual ingredients. Thus it is impossible to know exactly what you are buying.

You can, however, get some of this information at the National Library of Medicine Household Products Database (http://householdproducts.nlm.nih.gov). This online directory lists possible health effects of more than 2,000 ingredients found in 6,000 common household products. It also includes Hazardous Materials

Identification System (HMIS) ratings and brand-specific safety information provided by manufacturers. Although the hazard ratings are specific to workplace exposures, they also pertain to the ways consumers use these products at home.

For even more details, check with the U.S. Centers for Disease Control and Prevention (CDC), which assesses human exposure to environmental chemicals, including those found in household cleaning products. You can find the CDC's analysis in its National Report on Human Exposure to Environmental Chemicals (www.cdc.gov/exposurereport).

Armed with all this knowledge, what can you do to make cleaning your home as earth-friendly as possible?

- Simplify your shopping list
- Avoid antibacterials
- Minimize packaging and trash
- Shift your spending to safer products
- Make your own

Simplify Your Shopping List

You may be using a dozen or more different cleaning products, when one general-purpose cleaner will do for almost all jobs.

- **Use the products you already have;** then, rather than automatically replacing them, determine whether one all-around cleanser can replace several you used to buy.
- **Share products with neighbors.** Avoid having to stockpile lyes, solvents, petroleum distillates, and other toxic chemicals. Borrow what you need before buying it, and lend what you have to use up what you're storing.
- **Check labels for "signal words."** Manufacturers of cleaning products don't have to list the ingredients they put into their products. However, they must alert consumers to threats their products pose. Choose alternatives whenever you spot any of the following four signal words on a label: DANGER or POISON, which indicates that the product is highly toxic, corrosive, extremely flammable, or fatal; WARNING, which means a product is moderately toxic or harmful; and CAUTION, which shows that the product still should be avoided if a safer alternative is available.

- **Avoid aerosol products.** They disperse sprays so fine that their chemicals can be easily inhaled and absorbed into the bloodstream. Aerosols also ignite easily, and the cans may explode when subjected to high temperature or pressure.
- **Skip the smells.** Fragrances consist of phthalates that pollute air and water and often cause headaches, respiratory problems, and even anxiety. Buy "no fragrance added" or "fragrance free."
- **Make it childproof.** If you must buy hazardous products, choose childproof packaging. Make sure you have safety equipment and a first-aid kit on hand.

 thumbs down

Just Say No

- **"Corrosive" scrubs:** Corrosives can severely burn skin or eyes; if accidentally swallowed, they can scorch internal organs. Corrosive products can also react violently if they come in contact with other chemicals. Many corrosive products, like drain cleaners, oven cleaners, and some toilet bowl cleaners, are often marked DANGER.
- **Chlorine bleach:** Chlorine bleach may be found in laundry products, automatic dishwasher detergents, mildew stain removers, bath and toilet cleaners, and clothing stain removers. Its strong smell can irritate the lungs. People with asthma or chronic heart and lung problems should avoid it.
- **Ammonia:** Ammonia may be found in metal cleaners, glass cleaners, dishwashing liquids, and other products. Like chlorine bleach, it irritates the lungs and is better left alone by asthmatics or people suffering from respiratory or cardiac disease.
- **Phosphates:** Phosphates were once widely used in laundry detergents. They've been phased out in many states due to their ability to degrade water quality. The federal government's limit on the phosphorus content of laundry detergents is 5 percent by weight. However, there is no regulation on phosphates in dishwashing detergents, which may contain as much as 40 percent phosphorus. Phosphates also lurk in some toothpastes and other random cleaning products that whiten and brighten.
- **Fragrances:** Fragrances can be found in detergents, fabric softeners, dryer sheets, liquid soaps, and bleaches. The label may say "fragrance," or it may use words like "fresh mountain scent," "morning breeze," "ocean air," or some other lilting descriptor. Fragrances usually consist of phthalates, chemicals that cause ir-

ritation, allergic reactions, headaches, and even asthma, and can disrupt the reproductive systems of fish and frogs if they get loose in rivers and streams.

- **APEs/NPEs:** Alkylphenol ethoxylates (APEs) and nonylphenol ethoxylates (NPEs)
are surfactants, chemicals that make it easier for water to wash away dirt. APEs
and NPEs are frequently added to laundry detergents, stain removers, and other
cleaning products to increase their effectiveness. They're very good at evading
wastewater treatment, too, frequently ending up in streams and rivers, where
their hormone-disrupting traits are suspected of causing mutations among fish,
frogs, and turtles.

go green

Simple Green Cleaning Tips

- Avoid the need for dangerous cleansers by cleaning up a mess promptly.
- Remove shoes when you enter your house to reduce need for carpet cleaners.
- If you have it, use the self-cleaning feature of an oven—which relies on heat—
rather than oven cleaner.
- Don't mix cleaning products, especially chlorine bleach and ammonia, which can
form chloramine gas and cause coughing and choking. Chlorine bleach mixed with
an acid product like toilet bowl cleaner or rust remover could also form lethal gas.
- Use a microfiber cloth or mop to pick up dust, rather than a spray-on/wipe-off
furniture or floor cleaner that will pollute indoor air and leave a residue on
the furniture.
- Replace at least three commercial cleaning products with one general-purpose
cleanser or a make-at-home recipe (see pages 207–211).

thumbs down

Avoid Antibacterials

From glass cleaner and dust cloths to counter scrubs and soaps, germ-killing agents
are being added to cleansers at record speed. This, despite the fact that in 2005 a U.S.
Food and Drug Administration (FDA) panel concluded that there is no added bene-

Give Your House a Break: Cut Back on These Products First

PRODUCT	ACTION
Any cleaning product that adds fragrance or scent to its ingredients; usually laundry detergent, fabric softener, dish soap, furniture polish, air freshener, and dryer sheets	Choose "no fragrance added" alternative.
Any cleaning product that contains antibacterial agents; usually countertop cleaners, bathroom and kitchen cleaners, window cleaners, cleaning wipes, and throwaway cloths	Choose standard alternative.
Air fresheners and sprays	Open windows; use fresh flowers; eliminate source of foul odors; use potpourri.
Drain cleaners, oven cleaners, acid-based toilet cleaners	Clean regularly to avoid need for corrosive chemicals; flush drains with boiling water, clear with plunger, clean with baking soda and vinegar.
Throwaway dust cloths, treated throwaway towels, or cleaning cloths you use once and throw away	Use towels, rags, other cloths you can launder and reuse.

fit from using antimicrobial products over plain soap and water. In June 2007, *Scientific American* reported on the problems associated with antibacterial chemicals like triclosan and triclocarban and the increasing immunity people are developing to antibiotics. As we saw in Chapters 3 and 7, these synthetic chemicals are being added to cosmetics, personal-care products, and household cleansers primarily to give marketers another way to sell each product. They're not just building antibiotic resistance in humans, either. Because they are getting loose in the environment through wastewater, 60 percent of U.S. streams appear to be contaminated with antibiotics of some sort.

Consider the alternatives:

- Don't worry so much about germs. It's better to build up a tolerance for bacteria than to try to kill them all (something you'll never succeed in doing, by the way).
- Clean up using hot, soapy water rather than an antibacterial.
- When you shop, choose the standard version of a soap or detergent rather than the antibacterial option.
- Restrict use of antibacterial products to those recommended by a physician or health-care professional.

Minimize Packaging and Trash

Cleaning up the house can sure make a mess, depending on how you do the job. Bottles of soap, canisters of cleanser, packages of disinfecting wipes, and gobs of paper towels can add up to a bagful of trash unless we rethink not just the cleansers we buy but how we go about housecleaning itself.

Overall, packaging waste is increasing, much of it unnecessarily. According to Green Seal, an independent certification agency, up to 90 percent of most general-purpose cleansers is water. Packaging and shipping this excess water plus the cleaning chemicals it contains wastes energy and contributes unnecessary solid waste to our landfills. A better option is to buy a concentrated product that contains less than 20 percent water by weight. (The optimum dilution to look for when reconstituting concentrate is one ounce of the product to one gallon of water.)

Another new craze to hit the cleaning industry revolves around the world of wipes, disposable cloths, and paper towels. "Wipes" were first used to help mothers on the run clean their babies' bottoms. Now the same technology is being marketed for disposable cloth treated with glass cleaner, floor shine (like Swiffer), furniture polish, and "all purpose" wipe-ups. Extra-heavy paper towels are available for "clean and toss" duty.

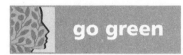

Don't Trash Your House When You Clean It

- **Buy laundry detergents and fabric softeners in concentrated packaging.** Brands to look for include: All Small & Mighty laundry detergent; Tide, Gain, Cheer, Era, and Dreft detergents, which are doubling their concentration under a "2X" line; and the less chemical intensive Method (available at Target) and Shaklee (available at www.shaklee.com).
- **Given the choice, buy products packaged in #1 or #2 plastics, the plastics most commonly accepted by community recycling programs.** Avoid PVC plastic (#3) whenever possible.
- **Choose boxes made from paper or cardboard that can be recycled.**
- **Recycle as much packaging as you can.**
- **Use washable, reusable towels, rags, and cloths rather than throwaway paper towels and chemical-laden wipes.** Even "green" wipes and paper towels get thrown away. Skip them in favor of reusables.
- **Buy bulk sizes** to reduce the number of packages you need to buy overall.

Shift Your Spending to Safer Products

Dozens of effective new cleansers, detergents, soaps, fabric softeners, and glass cleaners can help you green your cleaning. Most of these options will contain some combination of citrus, pine, natural oils, unadulterated minerals, water, and salts. To learn more about specific chemicals found in any one cleaner, read the excellent report "Household Chemicals," by Women's Voices for the Earth (www.womenandenvironment.org), or *Green Clean: The Environmentally Sound Guide to Cleaning Your Home,* by Linda Mason Hunter and Mikki Halpin.

Environmental Brand Stand

If you want to develop brand loyalties for ecologically sound cleaning products, get acquainted with the following companies. Most of their products are now available stream markets and at grocers like Whole Foods, at food co-ops, online, and ͏ngly, in big box stores like Wal-Mart and Target.

Ami (www.bonami.com). For more than 120 years, Bon Ami has manufac-͏ inexpensive, nontoxic cleanser free of chlorine, dyes, and perfumes. Made ͏lcite and feldspar minerals, Bon Ami's mildly abrasive properties allow it to ͏any surfaces without scratching, including tubs, tiles, and toilets; kitchen ͏and bath countertops; flatware and dishes; walls, floors, and furniture; pots and pans; and a variety of appliances and tools. It is readily available in most grocery stores, small markets, hardware stores, and online.

Seventh Generation (www.seventhgeneration.com; 60 Lake Street, Burlington, VT 05401-5218; 800-456-1191). This long-standing company's fragrance-free laundry and dish detergents and glass and all-purpose cleaning products helped set the standards other green cleaning companies have tried to emulate. Their vegetable-based laundry detergents are biodegradable and contain no chlorine, phosphates, artificial fragrances, or dyes. Household cleaners include degreasers; bathroom, shower, and toilet bowl cleaners; and carpet cleaner.

Bi-O-Kleen (www.bi-o-kleen.com/products.htm; P.O. Box 820689, Vancouver, WA 98682; 360-576-0064 or 800-477-0188). The company's all-purpose, kitchen, carpet, and dishwashing products are chlorine free, extremely concentrated to reduce packaging, contain no artificial colors or fragrances, and are based on no animal testing.

Shaklee (http://shop.shaklee.com/product/homecare1). These products, available strictly online, are free of many common cleaning chemicals, like chlorine, nitrates, and ammonia; their "starter kit" claims to eliminate 108 pounds of packaging waste from landfills and eliminate 248 pounds of greenhouse gas, the equivalent of planting ten trees. Shaklee's unusual cleaning products include recyclable vegetable-based dryer sheets that split in two in the dryer to "distribute softness throughout the load." Most products, like laundry and dishwasher detergents, laundry booster, and stain remover, can be bought in concentrated form to reduce packaging.

Ecover (www.ecover.com/us/en; to find a store in your area that carries Ecover, call 800-449-4925, Monday through Friday, 7:30 a.m. to 4:00 p.m. PST). These plant-based, biodegradable ingredients have been certified by an independent third party. Bottles and labels are made of recyclable plastic. Products include dishwashing liquid and powder, laundry powder, stain remover, nonchlorine bleach, toilet bowl cleaner, surface and glass cleaner, cream scrub and floor soap, and heavy-duty hand cleaner to remove paint, oil, and other difficult stains or substances from your skin.

Earth Friendly (www.ecos.com; 44 Green Bay Road, Winnetka, IL 60093; 800-335-ECOS (3267); fax: 847-446-4437).Sold also under the Ecos label, these plant-based products are free of petrochemicals and formaldehyde. Items include dishwasher liquids and powders; laundry detergents; carpet cleaners; spray starch, nonchlorine bleach; and several "Natural Spa" personal-care products, like hand soap and linen water that contain no parabens, dyes, or synthetics.

Citra-Solv (www.citra-solv.com; P.O. Box 2597; Danbury, CT 06813-2597; 203-778-0881; fax: 203-778-0911). Citrus oils, coconut, and vegetable-based cleansers plus nonchlorine bleach give Citra-Solv products their oomph. Look for dishwashing liquid and powders, window and glass cleaners, wood and furniture polish, spot removers, drain and pipe clearers, and nonaerosol air fresheners.

Method (www.methodhome.com; 637 Commercial Street, San Francisco, CA 94111; 415-931-3947 or 866-963-8463; e-mail:info@methodhome.com). Available at Target, Whole Foods, and an increasing number of grocery stores, Method's ingredients include biodegradable materials like soy, coconut, and palm oils. But what really sells Method are its stylish containers and bottles made from recyclable materials. Is it a cleaning product or a piece of sculpture? You decide, while you're appreciating the fact that none of the ingredients are tested on animals. Products include all-purpose cleaners, dish soap, liquid hand soaps and sanitizers, concentrated laundry detergents, baby detergents, dryer cloths, and a microfiber mop system that doesn't rely on chemicals to help pick up dust from under the couch.

Earth Choice/OdoBan (www.odoban.com/MenuEarthChoice.html). Available at Sam's Club, Earth Choice is specifically designed to help office managers implement environmentally preferable purchasing for their office cleaning supplies. Products include degreasers, carpet cleaners, bathroom cleansers, and stain removers.

You can also search out these specific scrubs and polishes:

All-purpose Cleaner

For countertops, tile or linoleum floors, walls, stove-top spills, microwave oven, stainless steel appliances, and plumbing fixtures:

AFM SafeChoice Super Clean
Begley's Best (www.begleysbest.com)
BioShield Vinegar Cleaner
Bon Ami Cleaning Powder

Bon Ami is probably the most affordable of these products, and you can buy it in almost every grocery store and in many hardware stores.

Remember to rinse with water after using any cleaning product.

Tough Cleaning Jobs: Graffiti, Adhesives, Grease, Ink

SoyClean (www.soyclean.biz) contains no hazardous ingredients as defined under the U.S. OSHA Hazard Communications Standard (29 CFR 1910.1200) or the Canadian Hazardous Products Act S.C. 1987, C30 (Part 1).

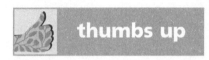

thumbs up

Restore Cleaning Products

The Restore company (www.restoreproducts.com) gets extra points for two reasons: its bottles can be refilled, and its website tells you exactly what's in its products. The company sells all-purpose cleaner, laundry detergent, kitchen and bathroom scrubs, degreaser, lime and scale remover, and EnzAway spot remover for pet stains. Restore offers shoppers a unique in-store system that allows you to refill your bottles and receive a one-dollar coupon to use on the purchase of the refilled product at the cash register. Refill stations are set up in Whole Foods, King Soopers, and various stores in Chicago and other retailers in Illinois, as well as outlets in Minnesota, Colorado, North Dakota, New York, Iowa, Wisconsin, Ohio, Indiana, and Nebraska. As for its full-disclosure policy, Restore tells shoppers what's in its products: "renewable, plant-based ingredients like soy, orange, coconut, and corn, and abundant minerals. We use no petroleum based ingredients . . . [and] Our renewable ingredients are gray water, septic and sewer safe. The ingredients are readily biodegradable and do not create toxic by-products. . . . Restore products contain no hazardous ingredients as defined by OSHA and contain no known or suspected carcinogens . . . [plus] Restore products are designed to be safer to use, and made within an acceptable pH range, so as not to burn your hands or poison your child." Procter & Gamble, are you paying attention?

big green purse

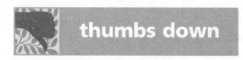

thumbs down

Dryer Balls and Sheets

Plastic dryer balls claim to be earth-friendly because they soften fabric "without chemicals." But they're made of polyvinyl chloride (PVC), among the least recyclable of plastics, and phthalates, two compounds that create undesirable environmental impacts. Because the dryer balls resemble toys, kids might be tempted to play with them or put them in their mouths. A better alternative is to use fabric softeners made by Seventh Generation or Ecover, or simply add 1/4 cup of baking soda to your wash cycle.

To avoid static cling, dry cotton clothes and synthetic clothes separately. Or, add 1/4 cup of vinegar to wash cycle to both soften fabrics and eliminate static.

Disinfectant

The only foolproof way to kill foodborne pathogens, such as salmonella or *E. coli*, is to wash all cutting boards, dishes, knives, and surfaces that have touched raw meat or eggs in hot, soapy water. If you're worried about germs spreading during flu season, focus your sanitation efforts on trouble spots like doorknobs, refrigerator handles, and telephone mouthpieces, and don't forget to wash your own hands frequently, also in hot, soapy water. Otherwise, during regular cleaning, focus on dirt, not disinfecting.

Drain and Toilet Bowl Cleaners

For clogged or sluggish drains, always use a plunger, a plumbing snake, or even a straightened wire hanger to bring up as much of the clog as possible. If that doesn't resolve the problem, Earth Friendly and Naturally Yours drain cleaners use enzymes, rather than caustic chemicals, to dissolve soap, grease, and grime. Install an inexpensive metal or plastic drain screen to prevent future obstructions, and flush regularly with a kettle full of boiling water.

Ovens

To save time and make cleaning easier, line oven bottom with aluminum foil; wipe oven walls and ceiling clean after each spill. Use the self-cleaning oven feature if available. For routine cleaning, try:

EnviroSafety Multi-Purpose Cleaner
Bon Ami (make a paste; leave it on; scrub off)

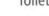

Toilets

If you clean once a week, you won't need harsh chemicals to remove toilet bowl rings and stains. Nonchlorine scouring cleansers include:

Bon Ami (www.bonami.com)
Ecover Toilet Cleaner (www.ecover.com/us.en)
Seventh Generation (www.seventhgeneration.com)

The following detergents are phosphate-free and contain no APEs or NPEs.

Automatic Dishwasher Detergent

BioShield Dishwasher Concentrate (www.eco-buildingproducts.com)
Ecover (rated highest of the most eco-friendly dishwasher detergents by *Consumer Reports*) (www.ecover.com/us.en)
Mrs. Meyer's Clean Day (www.mrsmeyers.com)
Seventh Generation Automatic Dish Powder Free & Clear (www.seventhgeneration.com)
Trader Joe's (available in their stores)

Note: If your glasses or dishes develop a foggy film, soak them in a mixture of two parts water and one part vinegar, or put vinegar in the rinse dispenser of your dishwasher.

Dishwashing Liquid

Earth Friendly Dishmate Hand Dishwashing Liquid (rated highest in a survey of *Green Guide* readers) (www.grassrootsstore.com)
Ecover Natural Dishwashing Liquid (www.ecover.com/us.en)
Method (www.methodhome.com)
Seventh Generation Dish Liquid (www.seventhgeneration.com)

Laundry Detergents—High-efficiency (HE) Machines

Bi-O-Kleen Laundry Powder (www.biokleenhome.com/products/household/laundry)
Ecos Liquid (www.ecos.com/pages/ecosliquid.html)
Ecover Biological Washing Powder (www.ecover.com/us.en)
Ecover Laundry Liquid (www.ecover.com/us.en)

Method Fresh Air 3x Concentrate HE (www.methodhome.com)
Seventh Generation Laundry Liquid Free & Clear (www.seventhgeneration.com)

If clothes seem stiff, add 1/4 cup of baking soda to the wash cycle. Dry clothes on medium-high, rather than the highest temperature setting.

Laundry Detergents—Standard Machines

The products below are all made with renewable, vegetable-based ingredients (corn, palm kernel, or coconut oil) and are either fragrance-free or scented with essential oils.

Bi-O-Kleen All-Temperature Laundry Liquid and Laundry Powder (www.bio kleen.com)
Cal Ben Seafoam Laundry Cleaner (www.calbenpuresoap.com)
Dr. Bronner's Liquid castile soaps (www.drbronner.com)
Dri-Pak Pure soap flakes (www.msodistributing.com/soapflakes.html)
ECOS Liquid Laundry Detergents and Delicate Wash (www.ecos.com)
Ecover Natural Laundry Powder and Natural Laundry Wash (www.ecover.com)
Mountain Green Skin Sensitive (www.mtngreen.com)
Our House Concentrated Laundry Care (www.ourhouseworks.com)
Seventh Generation Laundry powders and liquids (www.seventhgeneration.com)
Trader Joe's Next To Godliness (www.traderjoes.com)
Vermont Soap Aloe Castile Liquid Soaps in unscented and essential oil–scented varieties (www.vermontsoap.com)

Fabric Softeners

Ecover Natural Fabric Softener (www.ecover.com)
Seventh Generation Natural Lavender Scent Fabric Softener (www.seventh generation.com)

Bleaches and Stain Removers

Bi-O-Kleen Bac-Out Stain & Odor Eliminator and Spray & Wipe Cleaner (www.biokleen.com)
Bi-O-Kleen Oxygen Bleach Plus (www.biokleen.com)
Bio Pac Nonchlorine Bleach Powder (www.bio-pac.com)

Ecover Laundry Bleach and Natural Nonchlorine Bleach (www.ecover.com)
Naturally Yours All-Purpose Spotter (www.naturalyours.com)
Naturally Yours Natural Bleach and Softener (www.naturalyours.com)
Seventh Generation Nonchlorine Bleach (www.seventhgeneration.com)

Metal Polishes

Ecover Cream Scrub (www.ecover.com/us). It cleans chrome and stainless steel as well as kitchen and bath counters, floor tiles, walls, cupboards, and doorknobs.

Homewood Metal Polish (www.greenfeet.com). Lemon oil and minerals help scrub away tarnish on brass, copper, stainless steel, bronze, pewter, chrome, silver, and aluminum.

Howard Naturals Stainless Steel Cleaner & Polish (www.howardnaturals.com). This "smudge busting" pump spray demolishes food grime, fingerprints, and kitchen grease, in three scents: grapefruit-ginger, lemongrass-lime, and sage-citrus.

OurHouse Minerals & Metals Cleaner (www.ourhouseworks.com). Organic acid salts knock out mineral deposits on your brass, chrome, marble, copper, and stainless steel.

Twinkle Silver Polish Kit (www.drugstore.com). The kit contains no phosphorus, and the carton is 100 percent recycled cardboard.

thumbs down

Greenwashing Your Laundry

Laundry product manufacturers lure people in with unsubstantiated claims like "nontoxic," "hypoallergenic," and "natural." When these virtues aren't verified by third parties or extensive explanations on the company website, they're usually little more than marketing hype. The term "organic" on a cleaning product's label or in its title isn't meaningful, either, as there are no defined organic standards for cleaning products.

In another green scam, many spray fabric stain removers and spray starches come in aerosol spray cans labeled "no CFCs" (or chlorofluorocarbons, which deplete the ozone layer). That's true, but it misleads consumers into believing they are buying a more eco-friendly product when they may not be, as CFCs have been banned from all aerosols since 1978.

Choosing products in "recyclable" packaging is not the same as buying those in the preferable "post-consumer recycled" (PCR) bottles or boxes. Purchasing PCR supports companies that are providing a vital end-market for recycled paper and plastic and also completing the loop on using and reusing the products we buy.

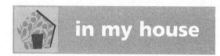

in my house

Common household cleaners can create chemical sensitivities when none existed before. I say this from experience. A few years ago, I was using a rented carpet shampooing machine and the standard shampoo that came with it to clean my living room wall-to-wall rug. It hadn't occurred to me to open the windows in the room or wear a protective mask. After all, I was just cleaning my carpet. After about half an hour of using the machine, I began feeling light-headed and nauseated. That feeling of discomfort intensified for the remaining sixty minutes it took me to complete the job. A few hours later, I felt like I'd come down with the flu: I ached from head to toe, my eyes were runny, and I was miserable. The symptoms lasted a couple of days. I did not develop a fever, which is how I knew I hadn't been hit by a virus. I did develop permanent sensitivity to chemicals. I'm now allergic to most fragrances. I can't wash my clothes or bed linens in detergent or fabric softener that contains fragrances, and all soaps I use must be fragrance-free. That's a big price to pay for a clean carpet.

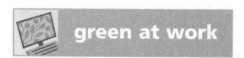

green at work

On the job, use the same products that you use at home.

- In your washroom, install pump dispensers of liquid soap that is fragrance-free and nonantibacterial.
- Have your workplace cleaned with earth-friendly products rather than those containing harsh chemicals.

Cleaning Up After Your Cleanser

The more toxic a product is, the more important it is for you to dispose of it carefully.

- Check labels for special disposal instructions.
- Find out which items your town or city accepts on hazardous-waste collection days and follow those guidelines. More specific advice on disposing of various hazardous materials can be found on the EPA's Household Hazardous Waste website or the Earth 911 website.
- **Whenever possible, recycle.** Unless you're dealing with hazardous chemicals, the empty plastic containers of cleaning products can often be recycled. Check to see that the number inside the arrows on the bottom of the container is accepted for recycling in your community.
- **Take hazardous leftovers to the local hazardous-waste facility or store them safely until your community arranges for a hazardous-waste pickup.** Do not dump toxic cleaning products (solvents, paint thinners, drain cleaners, lye, rust cleaner, etc.) down the drain, flush them down the toilet, or pour them down a sewer.

- Use nonantibacterial dishwashing liquid, phosphate-free dishwasher detergent, and a green all-purpose cleaner in the kitchen.
- Replace chemical air fresheners with cut flowers, potpourri, and fresh air.

 in my house

We clean almost everything using baking soda, vinegar, and water. We just keep a big box of baking soda and a gallon bottle of distilled vinegar in the upstairs bathroom cupboard as well as under the kitchen sink so they're always handy. For an occasional tougher stain on a countertop or wall, and for the toilets, I've taken a lesson from my mother. She's always used Bon Ami cleanser, a fragrance-free, ammonia- and chlorine-free, nonantibacterial scrub, and now, so do I. As a work-at-home mom, I cook three meals a day, so I wash a lot of pots and pans. I stick to nonantibacterial dishwashing liquid and a phosphate-free dishwashing detergent—though I always have to read the labels, since undesirable contents are sneaking in more and more as "standard ingredients" in my old standby products. We use a fragrance-free "high-e" detergent in our energy-saving washing machine. I'm not loyal to a particular brand right now; with so many new green innovations coming into the marketplace, I like to keep trying something new. We have given up fabric softeners and dryer sheets. The downside? Our towels are harder and scratchier. The upside? They're more absorbent. In the bathroom, the most frustrating problem is mold. It's so easy to squirt a chemical on this nasty black crud and zap it; it's a lot more work to scrub it. We try to squeegee the shower after every use, which helps. When mold does build up, Bon Ami is pretty effective, as is straight baking soda and a scrub bush.

Make Your Own

It's easy, cheap, and fast to make your own cleaning products with ingredients that are readily available and earth-friendly. You'll save time and money and be healthier, too.

BASIC INGREDIENTS

| Water | Lemon juice | Distilled vinegar |
| Baking soda | | |

BASIC TOOLS

Squeegee	Mop	Scrub brush
Cloth towels, rags	Broom	Scouring pad
Sponges	Bucket	Spray bottle

All-purpose Cleaner

- **Baking soda.** Dissolve 4 tablespoons of baking soda in 1 quart of warm water for a cleaning solution, or use baking soda sprinkled on a damp sponge. Baking soda will clean all kitchen and bathroom surfaces.

Drain Cleaner

- **Prevention.** To avoid clogging drains, use a strainer to trap food particles and hair, collect grease in cans rather than pouring it down the drain, and pour a kettle of boiling water down the drain weekly to melt fat, soap, or grease that may be building up.
- **Mild clogs.** Pour 1/2 cup of baking soda down the drain, followed by 1/2 cup of white vinegar and quickly cover. Let sit for a few minutes, then drench with a kettle of boiling water.
- **Severe clogs.** Depending on the size of the drain, use a plunger or plumber's helper. It may take a number of plunges to unclog the drain. *Do not use this method if you have used a commercial drain opener and it may still be present in the drain.* Use a flexible metal snake. The mechanical snake may be purchased or rented. Thread it down the drain to push the clog away. Alternatively, try a straightened wire hanger.

Toilet Bowl Cleaner

Use a toilet brush and baking soda or vinegar. To remove a ring, make a paste of borax and lemon juice, leave in place for two hours, then scrub and flush.

Furniture Polish

- **To Dust Varnished or Unvarnished Furniture**
  You can remove sticky fingerprints safely from wood surfaces with a lightly dampened cloth. Wipe furniture surface, and dry immediately with a separate clean, soft cloth. Use microfiber cloths for capturing dust.
- **To Polish Furniture That Has an Oil Finish**
  Mix two parts oil (preferably linseed or olive oil) and one part lemon juice. Apply and polish with a soft cloth. For added shine, buff with beeswax and a microfiber cloth or chamois.

Lime and Mineral Deposit Remover

Soften hard lime deposits around faucets for easy removal by covering the deposits with vinegar-soaked rags or paper towels. Remove after about one hour for cleaning. Vinegar shines chrome too.

To unclog metal showerheads, combine 1/2 cup of white vinegar and 1 quart of water in a saucepan you no longer use for cooking. Completely submerge the showerhead and boil for fifteen minutes. If you have a plastic showerhead, combine 1 pint of white vinegar and 1 pint of hot water in a large container, then completely submerge the showerhead and soak for about one hour.

Spot Remover

- **Blood or chocolate.** Rinse or sponge blood and chocolate stains immediately with club soda. Repeat as necessary. Wash as usual.
- **Ink stains.** To remove ink stains, put cream of tartar on the stain and squeeze a few drops of lemon juice over it. Rub into the stain for a minute, brush off the powder, and sponge with warm water or launder.

Aluminum Cleaner

To clean aluminum cookware, combine 2 tablespoons of cream of tartar and 1 quart of water in cookware. Bring solution to a boil and simmer for ten minutes. Wash and dry as usual.

Chrome and Stainless Steel Cleaner

Dip soft cloth in undiluted white vinegar and polish.

Brass Cleaner

Combine lemon juice and baking soda until you get the consistency of toothpaste. Rub onto brass with a soft cloth. Rinse with water and dry.

Unlacquered Brass

Clean and polish unlacquered brass with a soft cloth dampened with Worcestershire sauce.

Silverware Polish

Line a large, deep pan with aluminum foil. Put in silverware and cover with two inches of water. Add 1/4 cup of baking soda. Boil gently for several minutes. Tarnish from silverware will be absorbed by aluminum. Remove silverware from pan, then dry and wipe shiny clean. Do not use this method on antique silver knives. The blade will separate from the handle.

Silver and Gold

To clean tarnish off gold and silver (not silver plate), use toothpaste and a soft tooth-brush or cloth. Rinse with clean warm water and polish dry.

To Remove Stains

Soak fabrics in water mixed with either borax, lemon juice, hydrogen peroxide, or white vinegar.

HOUSEHOLD CLEANER	NONTOXIC ALTERNATIVE
Oven cleaner	Clean spills as soon as the oven cools using steel wool and baking soda; for tough stains, add salt (do not use this method in self-cleaning or continuous-cleaning ovens).
Glass cleaner	Mix 1 tablespoon of vinegar or lemon juice in 1 quart of water. Spray on and use newspaper or lint-free towels to wipe dry.
Rug deodorizer	Deodorize dry carpets by sprinkling liberally with baking soda. Wait at least 15 minutes, then vacuum. Repeat if necessary.
Plant sprays	Wipe leaves with mild soap and water; rinse.
Mothballs	Use cedar chips, lavender flowers, rosemary, mint, or white peppercorns.
Flea and tick products	Put brewer's yeast or garlic in your pet's food; sprinkle fennel, rue, rosemary, or eucalyptus seeds or leaves around animal sleeping areas.

Recipes and suggestions drawn from Dr. Wilma Hammett, extension housing specialist, North Carolina Cooperative Extension Service, North Carolina State University, Raleigh, North Carolina; from the Environmental Protection Agency's Consumer Handbook for Reducing Hazardous Waste; from the University of Missouri Extension Service (http://extension.missouri.edu/xplor/wasteman/wm6003.htm); from *The Green Guide*; and from the author's own trial and error.

big green purse

If you're hiring a cleaning service, try to find one that uses nontoxic products. Query your favorite search engine under the term "green housecleaning services." If you have a standard service clean your home, insist they use nontoxic, nonvolatile chemicals. Many housecleaning concerns will purchase industrial-grade cleansers or the cheapest product available; if necessary, provide cleansers yourself, along with cloth rags or towels rather than paper goods.

Safety Tips

- **If you are pregnant, minimize your exposure to household cleaning products as much as possible.** Most products have not been tested for their effects on unborn children.
- **Always read labels.** Buy the safest possible product.
- **Keep products out of the reach of small children.** Put children outside or in a separate room when cleaning.
- **Don't eat, drink, or smoke while cleaning.** Traces of chemicals can be carried from hand to mouth. Smoking can start a fire if the product is flammable.
- **Ventilate.** When cleaning, turn on fans and open windows.
- **Protect yourself.** Use gloves, goggles, and respirators that are appropriate to the task if the product presents hazards to skin, eyes, or lungs.
- **Clean up after using hazardous products.** Carefully seal products and properly refasten all caps.
- **Stow safely.** Store all hazardous products out of the reach of children and away from animals, preferably in locked cabinets or in cupboards with childproof latches.
- **Wash cleaning towels, cloths, and rags promptly.** Store cleaning chemicals in well-ventilated areas.

Greener Cleaning Wrap-up

- **Ignore alarming marketing messages.** Bypass antibacterial for soap and hot water.
- **Buy less.** Replace at least three individual products with one general-purpose cleaner.
- **Be safe.** Avoid products characterized by the words "Danger," "Poison," "Warning," or "Caution."
- **Read labels.** Choose "no fragrance added" and phosphate-free cleansers.
- **Buy products in concentrate form.** You'll save energy and reduce packaging.
- **Develop new brand loyalties.** Support manufacturers of green cleaners that go easy on you and the environment.

And if you can do only one thing, make your own general-purpose cleaner using baking soda and, occasionally, vinegar. You'll save time and money, protect yourself and the planet, and enjoy it all in a nice clean house.

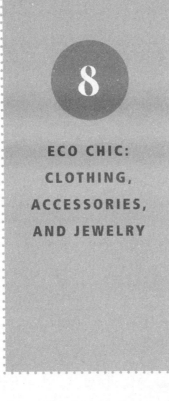

8

ECO CHIC: CLOTHING, ACCESSORIES, AND JEWELRY

WHETHER WE LOOK GOOD IN GREEN OR NOT, MORE AND MORE OF US ARE wearing it.

Soft organic cotton T-shirts. Bamboo-based business attire. Versatile vests spun from recycled soda bottles. Raw silk scarves. Linen shirts, slacks, and dresses. Shoes carved out of cork and padded with refurbished rubber. From top to toe, our wardrobes are getting earth friendlier; they're becoming snazzier, too. I wouldn't be surprised if Mother Nature herself was inspired to accessorize her fig leaf with a charming little handbag hewn from hemp.

She's probably also starting to breathe a sigh of relief. The apparel industry has never been a friend of the earth, given its often toxic impact on our natural resources. Every dollar we spend on clothing and accessories to green our wardrobe helps protect our air, water, wildlife, and wilderness. Yes, Mother Nature would approve.

Consider cotton, one of the most pesticide-intensive crops in the world. Approximately 25 percent of all insecticides and more than 10 percent of pesticides applied in the world are used to grow what its trade association calls "the fabric of our lives." It takes one-third pound of pesticides and fertilizers to produce enough cotton

213

for just one T-shirt. Pesticides endanger the farmers who apply them and the birds that come in contact with them. The chemicals that irrigate cotton fields can contaminate our drinking water, too. More pesticides are applied to the crop than the plants can possibly absorb; the excess runs off into streams, rivers, and lakes. Ninety percent of municipal water-treatment facilities lack equipment to remove these chemicals, notes the Organic Consumers Association. In the United States five of the top nine pesticides used in cotton production (cyanide, dicofol, naled, propargite, and trifluralin) are known carcinogens. Cotton even affects what we eat. By weight, 60 percent of harvested cotton is seed. This seed, which may contain residues of several different toxic chemicals, is fed to cattle and pressed into oils that are mixed into thousands of foods. When we gobble up potato chips and cookies, salad dressings and canned tuna, we may also be eating cotton—along with the sprays used to grow it.

Right now, less than 1 percent of the world's cotton crop is raised organically, but that will improve as consumer demand rises. The organic chemise we buy today can convince a grower to switch to organic farming tomorrow.

Our sartorial style can revolutionize other parts of the apparel world, as well. Nylon and polyester are made from petrochemicals, which means they're energy intensive and don't biodegrade. Manufacturing nylon creates nitrous oxide, a greenhouse gas at least three hundred times more potent than carbon dioxide. Creating polyester, reports Greenchoices.com, devours water and guzzles energy. Buying clothes that are fashioned from recycled synthetic fibers instead reduces pollution, saves energy and water, and even reduces landfill. Not bad for a jacket recut from a bunch of used plastic grocery store bags.

Once fabric is produced, it may be bleached, dyed, and "finished," processes that have their own environmental impact. Clothing dye can contaminate rivers and streams with heavy metals. Chlorine bleach can produce carcinogenic dioxin. Cottons marketed as "easy care" or "permanent press" may be treated with formaldehyde, another probable carcinogen, says the Environmental Protection Agency.

But these chemicals don't need to cause cancer to cause problems. People who are chemically sensitive may react to dyes and garment finishes by developing skin rashes, headache, nausea, muscle and joint pain, dizziness, and difficulty breathing. If the toxins escape into the environment, as they inevitably do when wastewater gets flushed back into the system, they foul rivers and streams and harm the fish, turtles, and frogs that live in them.

In addition to affecting our health, couture contributes to global warming and climate change. From the moment a cotton seed is planted or a polyester-destined drop of oil is drawn to the time you hang your purchase up in your closet, your outfit makes a climate statement. Growing fibers; manufacturing them into fabric; styling them into shirts, pants, dresses, T-shirts, and tops; shipping them to the stores and merchandise centers where they will be sold; and getting them into your dresser drawers requires fossil fuel combustion virtually every step of the way.

Even keeping our clothes clean takes a toll, whether we wash them at home, take them to a dry cleaner, or use a Laundromat. The resource costs—in energy, water, and wastewater discharge—add up. Dry cleaning is particularly insidious. Its wonderful convenience masks the fact that it relies on a toxic solvent called perchloroethylene, or perc, a chemical known to cause headaches, nausea, and dizziness. Perc has also been linked to reproductive problems, including miscarriage and male infertility, as well as disorders of the central nervous system. Both the International Agency for Research in Cancer and the EPA have labeled perc a probable human carcinogen. Right now, close to 60 million pounds of perc are used each year by the country's 35,000 dry cleaners. Not only do you shuttle perc into your home every time you carry in a newly cleaned suit or dress, but also at least 12 million pounds are released into the air annually, significantly contributing to local air pollution.

Our accessories don't let us off the hook, either. Making one gold ring, conservationists say, generates twenty tons of mine waste. Toxic chemicals like cyanide and mercury, which are used to leach gold out of rock, pollute drinking water supplies, contaminate farmland, pollute rivers and streams, and threaten the health of workers and communities. Gold and diamond mining operations can also displace people from their homelands and destroy traditional livelihoods. Conflict or "blood" diamonds have helped fund devastating civil wars in Africa, leading to human rights abuses and causing the deaths of millions. Tanning leather to make shoes and purses requires a host of toxic chemicals that pollute the air and water, kill aquatic wildlife, and endanger the health of people who do the tanning or live in the neighborhoods where the wastes are being discharged.

The Good News

Whew! All that doom and gloom is enough to make a girl shed her threads, join the nearest nudist colony, and live au naturel for the rest of her life.

On the other hand, if sporting your birthday suit day and night would make you blush, there is an alternative. You can dress from top to toe in organic clothing, easy-on-the-earth jewelry and handbags, and sustainably made shoes and still look great. That's where this chapter comes in.

It starts with an overview of earth-easy fabrics to look for, like organic cotton and fast-growing hemp. Thumb through the dozens of outlets noted here that sell women's, men's, and kid's ecologically sound clothes and accessories. Unfortunately, the majority of organic shopping outlets are online rather than in person, which is regrettable since so many of us still want to try clothes on before we buy them. One thing is clear: If manufacturers of organic clothing want to sell more than yoga wear and T-shirts to women, they're going to have to make it easier for us to try it before we buy it, at least until women feel comfortable with the sizes and styles they see on the Internet.

Wal-Mart's entry into the organic clothes world should change that: a 2007 survey shows that more women are purchasing lingerie at Wal-Mart than at Victoria's Secret; we'll probably snag more organic T-shirts there, too. No matter where you shop, it will help if you keep asking for organic outfits, whether you're buying a business suit or a pair of jeans. In the supply-and-demand equation, demand does wonders to increase supply, so ask, ask, ask.

In this chapter, you'll also find lists of nature-inspired jewelry designers, eco-chic handbags, and organic shoes. And because opportunities in the "recycled wear" department are increasing, I highlight them for you here. You'll even find a few suggestions to help you keep your eco-attire clean in green ways.

According to the Organic Trade Association, sales of organic fiber products jumped 22.7 percent in 2003, with women's clothing the fastest-growing category. You have more options to green your wardrobe than ever before. Have fun taking advantage of them.

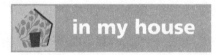

in my house

So far, my organic wardrobe includes a hemp sweater, cotton T-shirts, silk underwear, and socks made from bamboo. I bought the sweater for its color (a deep burnt orange) as well as its versatile style: it works with jeans as well as a business suit. I wasn't expecting this added bonus: it turns out that hemp is a great fabric to throw in a suitcase if you travel a lot, as I do. It never seems to wrinkle, and takes a lot of wear before it needs washing. I bought the sweater at a green festival, where I could try it on and make sure it fit. The socks I found on the rack at Meier's a "big box" store in Michigan. The T-shirts and underwear were easily ordered online, which is the only place I ever see organic clothes advertised. That's too bad. I'd buy more organic attire if I could sample it first. When I'm in a department store, especially if it's a chain, I always ask the manager where the "organic line" is. It usually takes her a minute to realize I'm not talking about fruits and vegetables.

Use Your Big Green Purse

Women spend an average of $1,069 on clothing for themselves every year, according to the Bureau of Labor Statistics 2004–2005 Consumer Expenditure Survey. Add another $823 to that if you shop for your husband, and several hundreds more for every kid you're outfitting. With anywhere from $3,000 a year or more in purse power, choosing clothing that makes a difference could go a long way toward greening apparel manufacturers and the clothing industry. We can also put the three R's to work—reduce, reuse, recycle—to improve our wardrobe's eco-impact.

- Reduce—Buy fewer, but higher-quality, clothes
- Reuse—Buy gently worn clothes, vintage garments . . . or swap
- Recycle your clothes
- Buy clothes made from organic, low-impact, or recycled materials
- Go Green and Clean

Reduce—Buy Fewer, But Higher-Quality, Clothes

The trend to "fast fashion," in which shoppers buy, then ditch, clothes for a newer style as if they were in a fast-spinning revolving door, works against our eco-ethic, but only if we give it ground.

The more earth-friendly approach?

- **Slow down.** Buy fewer clothes that will last longer. The way the fashion industry works, what goes around comes back around. You know from experience that today's designs will go out of style by the end of this season (if not sooner!). You also know that they'll come back into favor just about the time you've forgotten you even had them in your closet. Beat the industry at its own game by building on your wardrobe, not trashing it.

- **Invest in good clothes.** Buy brands that will last, even if you don't plan to wear them every single season. You'll save time and money—as well as resources—by not having to replace as many items every year.
- **Create a budget.** Know how much money you can or want to spend, and track your expenditures the way you do other household items. You'll limit the impulse buying that leads to overconsumption by becoming a master of the phrase, "It's not in my budget."

 in my house

We could all learn a lesson from my teenage daughter and her friends. To stretch their fashion budgets, stay on top of constantly shifting styles, and save time shopping, they borrow each other's clothes, jewelry, and accessories. Nothing seems to be off-limits—T-shirts, blouses, skirts, dresses, jackets, shoes, even bathing suits. When they need something different, whether for a special occasion or just a casual evening out, they raid each other's closets and avoid the mall.

 thumbs down

Catalog Catastrophe

American companies send out more than 20 billion catalogs a year, sixty-seven for every man, woman, and child in the United States. To produce these catalogs, reports Environmental Defense, companies use 3.9 million tons of paper annually, almost none of which consists of recycled fibers and very little of which is recycled after the fact. That means almost eight million tons of trees go directly from forest to landfill, making just a short stop in your mailbox as junk mail in between.

The pulp and paper industry ranks first in use of industrial process water, third in toxic chemical releases, and fourth in emissions of air pollutants known to impair respiratory health. Producing recycled paper causes 74 percent less air pollution and 35 percent less water pollution, and creates five times more jobs than producing paper from trees, according to the Center for a New American Dream. Want cleaner air and water? Cut back on the number of catalogs you receive.

Just as important, encourage catalog companies to print on recycled paper. Consumer pressure on Victoria's Secret, led by Forest Ethics (www.forestethics.org), convinced the lingerie company to reduce use of virgin fiber from North America's most pristine boreal forests and print catalogs on post-consumer recycled stock.

L.L.Bean, one of the country's largest clothing catalog mailing services, says you can help minimize the eco-impact created by catalogs if you:

- Eliminate duplicate catalogs (the same catalog coming to two people at the same address, or double catalogs coming to the same person).
- Limit the catalogs you receive (you can request only the major seasonal catalogs and skip all the in-between mini-promos).
- Keep catalogs to use as a reference throughout the season. Don't "order and toss."
- Remove your name from the lists a company shares with other mailing houses to prevent unsolicited catalogs from appearing in your mailbox.
- In stores, don't give out your street address when you make a purchase.
- Remove your name from a company's mailing list altogether and simply shop on-line (but when you do, indicate you do not want to receive catalogs by mail).
- Recycle the catalogs you do get.

I personally have found the most effective way to stop receiving a catalog is to contact the company by phone, using the toll-free customer service number. You can also try to remove your name and address online or by sending your catalog mailing label back to the company with a request to "cease and desist."

A new service, Catalog Choice (www.catalogchoice.org), makes it easy to cancel catalogs you no longer wish to receive. Once you create an online account, you can "find and decline" catalogs, using the Catalog Choice program. Catalog Choice contacts the catalog providers on your behalf, requesting that your name be removed from their mailing lists. The free service is a project of the National Wildlife Federation (NWF) and the Natural Resources Defense Council.

Reuse—Buy Gently Worn Clothes, Vintage Garments . . . or Swap

Buying used clothing offers another green alternative to new duds—and may ultimately conserve the most resources. Many secondhand clothes are in excellent condition, having been worn only one or two seasons before their owner decided to trade them in for a newer trend. These gems often sell for half their original cost, providing an inexpensive opportunity to acquire designer couture at reasonable prices while reducing the need to manufacture clothes "from scratch." At some shops, the proceeds even go to charity, giving you the chance to do well and do good at the same time.

Where to go?

- **Your neighborhood.** An estimated twenty thousand resale shops offer fashion values and let you sell the clothes you never want to wear again for money you can take away or spend on other items in their stores.
- **Minneapolis-based Plato's Closet** (www.platoscloset.com) offers the latest styles in name brands and discount prices. The company has opened some two hundred franchises since 1999 and planned to open thirty-five additional stores in 2007.
- **Crossroads Trading Co.** (www.crossroadstrading.com) is where shoppers can buy top-quality recycled and new fashions as well as receive cash or trade credit for items they sell to the store.
- **Buffalo Exchange** (www.buffaloexchange.com) has thirty national stores whose offerings feature designer wear, vintage, jeans, leather, great basics, and one-of-a-kind items.

You can also swap clothes with friends and family members who are as tired of their outfits as you are of yours. Host a swap party. Set as the price of admission three or four articles of clean clothing. Depending on your group, you can be formal and let everyone take turns picking items from racks you've arranged according to color, style, and size. Or people can genially wander about, peruse the offerings, and choose at ease.

big green purse

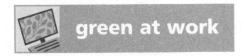

green at work

Buffalo Exchange

The green work ethic is alive and thriving at Buffalo Exchange, the Arizona company that encourages consumers to recycle their clothes rather than throw them away. In addition to its recycling mission, the company supports several nonprofit organizations. Buffalo Exchange collected more than a thousand used furs for Coats for Cubs, a program of The Humane Society of the United States (HSUS), from November 1, 2006, to April 22, 2007. The furs are being used as bedding to comfort orphaned and injured wildlife. (Furs can still be accepted by mailing them directly to the HSUS, Attn: Coats for Cubs, 2100 L Street NW, Washington, DC 20037.)

The company has also donated more than $250,000 to local nonprofit agencies through its Tokens for Bags program. When shoppers accept a token instead of a bag for purchases, the company donates five cents to a charity of the customer's choice.

For Earth Day 2007, Buffalo Exchange stores across the country raised more than $43,000 for the Center for Environmental Health through the sale of special one-dollar items.

Recycle Your Clothes

You've probably been recycling your clothes for years, though you may not think of it that way. But every time you donate your worn shoes, outdated dresses, and old blouses to the Salvation Army or Goodwill, each time you sell your used sweaters at a yard sale or give your kids' too-small T-shirts and shorts to the toddlers next door, you're extending the life of your attire and forestalling the need to manufacture anew, saving energy, water, and other resources.

Your effort is worthwhile. Clothes and shoes take up more space than any other nondurable goods in the solid waste stream, because, says the EPA, only 16 percent of discarded clothes and shoes are recycled. Despite the best efforts of charities and thrift stores, millions of tons of clothing are wasted every year.

My rule of thumb is, "Never throw clothes away unless they've been reduced to rags" (though that's when I use them to dust the furniture). Dozens of charities, like Purple Heart (www.purpleheartpickup.org), the Salvation Army (www.salvation

armyusa.org), and Goodwill (www.goodwill.org) will gladly take your clothes and get them to people in need. Other options:

- **Dress for Success** (www.dressforsuccess.org). This international not-for-profit organization promotes the economic independence of disadvantaged women by providing professional attire along with job counseling. Each woman "dressed for success" receives one suit when she lands a job interview; she can receive a second suit or outfit when she finds work. Since 1997, Dress for Success has served almost 300,000 women around the world. You can donate suits, blouses, pants, shoes, jewelry, briefcases, black tote bags, and other appropriate business apparel.
- **Soles 4 Souls** (www.soles4souls.org) Providing free footwear to people in need around the world, this nonprofit organization started after the Asian tsunami in December 2004, continued in the aftermath of Hurricane Katrina, and today distributes shoes worldwide. It also partners with Dress for Success to provide career footwear.
- **One World Running** (www.boulderrunning.com). This Colorado-based nonprofit organization ships donated running shoes, soccer gear, and baseball equipment to athletes in Central America, Haiti, and sub-Saharan Africa.
- **Nike's Reuse-A-Shoe** (www.nike.com/nikebiz/nikebiz.jhtml?page=27&cat reuseashoe&subcat=us-dropoff). The program grinds up and recycles discarded shoe material to build playground mats, basketball courts, and running tracks. Visit the website to find a drop-off spot near you.
- **Project Rejeaneration** (www.planetaid.org, info@planetaid.org). Del Forte Denim (www.delforte.com/rejeaneration) lets you recycle your jeans. When you no longer want them, send them back (in the bag they came in) and they'll be recast as a new piece of clothing. As a reward for recycling, you get 10 percent off your next Del Forte purchase (or you can donate your 10 percent to the company's Sustainable Cotton Project).

big green purse

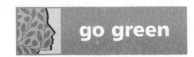 **go green**

Lasting Impressions

Buying clothes can consume a big chunk of your budget and take a lot of time, especially if you have kids and teenagers. "Out of style" clothes can end up in the trash even though they still have a lot of life left in them. How can you make clothes last longer?

- **Choose styles with staying power.** Traditional blazers, jackets, and sweaters endure and are worth some extra money. If you want to be trendy, buy fewer items, enjoy them while they're stylish, then "recycle" them at thrift shops or consignment stores once styles change.
- **Set your own trends.** Fashions are changing anyway. Don't be a slave to someone else's idea of what you should be wearing.
- **Buy gender-neutral attire.** Young children especially are usually willing to share shorts, T-shirts, and sweatshirts, or wear hand-me-downs.

Buy Clothes Made From Organic, Low-Impact, or Recycled Materials

Organic Cotton

A full range of organic cotton options is available, including:

- 100 percent organic
- organic/conventional cotton blends
- organic cotton blended with hemp, silk, wool, and polyester

Organic Exchange, a nonprofit organization that works with farmers to grow cotton organically, says that using any amount of organic cotton provides the growers with the "stability and momentum to convert more acreage to organic farming." As a consumer, aim for attire that is 100 percent organic, but fabrics that blend organic cotton with other fabrics are good options, as well.

Note: "Green" or "natural" cotton is usually unbleached, untreated, undyed, and formaldehyde free. However, it is not grown organically, and could still be heavily sprayed with pesticides during cultivation. Though an improvement, it is not as beneficial as organic.

Organic cotton must be certified by an independent third party or state agency to guarantee that no synthetic substances were used to grow or harvest the fibers. Cotton grown on land free of toxic chemicals for three years is certified as "organic," according to the Organic Trade Association. Cotton grown on fields that have been free of chemicals for less than three years is certified as "transitional organic."

Hemp

Hemp offers a terrific earth-friendly alternative to conventional cotton because it naturally resists pests, reducing the need for pesticides. Because it grows so densely, no herbicides are needed to control weeds. The plant requires about one-twentieth as much water to grow and process as cotton, and its naturally bright fibers demand little bleaching. Clothing made from hemp is strong yet lightweight, durable, and versatile. An acre of land planted with hemp can yield two to three times more fiber than the same area planted with cotton, minus the toxic chemicals.

Hemp is such an ideal ecofiber, it should be on the fast track to factories anywhere clothing and other textiles are made. But it's not. Because hemp is distantly related to marijuana, farmers are prohibited from growing the plant in the United States. Clothing manufacturers may import the fiber, since it's free of the levels of THC that make marijuana smokers high. You can buy clothes, as well as shoes, handbags, and even furniture, made from industrial hemp fabric. But it's against the law for American farmers to cultivate the actual plant.

Let's be absolutely clear: the only way you can get stoned on hemp is by enjoying the absolutely eco-friendly impact it has on the planet. If you want to smoke, inhale, or inject it, you're out of luck.

Bamboo

Bamboo is something of a miracle in the living world. One of the planet's fastest-growing plants, it can sprout one to three or four feet a day, depending on the species. It naturally resists pests and many bacteria. Manufacturers of bamboo clothing claim that because it is naturally antimicrobial, it will keep you odor free. When it is woven into fabric, it becomes as soft as cashmere. Its natural wicking properties keep you cool in summer and warm in winter. Bamboo may be combined with Lycra and/or cotton, depending on the garment being made.

Silk

For centuries, silk was created simply by feeding silkworms the leaves of mulberry trees. In recent years, the worms have been doused with the pesticide methoprene to disrupt their hormones, slow their growth rate, and extend the period of time during which they could spin silk.

Many consumers object to the inhumane treatment of silkworms. In addition to being flooded with chemicals, traditionally, the pupae are killed—either by baking or drowning—before they are allowed to emerge from their cocoons, so they won't break the long threads that make silk so beautiful.

The most eco-friendly silk comes from companies that have stopped using methoprene and that treat the animals more humanely.

Linen

Made from the flax plant, linen is among the oldest woven fibers in human history. Naturally lustrous and highly absorbent, linen is particularly desirable in spring and summer because it is so crisp and cool. The fact that it is two to three times stronger than cotton means it can last for generations. Another benefit: growing linen generally uses far less pesticides than conventional cotton does. If you like linen's natural ivory, tan, or gray colors, you won't have to worry about the wastewater dyed linen creates. If you prefer white linen, look for fabric that has been bleached using low-impact hydrogen peroxide rather than dioxin-creating chlorine. One trait no one much likes about linen is that it wrinkles easily and requires ironing.

Wool

In conventional wool production, sheep are given hormones and antibiotics to promote growth. They're "dipped" in organophosphate paraciticides to kill bugs that infest their wool. The wool is usually processed with toxic solvents and detergents. Increasingly, however, sheep are being raised organically, providing the clothing industry with organic wool to weave into apparel. To be certified organic in the United States, wool production must meet the same U.S. Department of Agriculture standards as certified organic meat, dairy, and other animal-fiber products.

Organic standards don't govern whether an animal is treated humanely. Australian merino sheep, whose wool is prized for its thick abundance, are subjected to "mulesing," a painful procedure that shears away chunks of skin and flesh from lambs' backsides in order to reduce maggot infestation in the folds of skin that produce the wool. As awareness of this cruel practice builds, "humane" wool is also becoming more common in the marketplace, along with organic.

 thumbs down

Leather

Many people have come to appreciate that wearing fur is inhumane and unnecessary. More and more shoppers are starting to focus on leather for the same reasons.

Leather is tanned animal skin. For some, it seems unnecessarily cruel to use animals for couture, especially when such a wide variety of alternatives exists. You can find a fabric counterpart for virtually every clothing item and accessory made from leather.

As far as the ecosphere goes, manufacturing leather makes a mess. (Stop reading here if you're easily grossed out, because converting an animal to textile is not nearly as pretty as the fabric it becomes.) Tanning animal skin removes hair and flesh so the skin can be stretched and softened. The process creates effluents— wastewater mixed with animal parts and the chemicals used to dissolve them. In developing nations, where much leather is made and environmental regulations are less stringent than in the United States, tannery effluents may be discharged directly into rivers or streams. They can smother aquatic life and render the water unsuitable for human use. Even if the effluents pass through a water-treatment system first, there's no guarantee that the toxic chemicals used in the tanning process, like chromium and selenium, will be removed.

Leather manufacturers in Italy and Mexico are beginning to replace toxic chemical solvents with more-benign substances, but they have a long way to go before their impact ripples through the leather industry. If you're set on leather:

- Select a product that's been tanned in the United States, where pollution-control regulations are stronger than in other parts of the world.

- Purchase beautiful goods made from faux or recycled leather.
- Shop at secondhand stores, where you can often find leather jackets, shoes, and purses whose beauty actually increases the more they're worn.

Other "Natural" Fibers

Remember that "natural" has no legal or federal definition. It can be used by manufacturers for marketing purposes no matter what they're selling.

Rayon, Tencel, and acetate are made from cellulose, a plant fiber derived from softwood trees like beech, tropical hardwoods, and even cotton fiber. To break down their tough cellulose cell structure into fiber, processing these fabrics requires many chemicals. Though they're sometimes marketed as "natural," they're not really earth friendly. Just getting to the cellulose wastes the organic matter they're derived from. According to the nonprofit consumer resource group Co-op America and its WoodWise guide, only "about a third of the pulp obtained from a tree will end up in finished rayon thread"; the rest is discarded.

When shopping for "natural" clothing, look for third-party verification for any environmental claims a clothing manufacturer makes. Get to know the manufacturer and what the brand represents by reading product descriptions on its website. Check in at www.biggreenpurse.com (search: clothing) for product updates and greenwashing alerts to help you get the most for the money you spend. And ultimately, support creation of sustainable clothing standards that encourage all manufacturers to achieve the same high degree of environmental performance.

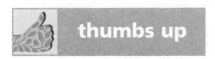
thumbs up

The New Green Clothes Closet

Vests and sweatshirts made from recycled soda bottles. Outdoor outfitter Patagonia's (www.patagonia.com) Synchilla fleece uses recycled soda bottles as its base material, with impressive results: since 1993, the company has diverted more than 40 million two-liter plastic bottles from landfills and saved about 11 thousand barrels of oil by making women's and men's sportswear from post-consumer waste. Patagonia's Common Threads Recycling Program asks customers to turn in their worn-out polar fleece garments (even those made by competitors) as well as Patagonia-brand cotton T-shirts and Capilene base layers so the company can convert them into new garments.

Pajamas and yoga pants made from organic cotton and soy. Gaiam (www.gaiam .com) offers organic cotton clothing, as well as an ActiveSoy collection that blends organic cotton and soybean oil.

T-shirts and polos made from energy-saving Ingeo. Dozens of online retailers distribute polos, long-sleeved shirts and T-shirts made from Ingeo (www.ingeofibers .com/consumer.asp), a high-performance, renewable, and biodegradable material that requires 68 percent less energy to make than polyester.

Hats and totes made from reclaimed cotton. Clothes Made From Scrap (www.clothesmadefromscrap.com) converts recycled soda bottles and reclaimed cotton—pre-consumer waste from cotton mills—into its sportswear. It also sells hats and totes made from 100 percent recycled plastic bottles.

Colors and Dyes

In addition to looking for organic clothes, search out those that are undyed or dyed with low-impact colorings.

- Undyed clothing options include color-grown cottons and linens and natural-color wools and alpaca. You can find cotton that grows in shades of blue, green, brown, and purple.
- Dirt dyes rely on minerals and irons in the earth. The "red dirt" T-shirts made in Hawaii and Georgia are examples of fabrics that absorb the beautiful sienna color of the earth they're soaked in.
- Low-impact, fiber-reactive dyes chemically bond directly to clothing fiber molecules, creating less wastewater runoff than other dyes. Fiber-reactive dyes contain no heavy metals or other known toxic substances, and meet European Union criteria for eco-friendliness. But note: all low-impact, fiber-reactive dyes are still made from synthetic petrochemicals.
- "Natural" dyes are not necessarily safer or more ecologically sound than synthetic dyes. They can be less permanent, more challenging to apply, and often involve the use of highly toxic mordants, heavy metals that help the dye bind to the fabric. On her website (www.pburch.net), Paula Burch, Ph.D., notes in All About Hand Dyeing that "some natural dyes, such as the hematein derived from logwood, are themselves significantly poisonous. Of course, the color pos-

sibilities are far more limited than synthetic dyes. It's funny how many people think that 'natural' means almost the same thing as 'safe,' as though they'd never heard of poison ivy or deadly mushrooms." As much care should be taken with natural dyes as with any of the common synthetics, Dr. Burch advises. "Unless a given dye, natural or not, has been tested for safety or is commonly used for food, it is important to follow these same precautions. Wear gloves, don't breathe the powdered form, and never reuse a dyeing pot for food preparation!"

If you have chemical sensitivities you may want to choose clothing treated with low-impact, fiber-reactive dyes or undyed, natural-color or color-grown fabrics.

What About "Miracle" Clothes?

You've seen them advertised. You may have bought them for yourself or your kids. They're the clothes that don't stain, don't wrinkle, and no matter how long you wear them they don't even smell. Are they a miracle that's going to cut your laundry loads in half? Or a marketplace mistake we need to rein in before too much damage is done?

Here's what we're dealing with. Innovations in chemistry have determined how to reduce textile fibers to sizes so small they make a human hair look like the transatlantic telephone cable by comparison. These "nanohairs"—one billionth of a meter in length; larger than atoms, but much smaller than cells—have particularly strong abilities to repel stains and prevent creases. They don't allow spilled wine or potato chip grease, for example, to soak into your clothing. They make jackets water repellent and keep trousers wrinkle free. Performance Khakis, "Never-Iron" Dockers, Eddie Bauer, Gap, Old Navy, and Perry Ellis are among the brands that offer nano appeal.

On the plus side, thanks to nanotechnology, our clothes will last longer and require less washing. Marketers looking to expand their profit margins are having a field day selling this new product to time-pressured women eager to tighten their clothing budget or save a few minutes doing laundry during a hectic day.

However, the Natural Resources Defense Council (NRDC) and other environmental and consumer groups worry that "while nanotechnology promises much, very little is known about the risks it may pose to people, wildlife, or the environment. The limited research on nanotechnologies indicates that there is a very real potential for harm. Likewise, there are no adequate federal or state regulations governing its use, so there is nothing holding back the nanotechnology industry from continuing to market products containing nanoparticles, which are likely to wind up in our bodies or the environment."

Like lead, asbestos, mercury, and dozens of other toxins, nanoparticles could be so insidious that, once they get into our environment, we can't get them out.

Studies in laboratory animals indicate that nanoparticles can cause inflammation, damage brain cells, and create precancerous lesions. Early research has also found that nanoparticles easily move from one area of the body to another, penetrating cells that normal-size versions of the same chemical may not be able to enter. Many scientists and environmentalists worry that nanoparticles that escape into the environment could harm wildlife and upset the balance of natural systems, much the same way parabens, phthalates, and other endocrine disrupters have affected fish, frogs, birds, alligators, and other animals that live in contaminated rivers and streams (see Chapter 3).

Normally, the federal Toxic Substances Control Act would be called upon to regulate nanomaterials. But since the law does not require manufacturers to provide safety data before registering a chemical, the burden is on the government—and consumers—to demonstrate that nanoparticles present a threat. The Environmental Protection Agency is developing a voluntary program to encourage the nanotechnology industry to adopt stringent safeguards. But voluntary regulations don't usually protect the public interest, as we've seen in the cosmetics industry (again, see Chapter 3).

Given how little we know about nanotechnology, and how much we've learned about the unpredictability of chemicals from our collective history with asbestos, lead, endocrine disrupters, and more, you can use your purse power to determine how nanotechnology evolves in the clothing industry.

- At the least, support efforts to require labels on apparel that contains nanomaterials or is made with processes that use nanotechnology.
- Require manufacturers to publicly disclose information on potential risks associated with nanotechnology.
- Support increased nanotechnology safety testing by independent or government laboratories.

Where to Shop

Dozens of online outlets offer the opportunity to Net-shop for earth-saving couture. Many of these retailers sell men's and children's styles as well as women's. Their designs don't tend to follow short-term trends; rather, they're reliably fashionable, often glamorous, and versatile enough to meet many of your lifestyle needs.

In 2003, organic fiber sales in the United States grew by about 23 percent over the previous year, to $85 million, according to the Organic Trade Association's 2004 Manufacturer Survey. Sales of organic women's clothing during that period grew by 34 percent, followed closely by increased purchases of infants', men's, children's, and teens' organic apparel. Now, with bamboo, recycled polyester, hemp, and new clothes made from old ones giving eco-chic additional appeal, you've got plenty to wear on the ecorunway. Take a look at some of the websites listed below.

One-Stop Shopping

Aventura (www.aventuraclothing.com). Halter tops, blouses, jackets, bottoms (dresses, pants, shorts, skorts, capris), accessories, beachwear/bathing suits.

Bamboo Clothes (www.bambooclothes.com). Men's T-shirts, tanks, sweaters, and boxer shorts; women's jogbras, panties, tops, bottoms, and shawls; socks; hand knitting yarn.

Bamboosa (www.bamboosa.com). Soft, protective, natural bamboo clothing for women, men, and baby; includes tees, tank tops, long-sleeved jerseys, sleep slip, yoga pants, men's tees, baby clothes.

Cottonfield (www.cottonfieldusa.com/home.php). Specializes in organically grown cotton clothing; sells women's tops, pants, skirts, dresses, jackets, sweaters, intimates, pajamas, and socks.

Dank Forest (www.dankforest.com). Hemp blouses, shoes, dresses, pants, shorts, and nightgowns, plus scarfs, shawls, and shoes.

Esperanza Threads (www.esperanzathreads.com). Organic cotton camisoles, blouses, dresses, jackets, cardigans, T-shirts, nightgowns; babywear; golf shirts, pants, sweats, T-shirts for men.

GoodHumans (www.goodhumans.com/Shopping/Clothing). Hemp hoodies and T-shirts, organic cotton socks, organic cotton pants, hemp dog collars, organic cotton yoga bras.

Maggie's Organic Clothes (www.organicclothes.com). Certified organic linen clothing plus organic cotton socks, tops, loungewear, T-shirts, and pants.

Of The Earth (www.oftheearth.com/links.cfm). This company manufactures organic fibers that are made into a variety of ecofashions. But the reason to visit their website is to click on the many links to other ecocouture companies. It's one-stop shopping at its earth-friendly best.

Rawganique Clothing (www.rawganique.com). Hemp and organic cotton blouses, dresses, shoes, underwear, T-shirts, hoodies, jeans.

Sahalie (www.sahalie.com). Hemp and cotton long- and short-sleeved T-shirts, dresses, pants, shorts, and shoes.

Sweetgrass Natural Fibers (sweetgrassfibers.com). Hemp-based women's tops, pants, skirts, dresses; men's tops, pants; baby and kid clothes; bargain bin.

Sportswear

Patagonia (www.patagonia.com). Organic cotton T-shirts, Synchilla sports gear made from recycled soda bottles; the Common Threads Garment Recycling Program encourages customers to return their worn-out Capilene® Performance Baselayers and other clothing for recycling.

Red Dog Sportswear (www.reddogsportswear.com). T-shirts, boxers, and briefs for men made from organic cotton.

REI (www.rei.com). "Ecosensitive" clothing line incorporates organic cotton, recycled polyester, hemp, and other earth-friendly fabrics into men's, women's, and kids' shorts, T-shirts, jackets, vests, hats, hoodies, skirts, gloves, and socks.

Pajamas

Deux Amies Collection (www.deuxamiesinc.com). Women's camisoles and pants in luxurious white, soft pink, or floral organic cotton; robes and nightgowns available in Heavenly Pink or Moonlight White.

Ecobodywear (www.ecobodywear.com). Nightgowns made from bamboo; robes, pajamas, and long johns.

Gaiam (www.gaiam.com). Organic cotton nightgowns in a variety of styles; cotton terry robes; pj bottoms.

Rawganique (www.rawganique.com). Hemp nightgowns.

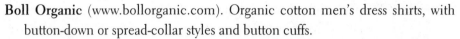

Business Attire

Boll Organic (www.bollorganic.com). Organic cotton men's dress shirts, with button-down or spread-collar styles and button cuffs.

Earth Speaks (www.earthspeaks.com). These jackets and coats should pass muster in most offices.

Linda Loudermilk (www.lindaloudermilk.com). Edgy pantsuits, dresses, tops you can wear if you want to make a bold ecostatement.

Margaret O'Leary (www.margaretoleary.com). Stylish dresses, sweaters, and jackets.

T-Shirts and Tank Tops

Bamboo Styles (www.bamboostylesonline.com). Tees for men and women.

Edun (www.edun.ie). Created by rock star Bono and his wife, Ali Hewson; edgy-style T-shirts, dresses, and sweaters, mostly for women but some men's tees as well.

Gap (call 800-GAP-STYLE to check individual stores). Unbleached, organic cotton men's T-shirts.

Natural High Lifestyle (www.naturalhighlifestyle.com). Tees, tanks, polos.

Turk + Taylor (www.turkandtaylor.com). For men and women.

Under the Canopy (www.underthecanopy.com). Tees, tanks, and tops made of 100 percent organic cotton jersey or soy.

Intimate Apparel

Blue Canoe (www.bluecanoe.com). Women's, lingerie, men's and women's yogawear.

Decent Exposures (www.decentexposures.com). Cotton bras.

EcoBodyWear (www.ecobodywear.com). Women's "boy shorts," bikini undies, bikinis with lace, and bras; men's briefs and boxers.

Gaiam (www.gaiam.com). Bras, camisoles, panties, thongs.

GladRags (www.gladrags.com). Reusable cotton menstrual pads and "moon cups" (to catch menstrual flow).

Rawganique (www.rawganique.com). Bras, camisoles, panties, men's and women's boxers.

Sustainable Skivvies (http://groovygreen.com/groove/?p=1260). Want even more options? Groovy Green's Sustainable Skivvies Web page links to more than a dozen additional brands offering intimate earth-friendly apparel.

Swimsuits, Flip-flops, and Beach Bags

EcoBodyWear (www.ecobodywear.com). Organic board shorts for men.

The Green Loop (www.thegreenloop.com). Click on "activewear"; you'll probably find options like Kelly B's one-piece and bikini suits.

Nautigear (www.nautigear.net). Totes, duffel bags, and shoulder bags made from recycled sail cloth.

Patagonia (www.patagonia.com). Women's Shore Thing sandals made with recycled rubber and nylon and a soft cork foot bed.

Rawganique (www.rawganique.com). Certified organic hemp swim shorts for men.

Reware (www.rewarestore.com). Solar beach bag to keep all your electronics (phone, iPod) charged if you can't bear to unplug at the shore.

Simple Shoes (www.simpleshoes.com). Toe Foo flip-flops for men.

Splaff (www.thegreenloop.com). Recycled rubber men's flip-flops.

Jeans

Certified Jeans (www.certifiedjean.com/index.html). Men's and women's jeans made from organic cotton grown in the United States, under U.S. labor laws. Not sold in suburban malls because, according to Certified Jeans, malls often contribute to the loss of wetlands, agricultural areas, and natural habitats.

The Green Loop (www.thegreenloop.com). This "warehouse" for ecodesigners often sells ecojeans on sale. That's a good thing, because jeans made from organic denim are pricey to say the least. Brands to check out: Del Forte, Loomstate, and Grace & Cello.

Rawganique (www.rawganique.com). 100 percent certified organic cotton jeans.

Socks

EcoBodyWear (www.ecobodywear.com). Organic cotton crew, quarter-length, and short-top socks.

big green purse

Maggie's Functional Organics (www.organicclothes.com). Organic cotton and wool crew, dress, and hiking socks; tights; baby and toddler tights.

Teko Socks (www.tekosocks.com). Socks made from wool, corn, recycled polyester, and organic cotton.

Shoes

Earth Shoe (www.earth.us). A wide variety of sandals, activewear, couture, boots, wide-width, and vegan options.

Green Toe shoes by *Simple* (www.simpleshoes.com). Eco-friendly sandals, flip-flops, and loafers that started life as recycled car tires, newsprint, and plastic bottles. Now they bring comfort to your feet, arriving on your doorstep in biodegradable cornstarch bags, no less. Plus, the company has a sense of humor. It would have to, to name its sandals Toe Jam, Toe Foo, and Toepeeka.

Nike (www.nike.com). One of the world's largest purchasers of organic cotton. Nike also incorporates recycled rubber into some of its styles.

www.alternativeoutfitters.com lists shoes made with synthetic or natural materials for the vegetarian in the family who prefers to live life completely "cruelty free."

Vegan Clothiers

Alternative Outfitters (www.alternativeoutfitters.com). Cruelty-free footwear, accessories, unisex items, T-shirts, outerwear.

Vegetarian Belts (www.vegetarianbelts.com/unisex.html) Unisex belts, women's belts, T-shirts, necklaces, bracelets.

The Vegetarian Site (www.thevegetariansite.com). Belts, shoes, wallets, clothing, and more.

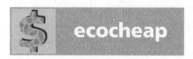

Green Clothes You Can Afford

You don't need to buy Stella McCartney's $495 organic cotton shopping bag to walk the ecorunway. Many organic cotton, hemp, linen, and wool clothes are competitively priced, both online and at the mall:

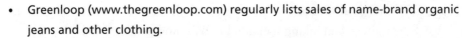

- Greenloop (www.thegreenloop.com) regularly lists sales of name-brand organic jeans and other clothing.
- The discount chain H&M has debuted a collection of organic cotton clothing for women, teens, and kids.
- REI offers a members co-op; dividends earned on purchases can help discount the price of other items you buy.
- Wal-Mart sells organic cotton yoga outfits, baby clothes, teen styles, and men's and women's tops.

What About Baby?

If you have babies or toddlers, you may be among the millions of parents who have become eager to dress their kids in organic clothes. The Associated Press reported in August 2006 that from 2004 to 2005 the organic fiber market for infants grew 40 percent, to $40 million, even as sustainable clothing sales for children and teens increased 52 percent, to $3 million. While those are still minuscule receipts compared to how much money parents spend on clothing overall, clearly organic is on the upswing, especially given parents' increasing concerns about exposing their kids to the fire retardants, insecticides, formaldehyde, polyvinyl chloride, and other chemicals that frequently taint kids' clothes. Some ecosafe places to shop:

Green Babies (www.greenbabies.com). The retailer's organic cotton clothing fits boys and girls from six through twenty-four months, and girls from size 2T through 6X.

Hae Now (www.haenow.com) Certified organic cotton fair trade T-shirts fit babies and toddlers as well as adults.

Hanna Andersson (www.hannaandersson.com). This Portland, Oregon–based baby and kids' clothing manufacturer tests its fabrics, buttons, and zippers to ensure that they're free of at least one hundred harmful chemicals. Their Oko-Tek Standard 100 is common in Europe; Andersson brought it to the United States in the hopes that other American clothiers would adopt the same approach.

See more listings in Chapter 10, Kid Stuff.

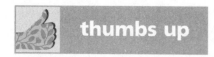

Carbon-Neutral Clothing

 Carbon Neutral Clothing (CNC) plants trees to offset the carbon dioxide created when clothing is manufactured. Look for the CNC logo among participating retailers and manufacturers, or find outlets online at www.carbonneutralclothing.com.

Skip the Sweatshops

Buying clothes that haven't been made in sweatshops is the equivalent of choosing fair trade coffee (see Chapter 5).It gives you a way to help adult workers earn a fair wage for their work while keeping children out of jobs they're too young to do. The following companies make an effort to pay their workers a fair wage for their labor. Many of these vendors offer clothes made from organic fabric as well.

Fair Trade Federation (www.fairtradefederation.org). This website offers a multitude of sweatshop-free manufacturers selling a wide variety of clothing and accessories.

Green Label Organic (www.greenlabel.com). These T-shirts are 100 percent organic, sweatshop free, and preshrunk. The low-impact reactive dyes include no plastics or phthalates. Available in men's and women's sizes; kids' coming soon.

The Green Loop (www.thegreenloop.com). The organic, fair trade ecofashion and personal-care products are made by designers from around the world. Fashions include blue jeans, T-shirts and tank tops, lingerie, swim and sportswear, business attire, and accessories, like purses and wallets. Check for frequent sales.

Indigenous Designs (www.indigenousdesigns.com). "Hand-made, premium fashion created with organic materials and fair trade practices" is how this company describes itself. Its modern styles don't make you think, "That's organic," despite the use of organic yarns and dyes. Look for mostly women's clothing: tops—tanks, tees, sweaters, polos, jean jackets; bottoms—skirts, shorts, capris, pants. Men's long- and short-sleeved tops and shorts, kids' overalls, and girls' dresses are available, too.

Justice Clothing Company (www.justiceclothing.com). Union-made, sweatshop-free apparel includes women's T-shirts, polo shirts, cardigans, tanks, cargo slacks, and lingerie. Men can shop for dress shirts, slacks, ties, underwear, casual gear, and jeans. They also sell outdoor gear "for everyone": scarves, stocking hats, gloves, jackets, and socks. Shoes, bedding, and bath products soon to come. "Justice" is encouraging manufacturers to switch to sustainable materials; check their product line to get the latest on their offerings.

Living Ethically Clothing / Shoe Company (www.livingethically.co.uk/Pages/Shopping/clothes.htm). This clearinghouse of ethically produced apparel and shoes is based in England but ships around the world. The shoes are stylish, as are many of the clothing and jewelry designs for men, women, and kids.

LotusOrganics.com (http://lotusorganics.com). The all-natural fiber clothing includes organic cotton, hemp, wool, and alpaca. LotusOrganics.com sells women's coats and jackets, exercise and yoga gear (the company specialty), intimates, pants, shorts, shirts, tops, skirts, dresses, suit pieces, and sweaters, as well as hats and scarves. Baby clothes (hats, pants, shorts, tees); and men's pants, shorts, sweaters, shirts, underwear, and pajamas are available, too.

No Sweat Apparel (http://nosweatapparel.com). This 100 percent sweatshop-free clothing line includes shoes, socks, outerwear, T-shirts, tank tops, sweats and athletic wear, polo shirts, jeans, and kids' clothes; all gear is produced by independent trade union members in the United States, Canada, and around the world. Some designs are available in organic cotton and hemp. See the website for store locations.

No Sweat Store (http://nosweatstore.com). If you prefer one-stop shopping, surf this online catalog of sweatshop-free, eco-friendly products. You'll find items from a variety of manufacturers, many of which start with organic fibers.

T.S. Designs (www.tsdesigns.com). Organic options include short-sleeved, ladies' cap-sleeved, and long-sleeved shirts; youth tees; slim-fit, junior fit, and baby tees.

Recycled Clothing

Some companies specialize in making clothing from recycled materials. REI and Patagonia focus on sportswear made from soda bottles and, to a lesser extent, plastic shopping bags. The following manufacturers offer additional options for your virtual shopping cart.

big green purse

Clothes Made From Scrap, Inc. (www.ClothesMadeFromScrap.com). T-shirts, caps, visors, vests, jackets, and aprons made from scrap cotton and recycled soda bottles.

Morning Star Trading Company (www.mstartrading.com). Tote bags, T-shirts, fleece vests and blankets, and a wide variety of promotional and specialty items fabricated from postindustrial cotton and recycled soda bottles.

RainBow Environmental Products (www.ecopromo.com). Anoraks, long-sleeved shirts, and jackets fashioned from the clippings, cuttings, and fiber by-products of U.S. and Canadian clothing mills.

Buying Organic in Your Neighborhood

Opportunities to buy earth-friendly apparel in the mall or at a local shop, though limited, are growing. Remember, the more often you ask the store manager for organic denim jeans or a sweater woven from hemp, the sooner she's likely to order it. Meanwhile, your best bets can be found at the following:

Bloomingdale's. The department store chain carries Edun brand organic cotton T-shirts; look for other brands, as well.

Eddie Bauer. The outdoorsy haberdasher sells organic shorts, tees, and polos for men. Women don't have much organic cotton clothing to choose from yet, apart from the Simple Satire shoe, which is made from recycled rubber and organic cotton.

H&M. Organic cotton dresses, tops, pants, and other casual and dressy attire fill the racks of this discount chain.

REI. This outfitter offers a good selection of organic cotton/Lycra blend and hemp shirts, women's beach pants, men's T-shirts, and men's and girl's hoodies.

Wal-Mart. Women strolling the aisles at Wal-Mart and its counterpart, Sam's Club, can pick up a T-shirt, pair of pants, or yoga outfit, head for the dressing room, and try on different sizes and colors until they find the right fit and hue. That convenience, plus a reasonable price, has already enabled millions of women to buy organic cotton ladies' apparel, plus organic baby clothes under the Baby George brand. Teenagers can buy green fashions, too.

Nordstrom. Look for organic cotton lingerie, shirts, and tops made by Eileen Fischer; and Edun brand organic cotton T-shirts.

Handbags

What would a book titled *Big Green Purse* be without a section on eco-chic hand-bags? After all, if we're going to shift our spending to make a difference, shouldn't we carry our money around in something that shows that we mean what we say?

Alchemy Goods (www.alchemygoods.com). Messenger bags, haversacks, totes, gym bags crafted from recycled vinyl mesh, rubber, and other materials.

Eco-Handbags.ca (www.eco-handbags.ca). Handbags, purses, clutches, totes, and messenger bags constructed from more materials than you may have known could be recycled, including candy wrappers, 35mm slides, chopsticks, juice boxes, and magazines. Check it out and be amazed—even if you don't need a new purse.

Ecoist (www.ecoist.com). Clutch purses, totes, wallets, and handbags fashioned out of movie billboards and discarded packaging. Ecoist plants a tree for every hand-bag sold.

Her Design (www.her-design.com). Stylish and versatile purses, clutches, computer totes, shoulder bags, and evening wear in organic cotton, silk, hemp, linen, and wool.

Vulcana (www.vulcana.com). Hobo bags, backpacks, clutch purses, and ex-pandable totes made from recycled car tires.

Vy & Elle (www.vyandelle.com). Messenger bags, totes for the gym or spa, and travel sacks made from billboard vinyl and sails.

World of Good (www.worldofgood.com). Bags crafted from discarded plastic, created by fair-trade artisans in New Delhi.

Go Green and Clean

What's the best way to clean your clothes, once you go to the trouble of greening them?

Home laundry

- **Launder as much as you can at home.** You'll avoid the toxic chemicals used in most dry-cleaning establishments.
- **Use an energy-efficient washer and dryer** (see Chapter 11). Phosphate-free detergents and chlorine-free bleaches, and energy- and water-saving methods (like washing full loads in cool water) will save you money as well as time.

big green purse

- **Avoid articles of clothing whose labels instruct you to "wash separately."** Since their dyes may run, they could be more trouble than they're worth. Save time, money, and energy by buying clothing you can clean with all your other apparel.
- **Read labels.** You often have the choice to hand wash or dry clean. Hand washing saves time and money (think: a quick soak in the sink, rinse, and hang up to dry in the bathroom versus a trip to the dry cleaner to drop off and a trip to pick up; dry cleaning dollars versus hand washing pennies), and there's no comparison on the eco-impact, especially when you use an environmentally benign soap.

Dry cleaning

As you add new clothes to your wardrobe, try to avoid items that require dry cleaning, which traditionally relies on a toxic solvent called perchloroethylene, or perc. Known to cause headaches, nausea, and dizziness, perc has been linked to reproductive problems, including miscarriage and male infertility, as well as disorders of the central nervous system. Look for these alternatives:

- **"Wet" cleaning:** This method uses water and nontoxic, biodegradable detergents to clean sensitive fabrics such as wool, silk, linen, and rayon. It is one of two processes considered environmentally preferable by the Environmental Protection Agency (EPA). It does not create toxic air or water pollution, nor does it appear to have negative health effects. Try it cautiously, however. A 2003 article on dry cleaning alternatives by *Consumer Reports* noted that wet cleaning methods might not work effectively on materials like lamb's wool and linen.
- **Liquid carbon dioxide (CO_2):** The other method the EPA considers preferable, liquid CO_2, is another alternative—if you can find it. Hangers Cleaners (www.hangerskc.com), a national chain specializing in CO_2 cleaning, won a National Environmental Award in 2002 from the National Pollution Prevention Roundtable for developing this technology. *Consumer Reports* rated CO_2 technology superior to both wet cleaning and perc, even though the detergents used in CO_2 cleaning emit some air pollutants. Cleaners using the CO_2 cleaning systems, which can be quite expensive, are starting to show up in some neighborhoods. If you can find one, give it a try and see how it stacks up against your other options.
- **GreenEarth:** This is the clever brand name for siloxane D5, a silicone-based

chemical that its manufacturer says degrades into sand, water, and carbon dioxide. However, the EPA is still assessing whether siloxane could cause cancer; a 2003 study showed an increase in uterine tumors among female rats that were exposed to very high levels of the chemical.

- **Petroleum-based solvents:** Petroleum products like Stoddard and DF-2000 may present a fire hazard and emit volatile organic chemicals that contribute to smog.

Cast a skeptical eye when dry cleaners claim to be green. To be sure, ask what processes and chemicals they use. Avoid perc as much as possible. If you use a traditional dry cleaner, air your clothes out when you bring them home to prevent indoor perc pollution.

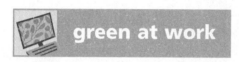

green at work

Make Every Day Casual Day

Dressy suits and standard business attire usually require dry cleaning to maintain their crisp, professional look. The earth (and your employees) will thank you if you institute a "casual dress code" on the job that encourages personnel to dress in wash-and-wear clothing every day, not just "casual Fridays" or during more laid-back summer months.

Jewelry and Accessories

Most metal mining has a devastating—and unnecessary—impact on the environment. There is enough gold above ground (already mined) to satisfy the jewelry industry demand for the next fifty years, much of it in the form of old or neglected jewelry. Likewise, you can find antique and vintage silver and gems in abundance, sparing the need for more mining and refining.

big green purse

make the shift

Earth-Friendly Jewelry

- **Shop at antique stores, estate sales, yard sales, and specialty shops** to find quality used jewelry you can polish to look brand-new.
- **Ask for diamonds mined in Canada,** where the human rights of miners are protected and diamonds are mined under stricter environmental laws than those that apply in Africa or other parts of the developing world.
- **Alternatively, choose diamonds that meet Kimberley Process Certification** (www.kimberleyprocess.com) provisions guaranteeing that the stones are not conflict, or "blood," diamonds.
- **Consider beautiful alternatives to diamonds,** like moissanite, which is made in a lab from synthetic silicon carbonite and is more durable than cubic zirconia.
- **Patronize companies that have pledged to support more environmentally benign gold mining practices:** Zales, Leber, Signet Group (parent firm of Sterling and Kay Jewelers), Helzberg Diamonds, Fortunoff, Cartier, Piaget, and Van Cleef & Arpels.
- **Buy jewelry at crafts fairs** from artisans who work with locally available materials—beads, glass, stone, stainless steel, and wood.

thumbs up

Green Jewelry That Shines

- **Brilliant Earth** (www.brilliantearth.com) jewelry features Canadian-mined diamonds in recycled gold bands, as well as other beautiful settings.
- **Earthwise Jewelry** (www.leberjeweler.com/earthwise) uses gold and platinum processed from reclaimed sources to make wedding and commitment bands, pendants, and rings. The collection also features colored gemstones mined and cut with a concern for environmental issues as well as fair-labor standards.
- **Eco-Artware** (www.eco-artware.com) offers all kinds of baubles, including cuff links, made from such recycled materials as typewriter keys and vintage watch parts.

- **GreenKarat** (www.greenkarat.com) sells rings, necklaces, earrings, pendants, and custom jewelry made from recycled gold.
- **Mercado Global** (www.mercadoglobal.org) features bracelets and necklaces woven from beads, crystals, and glass.
- **Porterhouse Crafts** (www.porterhousecrafts.com) sells silver jewelry refashioned from flatware.
- **Sarah Hood** (www.sarahhoodjewelry.com/jc_org.shtml) makes exotic bracelets and necklaces out of natural elements, like leaves, pods, and acorns.
- **Verde collection** (www.gwen-davis.com). This jewelry, fashioned from recycled and organic materials like bamboo, vintage beads, and antique Swarovski crystals, relies on a concept called "elemental design" to etch unusual images in bracelets, rings, necklaces, and earrings, then polishes the jewelry with beeswax.
- **World of Good** (www.worldofgood.com) distributes the works of 133 artisan groups in thirty-one countries.

Eco-Chic Wrap-up

- **Buy fewer, but higher-quality, clothes.** Ignore "fast fashion" and set your own style.
- **Recycle your worn clothing.** Contact Dress for Success, the Salvation Army, or local thrift shops.
- **Ease into sustainable apparel.** Start with organic cotton and hemp T-shirts, lingerie, socks, yoga wear, and fleece vests made from recycled soda bottles—all clothes that are likely to fit and that are easy to buy online or find at Wal-Mart, REI, and Patagonia.
- **Ask local stores to carry more organic options.** Meanwhile, find brands online you can trust for clothes that require a precise fit.
- **Create a line item in your clothing budget for eco-attire.** Shift at least 20 percent of the money you annually spend on garments to more earth-friendly options. Many ecologically sound clothes are competitively priced; you shouldn't need to spend more money once you find an ecobrand in your price range.
- **Cancel catalogs you barely or never read.** Shop online instead.
- **Launder your clothes at home.** Choose wet cleaning or liquid CO_2 over "perc" dry cleaning whenever possible.
- **Accessorize with care.** Choose jewelry made from recycled gold and silver or vintage settings.

And if you can do only one thing, simplify as much as possible. Mother Nature got it just about right with that fig leaf of hers. Set your own earth-friendly style and relax.

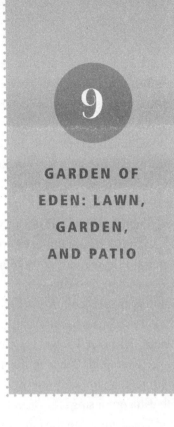

9

GARDEN OF EDEN: LAWN, GARDEN, AND PATIO

AT ITS BEST, NATURE IS BUSY, NOISY, DENSE, AND DIVERSE. IT BUSTLES FROM the jumble of animals and plants that buzz and bloom and whirl and unfurl as they go about the business of keeping the planet not only exciting but alive.

Ironically, the natural world sometimes bears little resemblance to the "natural" landscapes we try to create for ourselves. Often our "base" is the lawn, a monoculture that you won't find elsewhere in the environment because it consists of just one crop, free of weeds, other plants, insects, and wildlife. Maintaining this anomaly does not come cheap, especially in the ecological sense. The "perfect lawn" demands toxic chemicals, and they take their toll. Of the thirty commonly used lawn pesticides, thirteen are probable or possible carcinogens, fourteen are linked to birth defects, eighteen to reproductive effects, twenty to liver or kidney damage, and eighteen to neurotoxicity, according to the national Beyond Pesticides coalition. One study, published in December 2006 in the *American Journal of Epidemiology*, has connected residential pesticide use and breast cancer risk in women.

Pesticides are among the most common cause of childhood poisoning, too, according to 1995 data compiled by the American Association of Poison Control Centers. While poisoning from pharmaceuticals and cleaning substances is more common, poisoning by pesticides can be more serious. Between 1983 and 1990, reported the Natural Resources Defense Council, pesticide exposures were responsible for 4 percent of the total calls to poison control centers but for 12 percent of the total fatalities in those years.

One reason people are so vulnerable is because the quantity of chemicals we use to grow grass, flowers, trees, and maybe a few tomatoes is staggering. Homeowners apply ten times more chemical pesticides per acre just on their lawns than farmers do on their crops, according to the U.S. Fish and Wildlife Service. During a rain, runoff can carry these chemicals into streams or wetlands dozens of miles away. Air can transport lawn and garden contaminants over long distances, only to deposit them on land or water as acid rain or fog. Whether delivered via water or air, lawn and garden pesticides endanger wildlife.

Frogs, toads, and salamanders are particularly susceptible to the compounds in fertilizers and weed and pest killers. This is because amphibians breathe, at least in part, through their skin, providing an easier way for contaminants to enter their body. The U.S. Fish and Wildlife Service reports that amphibian eggs and larvae, including tadpoles, are especially vulnerable; frogs exposed during early stages of life can develop without eyes, or with extra or missing legs. Scientists have also documented the spread of fertilizer-caused "dead zones" in the Chesapeake Bay and the Gulf of Mexico that are completely inhospitable to fish and other marine life.

Even our pets face a risk. How much time does your dog or cat spend outdoors romping around the ground, where pesticide concentrations are highest? Animals can get sick themselves from pesticide applications, and make us sick, too by tracking lawn and garden chemicals into the house.

Lawns are also among the thirstiest features in our landscape. With some forty million acres of America carpeted in grass, turf is our largest irrigated crop, reports the journal *Environmental Management*. A staggering 60 percent of water consumed on the West Coast and 30 percent on the East Coast goes to watering lawns. Meanwhile, gasoline-powered lawn equipment causes nearly 5 percent of the country's total air pollution during the summer months.

The Good News

Increasingly, North American communities are restricting the use of lawn chemicals. In 2001, the Canadian Supreme Court ruled that communities can limit pesticides that are applied purely for cosmetic purposes. In the United States smaller municipalities in Massachusetts and elsewhere are lobbying their governments to adopt organic practices for public lawns and landscapes.

If you'd like to reduce the yard chemicals you use, too, this chapter can help.

The primary focus is on ways to shift your spending from chemical-intensive fertilizers, pesticides, and herbicides to earth-friendly alternatives that enrich the soil and create healthy plants. These pages offer fundamentals to help you grow organically as well as ideas for transitioning out of mundane lawn care so you can create an inspiring "naturescape" instead. Minimizing the chemicals you use is important especially for flowers you bring indoors and garden vegetables you eat. An added benefit: given the sometimes high price of organic grocery food, gardening organically offers a way to beat high prices and still get the quality food you want and deserve.

Be open to suggestions not just to maintain your lawn organically but to actually shrink it in favor of rock gardens, native ground covers, ponds, and waterfalls. You'll also find information about native flowers, bushes, and trees that help combat invasive species and promote biodiversity. This chapter offers ideas for saving water, too—and remember, any time you "save" one resource, you usually end up saving two others close to your heart: time and money.

Finally, because we use so much energy in the garden, this chapter suggests efficient alternatives to power tools, one of the biggest sources of air pollution in our communities.

Use Your Big Green Purse

Shifting your spending to more earth-friendly lawn and garden products encourages manufacturers to develop more benign options. Just as important, shifting the way you garden immediately improves the environment in which you and your family live. Here's how you can transform both your spending and your gardening techniques:

- Garden organically
- Plant native plants
- Minimize your lawn
- Save water
- Power down
- Reduce, reuse, recycle

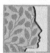

Garden Organically

Organic gardening involves a "whole system" approach to growing plants that begins with recycling natural materials back into the soil to maintain and increase soil fertility. Rather than apply chemicals to cure disease and control pests, you prevent problems by continually improving the dirt itself. No chemical quick fixes here: every year in an organic garden, the soil gets better, leading to healthier, stronger plants. By adding compost, and by mulching, a process of covering the top layer of soil with a couple inches of shredded wood bark, decomposed leaves, or grass clippings to retain moisture, you strengthen your soil and the fruits and vegetables you plant in it.

Rather than rely on synthetic pesticides and insecticides, organic gardening encourages ecological methods of pest and disease control. Using natural enemies of a pest, like ladybugs to keep aphids in check, is a common trick in a low- or no-chemical garden. Organic gardeners also strive to choose plants that are best suited to their soil type, climate, and growing conditions, including delicious or unusual "heirloom" varieties rarely found in the grocery store or the gardening center. A diversity of plants also attracts an abundance of birds and insects, bringing the garden to life in a busy and productive way.

go green

Why Garden Organically?

- Enjoy a wide diversity of birds, mammals, and garden insects.
- There's no need to buy, store, mix, water, or spray potentially dangerous chemicals.
- Eat delicious fresh food as soon as you pick it.
- Help save traditional plants by growing tasty heirloom varieties.
- Get closer to nature in your own backyard.
- Reduce pollution from commercial fertilizers.

WHERE TO START?

1. Cut back on fertilizers and pesticides.
2. Build and maintain healthy soil.
3. Plant right for your site.

1. Cut back on fertilizers and pesticides.

The term "pesticides" includes insecticides, herbicides, and fungicides. These chemicals kill insects, weeds, and fungal diseases. They're frequently nondiscriminatory: they can eliminate helpful earthworms and pollinating insects just as easily as the pesky slug that's chewing up your hostas—while putting you, your kids, and your pets at risk when you apply or store them. In fact, according to the Environmental Protection Agency (EPA), only between 5 and 15 percent of bugs in the garden are "pests." The rest, like ladybugs and praying mantis, are beneficial, feeding on the aphids, mites, and other intruders that wreak havoc on your flowers and vegetables.

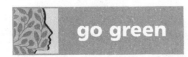

How to Minimize Pesticide Use

- **Spot treat problems.** A pest on one plant may not require you to douse the entire garden with chemicals.
- **Learn to live with some pests.** Aim to keep bugs in check, rather than eradicate them completely.
- **Mulch to control weeds.** When weeds appear, use tools, rather than herbicides, to remove them.
- **Rotate crops.** Vary what you plant so pests don't return.
- **Choose easy-care plants.** If a plant or tree continues to attract bugs or disease, replace it with a less troublesome variety.
- **Don't overdo it.** Read the directions on the package closely, being careful not to exceed the amount of chemical recommended for use.

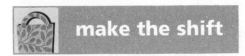

Organic Pest-Control Options

To reduce the number of persistent toxic chemicals you use, shift to more-benign alternatives, available in most garden centers:

To control pesky insects, use:

Insecticidal soap: Natural insecticide that can be used up to harvest time for control of aphids, worms, scale insects, spider mites, and other common insects.

Thuricide: Contains BT, a bacteria that attacks certain worms, loopers, caterpillars, and other insect larvae. May be applied until harvest.

Sticky whitefly traps: A simple hanging glue trap that attracts and traps whiteflies.

Diatomaceous earth: Ground skeletons of certain sea organisms. Effectively controls many crawling insects by piercing their outer shell or skin (though may also harm beneficial insects). May be used as a powder or mixed with water and used as a spray.

Tree tanglefoot: A sticky paste or putty used as a band application on tree trunks. Effective on a variety of climbing insects.

Beneficial nematodes: Microscopic roundworms used to control grub worms and other harmful insect larvae. Available in a powdered form to be mixed with water and sprayed on lawns and soil areas.

Ladybugs: Beneficial insects that feed on aphids, scale insects, thrips, and mealybugs. Available in live form for release in yards and greenhouses.

Praying mantis: Beneficial insects that eat aphids, caterpillars, grasshoppers, beetles, mosquitoes, and other pests. Available as egg larvae to be set out in yards and greenhouses.

Fungicides, Algaecides, Bactericides, Herbicides

Safer garden fungicide: Liquid sulfur product that controls powdery mildew, black spot, and rust on ornamentals, flowers, and vegetables. May be used up to the day before harvest.

Bordeaux mixture: A natural fungicide containing copper and lime; use as a foliar spray to control anthracnose, leaf spot, and various blights on ornamentals, fruits, and vegetables.

Copper fungicide: In liquid form, this trace mineral is an effective control for powdery mildew, black spot, leaf spot, anthracnose, and various blights on ornamentals, fruits, and vegetables.

Vinegar: Use to acidify soil, kill weeds, attack fungi, and disperse fire ants.

Corn gluten meal: An organic fertilizer consisting of trace elements including sulfur; can suppress weed seeds as they start to germinate.

2. Build and maintain healthy soil.

A teaspoonful of healthy soil contains about four billion organisms. This community of beneficial soil creatures, says the EPA, keeps our landscape healthy by recycling nutrients and making them available to plants, storing water until plants need it, and protecting plants from some pests and diseases.

One of the first mistakes gardeners make is to fertilize their plants regardless of the health of their soil. Instead, before you drop a seed in the ground:

- **Test your soil** to determine how much nitrogen, phosphorous, potassium (N-P-K), and lime it needs, if any. You can obtain a test kit from your county extension office or local garden-supply store. It will take a couple of weeks to get the results.
- **Determine what extra nutrients your soil needs,** if any. Familiarize yourself with your plants' nutritional requirements. Bushy, fruit-bearing produce items like tomatoes and beans demand different amounts of N-P-K than root crops like carrots and radishes. Rather than broadcast fertilizer, feed plants according to their needs.
- **Add compost.** Buy it at farmers' markets or gardening stores, or make it yourself from kitchen scraps and yard waste.
- **Mulch** to retain water and keep weeds under control. If you buy commercial fertilizers, use the "slow release" variety that will build a strong root structure.

It's worth saying an extra word about compost. Composting is nature's way of turning kitchen and yard waste into organic gold. Through good old-fashioned biological processes, composting converts table scraps, leaves, weeds, and other organic matter into rich, crumbly, soil-like material that attracts healthy worms, fights disease, and improves the fertility of the soil. Composting saves you money by reducing the need to buy chemical fertilizers. Composting can save communities money, too. Yard trimmings and food waste together constitute 23 percent of the U.S. municipal solid waste stream. That's a lot of garbage going to landfills when it could become environmentally beneficial compost instead.

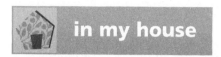

in my house

We compost all our kitchen waste (except for meat and fish scraps). It's just as easy to scrape leftovers from the dishes into a composting bucket as into the garbage disposal. Every couple of days we carry the bucket out to our compost bin, which is one of those convenient barrels that spins on an axle to keep the air circulating so the material will decompose. We take a break during the winter when it's cold outside and we figure we should stop adding to the bin for a little while to let the organic matter inside finish breaking down. In the spring, we are always amazed. Our ten months' worth of kitchen waste decomposes into only about a wheelbarrowful of rich organic material. What a great and economical addition to the garden!

ecocheap

Make Your Own Compost

Homemade compost provides an absolutely free way to obtain fertilizer and soil amendments. It also reduces the amount of trash you throw away, since you're spared the plastic bags used to package commercial compost. You can visit www.epa.gov/compost to learn how to build a compost pile in a back corner of your yard. You can also buy an easy-to-use compost bin or tumbler from a garden retailer like Gardener's Supply Company (www.gardeners.com). If you pay to dump your trash at the local landfill, the cost of the bin pays for itself in no time in reduced dumping fees and savings on purchased compost.

If you don't want to compost outside, you can set up a worm bin and compost indoors. To learn more, see *Worms Eat My Garbage: How to Set Up & Maintain a Worm Composting System* by Mary Appelhof. For directions on how to build a worm-composting bin, visit www.biggreenpurse.com (search: compost).

3. Plant right for your site.

Picking the right plants for your yard is a lot of fun. It's also essential if you want organic gardening to succeed. I tried for years to grow rhododendron in my backyard, but they continually succumbed to a fungal disease called phytophera that could only be controlled with a chemical I didn't want to apply in my organic garden. I

big green purse

finally gave up and planted Annabelle hydrangeas instead. All these wonderful flowering bushes need is water.

How do you pick the right plant?

- **Get lists of species that grow well in your climate** from your county extension agent, the local gardening club, the nearest gardening center, or the nearby botanical garden.
- **Inventory** the available light, water, soil quality, and space so you can buy appropriately.
- **Choose hardy fruit and vegetable varieties,** so you can skip pesticides.
- **Avoid invasive species,** nonnative plants that will take over your garden and spread out of control.
- **Adopt "companion planting,"** the practice of growing different plants together to benefit the entire garden. For example, if you grow garlic close to your roses, you'll keep many pests away. Marigolds are good companions to tomatoes for the same reason.
- **Plant to attract wildlife** such as birds, and bees, butterflies, and other beneficial insects. Install a birdbath or small pond. Leave some dead trees or bushes for birds and animals to nest in.

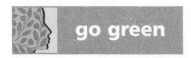

Plant a Beneficial Border

You can control pests by planting flowers that lure ladybugs, lacewings, ground beetles, and other beneficial insects. *Organic Gardening* magazine says the following ten make the best border:

1. **Bachelor's buttons or cornflower (*Centaurea cyanus*):** A beautiful blue wildflower whose nectar will attract ladybugs, lacewings, and beneficial wasps, it should be directly seeded into the soil. The flower will reseed "energetically."
2. **Sweet alyssum (*Lobularia maritima*):** A low-growing white annual, it smothers weeds and attracts aphids. Start with seeds or buy bedding plants.
3. **Borage (*Borago officinalis*):** The bright blue clusters of edible flowers on this annual herb lure pests away from more desirable garden plants.

4. **Cup plant (*Silphium perfoliatum*):** This six- to eight-foot-tall native perennial has bright yellow flowers and leaves whose cups collect dew and rainwater, perfect for quenching the thirst of small birds and beneficial insects.

5. **Anise hyssop (*Agastache foeniculum* or *A. rugosa*):** With purple or violet flowers and licorice-scented leaves, the perennial summer bloomer draws butterflies and other pest-eating beneficial insects.

6. **Golden marguerite (*Anthemis tinctoria*):** These bright yellow, two-inch daisies thrive in poor soil and attract five kinds of beneficial insects.

7. **Fennel (*Foeniculum vulgare*):** Long-lasting fennel flowers are extremely enticing to all nectar-feeding beneficial insects, as well as the anise swallowtail butterfly. Plus, it's tasty in salad and other recipes.

8. **Mountain mints (*Pycnanthemum virginianum* and *P. muticum*):** These natives make excellent border plants while warding off pests; they can be invasive, however.

9. **Pussy willows (*Salix species*):** Willows are particularly valuable because they produce pollen in early spring, when many beneficial insects are emerging and need food.

10. **Ornamental grasses:** All clump-forming grasses provide excellent summer shelter and overwintering sites for ground beetles, ladybugs, and other beneficials.

Source: OrganicGardening.com

Plant Native Plants

Native plants are those that grow naturally in the region where they evolved. They are hardy because they have adapted to local growing conditions: climate, rainfall, soil quality, available sunshine, pests, and predators. Native plants benefit a landscape because, once established, they usually require minimal pesticides, fertilizers, and even water. Plus, they attract a variety of birds, butterflies, other insects, and other animals.

In North America, plant species are considered native if they were growing here prior to European settlement. Today, approximately 25 percent of flowering plants in North America are nonnatives or alien species, most of European or Asian origin.

Native plants can prevent the spread of alien or invasive species by helping keep ecosystems diverse, healthy, and intact. They also provide familiar sources of food and shelter for wildlife, especially as more and more development occurs and wildlife habitat is destroyed. Natives help conserve soil and water since they thrive in the climate and terrain in which they're planted. Overall, planting native species is a simple step you can take to strengthen and rebuild the natural world.

To find a native plant society in your region, contact the Native Plant Information Network at http://wildflower.utexas.edu.

To determine what natives to plant in your landscape, visit PlantNative at www.plantnative.org.

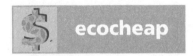

Swap Plants

For an inexpensive source of plants native and otherwise, join your local horticulture or native plant society. Trade plants with other members. Or organize a swap in your neighborhood. Here's how we do it at the Takoma Horticulture Club:

- We hold two official swaps, one in the spring, and one in the fall.
- Every person who attends brings something: a plant, a garden tool, gardening magazines, or another useful item to swap. Most people bring more than one plant, since the events provide the impetus to divide perennials that are getting overgrown.
- We each take a turn briefly describing the merits of what we have brought and the care it requires.
- After all plant presentations have been made, the "floor is open" and people make a dash for the specimens they want to take home.
- There are usually so many plants to swap, you can always leave with a new and different addition for your garden.

Patio and Porch Gardens

If you opt to garden on your porch or patio rather than in your yard, follow a few special rules, courtesy of the Iowa State University Extension Service:

- Use almost any type of container, as long as it provides good drainage through holes in the bottom or around the sides near the bottom. Avoid containers that have been pressure-treated with arsenic.

- Give fruit-bearing plants like tomatoes, bell peppers, eggplant, and cucumbers more sun than lettuce, cabbage, spinach, parsley, and other leafy vegetables.
- Water frequently and deeply so that moisture reaches the bottom of the container and excess runs out through the drainage holes. Never allow the soil to dry out completely between waterings, as the plants may drop their fruit and flowers if they become too parched.
- Fertilize somewhat more frequently than in-ground gardens if you use soil-less potting mix, since you'll need to add nutrients that otherwise would be provided by the soil. Brew an enriching "tea" by steeping compost in water; otherwise, fertilize organically.
- Make your own organic potting soil. Search "organic potting soil recipes" on the Internet to find a mixture that appeals to you. Most will include compost, sharp sand, sphagnum peat moss, and nutrients to feed your plants.
- You can buy ready-made organic soil-less potting medium at many garden centers, as well as at retailers like Home Depot and Lowe's.

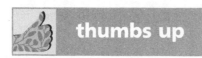

thumbs up

Organic Fertilizer and Fresh Air

Plantea (www.plantea.com) offers a mixture of twelve certified organic ingredients, including kelp, rock phosphate, bonemeal, greensand, dried herbs and parsley, and beet powder, in an organic tea bag. After brewing the tea for at least half an hour, pour it on the soil around your plants or dilute it and spray it on their leaves. Then wait for your cherry tomatoes, cucumbers, and peppers to grow.

And when it's time to bring those patio plants indoors . . .

Common houseplants have the ability to reduce carbon dioxide and vapors from toxic, irritating volatile organic compounds (VOCs). Research conducted by Bill Wolverton, Ph.D., for the National Aeronautics and Space Administration measured how well a single plant works to clean the air in a sealed chamber. Extrapolating from these results, Dr. Wolverton says that three plants per one hundred square feet in a home or office will improve air quality. Some of the best overall plants are the areca palm, lady palm, dracaena, chrysanthemum, and my favorite, the peace lily. You can read all about it in *How to Grow Fresh Air: 50 Houseplants That Purify Your Home or Office,* by Bill Wolverton.

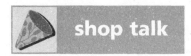

At the Garden Center

Gardening centers can do a lot to promote organic gardening and landscaping. When you shop for plants and gardening supplies, ask garden businesses to:

- Stock more plants that are native to your region of the country.
- Educate customers about invasive species and provide tips to help gardeners contain invasives in their garden or landscape.
- Use recyclable materials in their pots, flats, and carrying boxes.
- Stock plastic pots made from #1 or #2 plastic so they can be more easily recycled in community recycling programs.
- Promote native plants, organic gardening, and water conservation on the company website.

Minimize Your Lawn

Organic products are making inroads into the $35 billion lawn- and garden-care industry, giving you plenty of marketplace choices that will make a difference to your grass. A 2005 survey of two thousand adults by the Natural Marketing Institute found 20 percent of consumers had bought some kind of environmentally friendly lawn-and-garden product. According to CNN, market researchers Freedonia Group estimate a 10 percent annual growth for the organic fertilizer market, twice the projected growth for all lawn and garden goods.

If you want to grow a lawn, natural care will minimize your use of fertilizers and pesticides.

- **Build healthy soil using organic fertilizers.** Grass grows best where soil organisms like earthworms recycle plant material so nutrients are slowly released in the root zone of the grass. You can help by applying slow-release organic fertilizers rather than commercial fertilizers that boost plant growth rapidly. In addition, consumers often apply too much fertilizer, sending polluting phosphorus and nitrates into groundwater, streams, rivers, and lakes. Choose composts and pasteurized manures, which will release nutrients gradually and reduce runoff.

- **Aerate.** Aerating the soil strengthens the lawn's root system by increasing the amount of air, water, and nutrients that can reach the plant's roots. The practice loosens compacted soil, removes thatch buildup, and wards off pests, too. To aerate, remove small cores of compacted soil or punch small holes in the soil at regular intervals. You can do this by hand with a pitchfork, or you can rent a machine to make the job easier.

- **Mow high, mow often.** Mowing your lawn at a higher level encourages grass to develop a deeper root system as well as to tolerate drought, heat, shade, disease, and pests. Recommended mowing heights are 3 inches for tall fescue, 2 1/2 inches for perennial ryegrass, and 1 inch for bent grass. Mow often when the grass is growing fast, but cut no more than one-third of the length of the grass blades so the grass is not stressed.

- **Grasscycle.** Grasscycling is the simple practice of leaving clippings on the lawn when you mow. It's one of those easy yard chores that saves both time, because you don't have to bag the clippings, and money, because you don't need to buy fertilizer: the clippings decompose and return nutrients to the soil to help keep the grass growing. Grasscycling benefits your community, too. It's estimated that grass clippings make up about half of all yard trimmings that are thrown away over the course of the year. Leaving the clippings on the grass reduces pressure on shrinking landfill space. Just mow, and go.

- **Water deeply and infrequently.** Frequent, light watering creates a shallow-rooted lawn. Overwatering leaches grass nutrients, promotes certain weeds, and starves grass roots of oxygen. Soak your lawn to the roots but not to the point that the lawn remains soggy.

- **Remove excess thatch.** Thatch is the partially decomposed grass stems, roots, and leaves found between the green part of a lawn and the surface of the soil. About a half inch of thatch helps reduce soil compaction and prevent some weed seeds from germinating. Thicker thatch can make your lawn more vulnerable to drought. To reduce thatch, pull a thatching rake across the lawn to draw up the debris.

- **Have realistic expectations.** Your lawn doesn't have to be perfect for it to serve your purposes. In fact, it should harbor some weeds and insects. Remember, it's an ecosystem—it should host a variety of animals and plants. If you notice that your yard is too shady or dry for grass, consider native plants, paving stones, and other landscape alternatives.

big green purse

- **Mow to have low impact.** Pollution-free alternatives to gas-powered lawn mowers reduce smog and minimize the CO_2 emissions that cause climate change. Electric mowers use either a rechargeable battery or an electric cord. Have a smaller lawn? Try a manual push, reel mower (see pages 271–272).

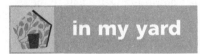

Though half of our yard is landscaped with weedy grass, hedges, and flowers, the other half consists mostly of native trees, ground cover, and bushes. To make the native area attractive to birds and insects, my son and I also installed a small pond, a task that sounded daunting until we found a cheap and ready-made liner at Home Depot, and a simple fountain pump at our local garden-supply store. We worked together one afternoon to dig out the hole for the pond liner. Once we nestled it into its spot, we surrounded it with large rocks we selected from the local quarry. Now, when it's filled with water, the pond looks like it's always been there. There's nothing more relaxing in the summer than sitting on the porch, listening to the fountain gurgle. It can make us feel like we're a million miles away, rather than practically in the heart of Washington, D.C.

Fertilizers

Plants need appropriate pH levels to grow. The pH scale ranges from 0 to 14. Acidic soils have smaller pH numbers, while alkaline substances have larger ones. A pH of 6.5 is considered the point where the nutrients plants need to grow—nitrogen, phosphorous, potassium, and various trace minerals—are most easily available. When choosing grass varieties for your garden, determine what pH levels they require. Test your soil to know what you need to add and to avoid overfertilizing. Soil test kits available at Lowe's and other garden centers allow you to analyze your soil's pH on the spot.

Your local county extension office can also evaluate your soil sample for pH and nutrient levels, usually for a small fee. Most offices provide a sterile container for your sample and a form so you can answer questions about your garden, where you live, and the plants you wish to grow. The soil analysis usually takes a few weeks. It will include detailed results and suggested amendments specific to your region.

When you choose a fertilizer, pick the most organic option available, whether organic cottonseed meal, blood meal, fish emulsion, or manure. Compared to synthetic fertilizer formulations, which are designed to pack a short-term punch and deliver quick results, organic fertilizers contain relatively low concentrations of actual nutrients and often take longer to work. That, in fact, is their advantage. They increase the organic content and consequently the water-holding capacity of the soil, while improving the soil's physical structure, allowing more air to get to plant roots. And because organic nutrients work slowly, they're less likely to contribute to water pollution than fast-acting synthetic fertilizers.

For these reasons, the U.S. Fish and Wildlife Service recommends applying organic fertilizer rather than synthetic. The fertilizer should be applied when soil is moist. Lightly water to help fertilizer move into the plant's root zone and keep from blowing away. Make sure to check the weather forecast to avoid applying before a downpour or rainstorm, which may wash fertilizers into storm drains or nearby streams.

make the shift

Eco-Friendly Fertilizers

When shopping for fertilizer, look for:

Natural organic fertilizers. These include manures, composts, and agricultural by-products that might otherwise be wasted. Natural organics contain relatively low amounts of nutrients that act slowly and minimize runoff. Some options include alfalfa, blood meal, bonemeal, and soybean meal.

Slow-release fertilizers. If you have to choose a nonorganic fertilizer, choose a slow-release product. It's more concentrated than the organic alternative, but won't create as much chemical runoff as a fast-release fertilizer. Neither will it work as quickly, though that will probably lead to healthier grass. Because they are quick to act, fast-release fertilizers need to be reapplied more frequently than either slow-release or organic fertilizers, adding to the time and expense required to keep your lawn green.

Caution, not danger. Whatever you buy, look for warning signs on the label. Remember that "warning," "poisonous," "danger," and "caution" signify products that pose the greatest threats to people, wildlife, and the environment. If you must choose a nonorganic product, look for one that urges "caution" rather than any of the other signal words.

 thumbs up

Corn Gluten Meal for Pest Control

Increasingly, consumers and lawn-care professionals are turning to corn gluten, a by-product of the manufacturing process of corn syrup, to reduce chemical use on American lawns. The organic material curbs chickweed, crabgrass, clover, and other weeds. Used at a concentration of twenty pounds per one thousand square feet in the second or third week of August, corn gluten meal will virtually eliminate clover for several years, with no harmful side effects to animals, people, air, or water, according to Nick Christians, a turf grass professor at Iowa State University.

 thumbs down

Some Chemicals to Beware

Many communities are banning or minimizing use of harsh lawn chemicals. In Massachusetts, the cities of Needham, Newton, Wellesley, and Weston have moved toward organic lawn-care practices and are encouraging residents to do the same. The Needham Health Department is urging homeowners to drop chemicals altogether in favor of organic lawn-care practices. Newton is practicing "integrated pest management"—a predominantly organic technique that allows the short-term use of chemical herbicides and pesticides to treat stubborn problem areas. Meanwhile, the Canadian Supreme Court has banned the use of "cosmetic" pesticides, harsh chemicals whose only purpose is to enhance a lawn's physical appeal.

The chemicals that concern them?

Bifenthrin, the key ingredient in many grub- and insect-control products, is listed by the EPA as a possible carcinogen and is toxic to fish. It is already banned in several counties in southern New York State. *Organic approach for grub control:* milky spore, a fungal disease that attacks grubs naturally.

2,4-dicholorophenoxy acetic acid, or 2,4Dcq, a weed killer, is linked in some studies to increased cancer risk, though not classified as a carcinogen by the EPA. *Organic approach for weed control:* corn gluten.

Benomyl (a fungicide), carbaryl, ethoprop, and bendiocarb (insecticides) have been found to reduce beneficial earthworm populations by 60 to 90 percent, according to the Buxton, Kentucky, Turfgrass Research Progress Report. Earthworm castings are rich in organic matter and nutrients. They aerate the soil and can return leached nutrients to the soil surface. *Organic approach:* beneficial insects, organic fungicides, native plants resistant to fungus.

Lawn Services

Given how time-pressed many families are today, it's no wonder the lawn-service industry is thriving. At least ten million single-family households in America spend a total of more than $3 billion annually on lawn services, and the number is growing.

Unfortunately, natural lawn-care services aren't springing up quite so fast. One company dominates the national market: NaturaLawn of America. Its seventy-one operating franchises in twenty-five states offer an organic-based fertilization program used in conjunction with a specially designed Integrated Pest Management (IPM) program. The IPM program focuses on preserving the natural enemies of turf pests; introducing newly developed, pest-resistant turf varieties; and providing continuing consumer education on how to mow and water to minimize pests and disease. NaturaLawn claims its IPM system has reduced weed and insect lawn chemicals by more than 80 percent compared to traditional chemical lawn care. The company offers two different programs. IPM is a mainstay, but a no-herbicide approach is available for those who prefer to avoid toxic chemicals completely.

To find other natural lawn-care services in your community, visit the website of Safety Source for Pest Management (www.beyondpesticides.org/infoservices/pcos/findapco.htm), a directory of 225 companies in forty states and the District of Columbia that offer least-toxic lawn-care services.

If you must hire a conventional lawn service, protect yourself from rampant chemical spraying by first scheduling a site visit to review the state of your lawn. You'll want to know:

- What products does the company use to fertilize, treat pests, and otherwise green up your grass?

- Does the company monitor for pests, or simply spray on a schedule?
- Does it try to address problems, or just treat the symptoms?
- Does it test soil annually?
- Does the company keep records of its results, so it can improve your soil quality over time?
- Does it train you in organic lawn management?
- Is most of the company's business in natural lawn care or chemical applications?
- Does the company use organic or least-toxic, slow-release fertilizers to minimize runoff?
- Does it post warning flags to alert parents to keep children, as well as neighbors and pets, off the treated lawn while it poses a safety threat?

Want more ideas? Check out *The Wild Lawn Handbook: Alternatives to the Traditional Front Lawn*, by Stevie Daniels. Stepables (www.lawnalternatives.com) specializes in ground covers (like "*Leptinella gruveri*," or "miniature brass buttons") that tolerate foot traffic as well as their grassy cousin.

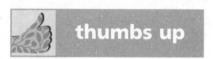 **thumbs up**

Ecolawn

Like the idea of a place in the yard to throw the Frisbee with the kids or the dog, but tired of intensive mowing, spraying, fertilizing, and watering? Consider sowing your landscape with an "ecology lawn mix." The turf mixture combines grass, sweet clovers, wildflowers, and herbs, just like the low-maintenance "herbal lawns" of olde England. Created by Oregon-based Nichols Garden Nursery (www.nichols gardennursery.com), ecolawns remain attractive between mowings and are both drought and shade tolerant.

What About Trees?

In addition to converting more of your landscape to bushes, shrubs, and gardens, consider adding trees. Trees are the first line of defense from the familiar heat island effect that can bake cities, where "the sun beats down on bare pavement—particularly dark pavement—and that energy is absorbed and then reemitted," says

Lawn Alternatives

Given all the chemicals, water, pollution, and time associated with maintaining a lawn, you may decide to replace your high-maintenance, pesticide-intensive grass carpet with a simpler, more earth-friendly alternative.

Consider these options:

- A natural meadow requires no feeding or watering after the seeds and young plants are established, and needs mowing only once a year. Meadows, which grow best in full sun, attract a bevy of beautiful plants—goldenrod, asters, coneflowers, bee balm, and phlox—as well as butterflies, dragonflies, and bumblebees.

- Evergreen ground covers like partridgeberry, wintergreen, creeping thyme, and bugleweed demand no mowing or fertilizing.

- Prairie and native grass lawns can be grown in many parts of the United States.

- Rock gardens, fountains, and ponds are aesthetically appealing and provide a reliable water source for birds and bees.

If you can't bear to give up your entire lawn, convert some portion of it. Enlarge your gardens and planting beds, extend paths and walkways, and let sections in the backyard "go wild." Putting in a playing field, like a volleyball or badminton court or a horseshoe pit, will minimize the amount of lawn you need to maintain, too.

Kathy Wolf, a University of Washington research scientist. Cars continue producing air pollution after they are parked as the gasoline left in hoses and elsewhere evaporates. Hot cars on bare lots produce more pollution than cooler cars under trees. Parking in shade will save you gas money as well as reduce the amount of smog-causing gasoline vapors wafting into the atmosphere, another study showed.

Major U.S. cities are launching aggressive tree-planting efforts to reduce temperatures. Los Angeles intends to plant 2 million trees over the next three decades. Chicago has already planted 500,000 trees the past twenty years, benefiting from city-scale studies that have shown a nine-degree difference between less-vegetated urban centers and leafy suburban neighborhoods.

If you plant three trees on the west side of your home, you can trim your air-conditioning bill by at least 30 percent. You'll also be helping clean up the air and cool the globe. Because they use carbon dioxide as they grow, trees offset and even reduce CO_2 emissions. According to the National Wildlife Federation, between 60 and 200 million spots around our homes and in our towns and cities are suitable for trees, offering the potential to offset America's CO_2 emissions by 33 million tons of CO_2 a year, and save Americans $4 billion annually in energy costs. Planting trees around your home also enhances your property values significantly. Plus, what better place is there to hang a swing for your kids' endless summer enjoyment?

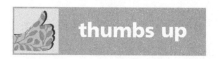

Arbor Day Foundation

Eager to plant a tree but don't know what variety to choose, or how to keep it growing once you get it in the ground? The Arbor Day Foundation has all the answers at www.arborday.org. **Bonus:** If you join the foundation for as little as ten dollars, you'll receive ten free trees.

Save Water

During the summer, half of all the water you use you pour on your lawn and garden. A thousand-square-foot lawn requires 10,000 gallons of water per summer just to remain green, reports *U.S. News & World Report*. In the West, some rivers are running dry just to quench the great thirst lawns work up day after day.

What I hate most about watering is how much time it takes. Given everything else I have to do, setting out sprinklers, moving them around to cover the entire yard, and keeping track of how long the water is on adds a level of stress to gardening that diminishes the pleasure of putting a hoe into the soil in the first place.

Fortunately, technology has come to the rescue. You can save a tremendous amount of water and time by using hose timers, drip irrigation, and soaker hoses. But even before you turn to hardware, you can make your landscape more water efficient:

1. **Turn your soil into a sponge.** Add compost, chopped-up leaves, decomposed manure, or other organic material to improve texture and the soil's ability to retain water.
2. **Water the roots.** Drip irrigation delivers 90 percent of the water directly to your plants. Soaker hoses in borders and beds work well, too.
3. **Mulch two to three inches.** You'll keep water in the soil and weeds out.
4. **Water in the morning or early evening.** You'll lose less water through evaporation.
5. **Use "free" water.** Collect rainwater in barrels or cisterns for your garden and container plants.
6. **Put a timer on your tap.** Easily control how much and when you water.
7. **Reduce your lawn.** Plant drought-resistant ground covers and low-maintenance perennials instead.
8. **Plant carefully.** Choose native plants that thrive in the amount of rainfall your area normally receives; group plants with similar water needs together.
9. **Water less often but thoroughly when you do.** Watering too lightly encourages the plants' roots to stay at the soil's surface, making them vulnerable to drought.
10. **Take care of your plants.** Weeding, thinning, pruning, and controlling pests will keep your plants resilient and needing less water.

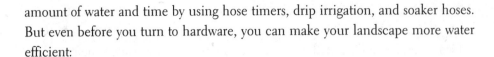

thumbs up

Get "Free" Water

According to Gardener's Supply Company, just a half inch of rain falling on a thousand-square-foot roof will yield three hundred gallons of water. How much water might your roof provide? For a modest-sized house, say 30 x 36 feet, with a typical two-foot roof overhang, a half inch of rain would yield about 408 gallons of water. That's enough to fill six standard-size rain barrels. You can attach a spigot and hose to the bottom of the barrel if you want to water a large garden or lawn. You can also fill watering cans from the top of the barrel. Keep a tight-fitting lid on the

big green purse

barrel to prevent mosquitoes from breeding. Interested? Take a look at the options available at www.gardeners.com.

Water-Wise Technology

Low-tech landscape tools can be real water- and time-savers. Check to see what's available at your local garden-supply center, or try these aids:

- **A home drip-irrigation system** from DripWorks (www.dripworksusa.com). For an easy-to-understand guide, download "Drip Watering Made Easy" at www.raindrip.com.
- **Water timers** so you can turn the water on and off automatically; available at Lowe's, Home Depot, and most garden-supply outlets.
- **Soaker hoses** that allow you to water easily around bushes, trees, and flower and vegetable beds; available from Moisture Master (www.mrdrip.com/moisturemasture), or check with garden-supply stores and home centers in your neighborhood.
- **Oscillating sprinklers** from Red Hill General Store (www.redhillgeneralstore.com). Oscillating sprinklers apply water more evenly than overhead sprinklers and can be easily adjusted to cover square or rectangular areas.
- **The Noodlehead sprinkler** (www.noodleheadsprinkler.com), which emits large drops of water close to the ground to minimize evaporation.

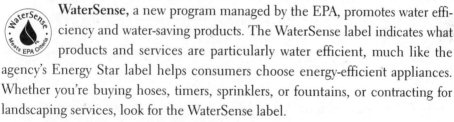 **WaterSense,** a new program managed by the EPA, promotes water efficiency and water-saving products. The WaterSense label indicates what products and services are particularly water efficient, much like the agency's Energy Star label helps consumers choose energy-efficient appliances. Whether you're buying hoses, timers, sprinklers, or fountains, or contracting for landscaping services, look for the WaterSense label.

For more information, see www.epa.gov/watersense/.

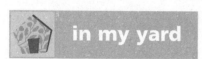

A couple of years ago, my husband installed a drip-irrigation system throughout our entire yard. We have an extensive perennial garden, and it was taking me hours to water it, especially in the heat of the summer. In fact, it was the gardening job I

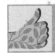

hated most. I'd inevitably get eaten up by mosquitoes while I watered plant by plant or moved various sprinklers around. It took him one weekend to figure out what configuration of hoses and nozzles we needed, and two weekends to install everything. The system works like a charm. It saves me a tremendous amount of time and hassle, and some money too, as I'm not wasting water on anything but the plant roots. I'm putting in a couple of rain barrels next, simply because the idea of getting "free" water is too good to pass up. As for my lawn, I never water it. I grow some combination of drought-tolerant grasses and various weeds that when kept about three inches tall never seem to turn brown no matter how little water (or fertilizer) they receive.

thumbs up

Xeriscaping

Xeriscaping derives from the Greek *xeri*, or "dry," and *scape*, meaning "a kind of view or scene." In plain English, xeriscaping simply means landscaping with drought-tolerant plants to conserve water. A xeriscaped yard usually requires less fertilizer and reduces pest control because the plants are growing in greater harmony with nature. Plants in a xeriscape are usually, though not necessarily, native to the region. Learn more about xeriscaping and how it can enhance your landscape from Earth Easy (http://earth-easy.com/grow_xeriscape.htm) or the U.S. Environmental Protection Agency's Water Efficient Landscape Planner (www.epa.gov/grtlakes/seahome/landscp.html).

If you insist on having a lawn, follow these watering suggestions from Sydney Water, in Sydney, Australia:

- **Add compost** to your soil before planting your lawn, or use a good-quality mix if you are buying soil.
- **Choose slow-growing, water-efficient lawn varieties** that are best suited to your soil. They have deep roots for drought tolerance and need less mowing than other varieties.
- **Avoid planting** on slopes or in hard-to-reach places that are difficult to water and maintain.
- **Apply a weed-free, sand-based, organic top dressing mix** to establish your new lawn and minimize the amount of water it requires.

- **Water your lawn for longer periods of time, but less often,** to encourage deeper roots and drought tolerance. A good soaking every now and then is ideal.
- **Choose slow-release fertilizers** based on well-decomposed animal manure or organic matter. The less water you use, the less fertilizer you need.
- **Aerate the soil** occasionally with a garden fork to help water soak in.
- **Don't cut your lawn too short.** Mow only the top third of the grass blades. You can reduce water loss even further by leaving your lawn clippings as mulch on your lawn or garden. Grass clippings are also great to add to your compost bin.
- **Design your driveways and paved areas** to drain toward a lawn or garden bed and away from the street, especially if your soil is sandy.
- **Use sod rather than seed to start a new lawn.** Turfgrass sod requires 15 to 60 percent less water to establish a lawn than does seeding. Avoid bluegrass. Instead use fescues, ryes, and buffalo grass. Better yet, use a ground cover, which requires less water than turf.

Power Down

Emissions from lawn mowers, snowblowers, chain saws, leaf vacuums, and other gasoline-powered lawn and garden tools create nasty, dirty air. From carbon monoxide, a colorless, odorless, poisonous gas, and global warming hydrocarbons, to the nitrogen oxides that contribute to smog, lawn and garden tools account for almost 5 percent of urban air pollution. John Millett of the U.S. Environmental Protection Agency says that one power mower alone emits as much hourly pollution as eleven cars, while a riding mower produces as much as thirty-four cars. Multiply that by the more than three billion hours per year Americans spend using lawn and garden equipment, and the air-quality impact of maintaining our landscapes begins to look more like a black cloud than a green halo.

What to do?

- **Use manual tools,** especially for smaller jobs.
- **Reduce mowing time** by planting slow-growing turf grasses or grass/flower combinations.
- **Decrease lawn area** to reduce the amount of mowing needed overall.
- **Avoid spilling gasoline.** Spills pollute the air and groundwater, too.
- **Maintain your equipment,** changing oil and cleaning filters to minimize air pollution.

- **Use electric or battery tools,** which generate less pollution than gasoline-powered machines.

Try Electric or Manual Tools over Gas-Powered Ones

According to Green Seal, the nonprofit certification agency, the average gasoline mower tested by the EPA emits more than 9,000 times more hydrocarbons than its electric equivalent. If just 20 percent of U.S. homeowners switched to electric mowers, 84,000 fewer tons of carbon monoxide would be emitted into the air each year. Other benefits:

- Electric lawn mowers cut noise pollution by 50 to 75 percent. Push mowers are even quieter.
- Push mowers generate virtually no environmental impact; an electric mower, which uses about three dollars in electricity each year, can save you 73 percent in total energy costs.
- Electric and manual leaf blowers and hedge trimmers offer similar benefits over their gasoline counterparts.
- If you opt for an electric lawn mower, you can choose between a corded model and a cordless one with a battery. Other cordless power tools include weed and grass trimmers, hedge trimmers, and grass shears.
- Manual tools include rakes, brooms, pruning shears, shovels, and push mowers.

The EPA notes that each year homeowners spill seventeen million gallons of gasoline when refilling lawn and garden machines, six million more gallons than the *Exxon Valdez* dumped into Prince William Sound in 1989. If you use gasoline-powered equipment, the Edison Electric Institute recommends the following:

Perform routine maintenance as recommended in the owner's manual. Change the motor oil, clean or replace air filters, and get periodic tune-ups to reduce air pollution and improve energy efficiency.

Use the proper fuel/oil mixture (as indicated in the owner's manual) for equipment with two-stroke engines. An improper mixture will decrease efficiency and increase pollution. (Four-stroke engines do not use a fuel/oil mixture.)

Maintain sharp blades on cutting tools so you spend less time running the motor.

Clean the underside of your lawn mower's deck to reduce resistance and maximize efficiency.

Avoid spilling gasoline, which contributes to air pollution when the gasoline evaporates. Use a funnel to pour gas into the tank, and be sure not to overfill.

If you buy new gasoline-powered equipment, choose models with a four-stroke engine. Two-stroke engines use more energy and create more pollution.

Lawn Mower Tips

Gasoline-powered lawn mowers are the environmental Godzillas in the landscape toolshed. Consider these alternatives to help tame the beast.

Mulching mower. To fertilize your grass and reduce the amount of nitrogen that ends up in waterways, get a mulching lawn mower. These mowers pulverize the grass and cycle it back to the lawn as a fine powder. Since grass is already 10 percent nitrogen, you'll be returning to your lawn some of the food it consumed while it was growing. "If you mulch your grass clippings year-round, you can put one pound less fertilizer on your lawn," says Adria Bordas, horticulture extension agent with Fairfax County Cooperative Extension.

Push mower. You'll generate no air pollution, and use about a thimbleful of oil to keep the machinery working if you choose a push mower. Make sure you try the grass catcher before you buy. It should be easy to remove, empty, and replace. You may need to mow more frequently, since many push mowers can't handle grass taller than three inches; check the cutting height adjuster for ease of operation. You'll have to keep the blades sharpened and rust free for these mowers to maintain effectiveness.

Electric lawn mower. You can choose between a corded model and a cordless one with a battery. A battery model suits smaller lawns better than larger ones, as the battery may not last as long as it takes to mow a large greensward. You'll also have to recycle the battery when it's reached the end of its life. In general, electric mowers offer many environmental benefits over their gas counterparts: they create no emissions, run cleaner, need less maintenance, and, with no pull cord, are easier to use. They're also cheaper to run. According to the Electric Power Research Institute, an average electric mower uses the same electricity as an ordinary toaster, costing just five dollars per year.

Corded mowers are restricted by their one-hundred-foot cord length and the run time of their battery charge, either thirty or sixty minutes. You also run the risk of running over the cord, though top models guide the cord to the side of the handle to prevent problems. Cordless mower batteries are made of lead acid and must be disposed of at a recycling facility.

Look for alternatives to the gasoline lawn mower at:

Black & Decker (www.blackanddecker.com)
Clean Air Gardening (www.cleanairgardening.com)
Neuton (www.drpower.com)
Sunlawn (www.sunlawn.com)

If you don't want to shop online, you can buy a wide variety of electric tools and mowers at any Lowe's, Home Depot, or Target, as well as your nearest gardening center.

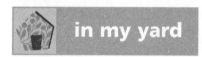

in my yard

We're pretty good about powering our lawn and garden tools with our own sweat and grunts, but we're not perfect. We had to abandon our push lawn mower a few years back in favor of an electric mower because it was just too much work to keep the push mower's blades sharp enough to do the job. Somehow, they seemed prone to rust, and we didn't have time for the maintenance. Besides, as righteous as it made us feel to push that dull little mower back and forth across the lawn all summer long, we finally had to acknowledge that mowing actually means "cutting," not rolling the grass down flat under the blades, which was the effect we were having with our dutiful but dudly mower. We trim our hedges with clippers, not an electric buzz saw. Most of the time, we cut branches and small trees with an axe or handsaw. We've had a gas-powered chain saw for years, and we use it so rarely, I just haven't seen fit to replace it with an electric one. I've also drawn the line at leaf blowers. Raking leaves in the fall is a family ritual. Somehow, it wouldn't be the same if the four of us were all out in the yard with noisy leaf blowers instead of dueling rakes and the conversation that inevitably arises when we're working together to make our leaf pile the biggest one in the neighborhood.

Lounging Around: Outdoor Furniture

Six billion acres of rain forest once covered the globe. Only 2.5 billion acres remain today, according to the National Wildlife Federation. Deforestation of tropical rain forests from illegal and unsustainable logging poses a major threat to global biodiversity and contributes mightily to greenhouse gas emissions. Since the United States is one of the largest consumers of outdoor furniture made from tropical wood sources, one way we can protect forests is to buy patio and garden furniture made from sustainably grown wood, or from alternative materials. Some options:

- The NWF is working with garden furniture retailers and manufacturers to help ensure that the tropical wood they use is legally harvested and procured and, ideally, certified under the Forest Stewardship Council (FSC) system. Look for the FSC logo whenever you purchase patio furniture made from tropical wood.
- Choose furniture made from high-quality recycled plastic. Available through Atlantic Plastic Patio Furniture Company (www.plastic-patio-furniture.com) or By the Yard (www.bytheyard.net), which makes its benches, lounge chairs, and Adirondack-style chairs from recycled plastic jugs. The advantages of plastic? It doesn't require painting, staining, or refinishing. Tailwind furniture (www.tail windfurniture.com), another manufacturer of recycled plastic patio furniture, also carries a line of kids' furniture.
- Modern Outdoor (www.modernoutdoor.com) retails a very high-end Etra collection, which includes chairs and benches and is made from Ipe (pronounced ee-pay), a tropical wood grown in sustainably managed forests in Brazil that resists rotting, scratching, and mold. It's reputed to be three times as tough as teak and requires no protective stains or other chemicals.
- PatioFurnitureUSA.com is a source for the Lutyens garden bench, crafted from eucalyptus trees managed according to principles dictated by the Forest Stewardship Council.

Outdoor Lighting

Solar landscape lights use photovoltaic cells to transform sunlight into electricity that powers an energy-efficient LED bulb. Because they have no electrical wires or outlets, they're completely weatherproof. They can be installed on walkways, garden paths, fences, walls, and porches. They usually come in a variety of finishes: black, silver, copper, brass, verdigris, brown, white, and wood.

Look for options online at:

- **The Backyard Bird Company** (www.backyardbird.com/solali.html) includes solar rock lights and sets of four and six solar garden lights.
- **Backyard City** (www.backyardcity.com/outdoor-lighting/Solar-Lighting.htm) features spotlights, solar-lighted planters, and stained-glass lanterns.
- **The Solar Light Store** (www.solarlightstore.com) sells hanging lanterns, deck lights, spotlights, and path lights.
- **Sunrise Lighting** (www.sunriselighting.com/docs/solar/) offers a wide variety of pole, column, and wall-mounted solar lights.

Reduce, Reuse, Recycle

Gardening can be a messy affair. In addition to stacks of plastic pots, a season of digging around in the dirt usually generates plastic flat trays from six-packs of annuals, plant-marker sticks, empty plastic mulch bags, pesticide and fertilizer canisters for the nonorganic gardener, old hoses, rusty tools that can't be repaired, and much more.

Nursery pots, flats, and cell packs alone use up to 320 million pounds of plastic a year, reports the Pennsylvania State University College of Agricultural Sciences. Most of that ends up in a landfill or hazardous waste incinerator because they're made from the kind of plastic (#4, 5, or 6) that is not easily recycled by community programs.

But there are better alternatives that let you reduce, reuse, and recycle your garden goods:

- **Cart your empty pots and flats to the local farmers' market.** Some grower will be happy to take them off your hands rather than buy new ones herself.
- **Buy organically grown, biodegradable pots** made from peat or paper that can be planted right in the soil.
- **Grow your own plants from seed or cuttings** to reduce the number of pots you buy.
- **Have mulch delivered in bulk** to reduce or eliminate the number of plastic bags you trash.
- **Buy fertilizer and other garden products in concentrate form** to minimize throwaway bottles.
- **Plant mostly perennial beds;** devote annuals to decorative planters, limiting the number of potted plants you buy every year.

- **Start your own seedlings.** Reuse pots and flats from your own gardening ventures.
- **Ask nurseries and home garden centers** if they will take their pots back to reuse or recycle.
- **Urge your community recycling program** to accept #4, 5, and 6 plastics for recycling.

Online Product Resources

Fertilizers

Clean Air Gardening (www.cleanairgardening.com) offers organic fertilizer for fruit, trees, flowers, and vegetables, plus reel push mowers, recycled plastic compost bins, polywood furniture made from recycled milk cartons, and rain barrels.

CockaDoodle DOO (www.purebarnyard.com) is a brand of organic fertilizer, weed control, potting soil, and topsoil based on poultry manure, corn gluten meal, seafood compost, and sphagnum peat moss.

Dirt Works (www.dirtworks.net) features organic fertilizers, including products made from bat guano, poultry manure, bonemeal, and worm "tea."

Extremely Green (www.extremelygreen.com) sells fertilizers, organic compost, soil amendments, traps and baits, and many other products for the organic landscape.

Heirloom Seeds (www.heirloomseeds.com) includes tomato and vegetable fertilizer, all-purpose fertilizer, earthworm castings, and slow-releasing Sunleaves "soil sweetener."

Miracle-Gro Organic Choice (www.miraclegro-organics.com) products include all-purpose plant food, blood meal, fertilizer, bonemeal, garden soil and potting mix made from natural, low-odor fertilizer, high-quality sphagnum peat moss, composted bark, and a wetting agent derived from the yucca plant. Miracle-Gro Organic Choice Garden Soil also contains composted manure.

TerraCycle (www.terracycle.net) makes affordable, potent, organic products by feeding organic waste to millions of worms. The worm poop is then liquefied into a powerful organic plant food and bottled directly in used soda bottles. Available online as well as at Home Depot, Target, Whole Foods, Ace Hardware, and other retailers.

Organic and Heirloom Seed Companies

High Mowing Organic Seeds (www.highmowingseeds.com) offers 250 varieties of vegetables, flowers, and medicinal and culinary herbs.

National Sustainable Agricultural Information Service (http://attra.ncat.org) provides a state-by-state listing of organic seed companies and short descriptions of their offerings.

Native Seeds (www.nativeseeds.org) features seeds for such unusual heirloom plants as sorghum, chickpeas, maize, fava beans, black-eyed peas, and amaranth.

Seeds of Change (www.seedsofchange.com) sells an extensive range of open-pollinated, organically grown heirloom and traditional vegetable, flower, and herb seeds.

Garden Supplies

Clean Air Gardening (www.cleanairgardening.com) is a source for organic pest control, energy-saving lawn and garden equipment, compost bins, and rain barrels.

Extremely Green (www.extremelygreen.com) sells organic lawn-care kits, fertilizers, pesticides, soil-test kits, grass seed, mulch, and compost.

Fiskars Brands, Inc. (www.fiskars.com) manufactures pruning and digging tools, garden hoses, rakes, and brooms.

Gardener's Supply Company (www.gardeners.com) sells solar landscape lights, compost bins, tools, pots and planters, efficient watering hoses, and other paraphernalia.

Gardens Alive! (www.gardensalive.com) is a mail-order company dedicated to control of garden pests, offering IPM (see page 264), fungicidal and herbicidal soaps, grass seed, White Dutch clover, and more.

Peaceful Valley (www.groworganic.com) offers more than 4,500 products, including organic fertilizer, organic seeds, heirloom seeds, natural lawn-care products, compost and composting supplies, natural pest control, garden tools, and accessories.

Planet Natural (www.planetnatural.com) provides earth-friendly products ranging from hoes and compost tumblers to seed starting kits, organic fertilizers, organic weed control, ladybugs, natural pesticides, and heirloom flower and vegetable seeds.

Wildflower Farm (www.wildflowerfarm.com) features nursery-grown, native

North American perennial wildflowers, native grasses, and an "ecolawn" that requires very little mowing and watering.

Also check Target, Home Depot, and Lowe's for organic-gardening supplies.

Lawn Care

Extremely Green (www.extremelygreen.com) sells organic lawn fertilizers, pest- and disease-control methods, seed, and tools.

Gardens Alive! (www.gardensalive.com) markets organic soil amendments and nematodes to combat lawn grubs.

Peaceful Valley (www.groworganic.com) has put together a colorful herbal lawn mix that includes chamomile, alyssum, creeping daisy, thyme, and Johnny-jump-ups.

Garden of Eden Wrap-up

- **Garden organically.** Eliminate pesticides and herbicides from your landscape.
- **Compost.** Build the health of your soil naturally and save money on fertilizers.
- **Plant natives.** Restore balance to your landscape while reducing the need to fertilize and water.
- **Minimize your lawn.** Replace turf with flowers, bushes, trees, ponds, paving stones, and sculpture.
- **Save water.** Install drip-irrigation hoses, use water timers, and plant native species and drought-tolerant plants.
- **Save energy and clean up the air.** Shift to hand-, battery-, or electric-powered tools, especially lawn mowers.
- **Reduce the amount of garden trash you create.** Reuse and recycle pots, plant mostly perennial beds, and seed plants in reusable flats or directly in the ground.

And if you can do only one thing, replace your commercial fertilizer with organic compost you make or buy. You'll rebuild your soil, strengthen plants against pests and disease, and eventually restore your landscape so that it looks like the Eden you want to come home to every day.

10

KID STUFF: BABIES' AND CHILDREN'S FOOD, GEAR, AND TOYS

CHILDREN FACE SERIOUS RISKS FROM DAY-TO-DAY ENVIRONMENTAL THREATS. Their chances of suffering from asthma are increasing due to indoor air pollution, automobile emissions, and global warming. The chemicals in personal-care products may affect kids' reproductive ability. Pesticides sprayed on food could skew children's nervous systems or impede their ability to learn. Even their playthings can pose hazards. Anyone following the news will have heard about the discovery of lead paint in toys from China, as well as hormone-disrupting phthalates in teething rings and baby bottles.

But the news isn't all bad. We help protect our sons and daughters every time we shrink the size of our "environmental footprint." How? Consuming less while using our purse power to make manufacturing greener helps restore the planet and benefits kids of all ages. Getting our children interested in the outdoors can give them a lifelong connection to the restorative power of nature. Education plays a role, too: when we teach kids about their world, we give them a chance to create a better world for their own offspring.

That world will inevitably require thoughtful family planning. According to the U.S. Census Bureau, the nation's population is projected to increase to 392 million by 2050—more than a 50 percent surge over 1990 levels. During the same time frame, estimates the United Nations, the world population is likely to swell by 2.5 billion, to a total of 9.2 billion. The impact of so many people on the earth's "carrying capacity"—the number of people who can be supported without reducing the ability of the environment to sustain quality of life over the long term—will be unprecedented.

The effects of a burgeoning population are already being felt across the globe—severe pollution, water shortages, increasingly crowded living conditions, disappearance of prime agricultural land. We're losing wilderness and scenic countryside in clashes with urban and suburban sprawl. Population growth especially in industrialized countries like the United States is generating disproportionately large per person quantities of the greenhouse gases that cause global warming. The quality of our daily lives actually deteriorates as population grows, reports Population Environment Balance, a nonprofit organization dedicated to stabilizing the population of the United States.

A full-scale discussion about population is beyond the scope of this book. But it's important to note that children are usually the ones most jeopardized by the problems created when the environment is degraded due to demands people place on it. As we think about the future we want to leave for our children and theirs, let's find opportunities for thoughtful consideration of this critical issue.

The Good News

One of the best gifts we can give our children is a personal, spiritual connection with nature. Resolve early on to pursue this; at times, it will be a struggle. These days, the average age at which kids begin using electronics is 6.7, with tykes as young as four and five playing computer games and answering their own cell phones. Indeed, a Kaiser Family Foundation study found that the average American child spends forty-four hours per week (more than six hours a day!) staring at some kind of electronic screen. Other research has linked excessive television viewing to obesity, violence, and lower intelligence in youths. Still, even if kids are already way more into *Grey's Anatomy* than insect anatomy, you can interest them in the natural world. This chapter begins with tips for unplugging the Xbox so you can swap screen space for green space.

Since kids use so much stuff, these pages also include suggestions for reducing, reusing, and recycling the piles of clothes, toys, furniture and other gear children leave in their wake. You get enough information to take a stand on the diapers debate (or maybe to reinforce the position you've already staked out). There's a rundown on some of the safety concerns posed by baby bottles, toys, and other plastic gear. You're reminded why you can—and should—go easy on kids' perfume, lotion, and powder (hint: it's not just because most babies naturally smell so sweet). From breast milk to canned food, you get the lowdown on packaging and ingredients. In all categories, you'll find opportunities to shift your spending and prod manufacturers to improve their products.

The chapter ends with ideas on where your children can go to college to study environmental sustainability and maybe help solve the problems we've created for them. Of course, if we follow the ideas suggested in this book, their job will be a little easier. And that, after all, is the point, isn't it?

Use Your Big Green Purse

Given how much money we spend on our children, our purses could green every industry you've read about in this book. But we're not doing our job if we focus only on spending without showing our offspring how to live more earth-friendly lives, too. As our children's first teachers, what lessons do we want them to learn?

- Connect with nature
- Control consumption
- Keep baby clean—not sanitized
- Focus on food
- Keep toys safe
- Educate and engage

Connect with Nature

Given kids' obsessions with television, computers, video games, and other electronics, it's increasingly difficult to pry them away from their screens in favor of fresh air. But they face what author Richard Louv calls "nature deficit disorder" if we don't.

This lack of connection to the environment, Louv says, exists in kids, families, even whole communities. In part, Louv blames the incredible time pressures to which we submit ourselves and our children. Given everything we try to cram into our lives—work, school, sports teams, music lessons—nature is getting the very short end of the stick.

But Louv, writing in *Last Child in the Woods: Saving Our Children from Nature-Deficit Disorder*, also attributes the problem to the increasingly dominant role technology plays in our lives. "Children prefer to connect to electrical outlets" rather than to the world around them, he observes, and the health fallout is substantial. Two-thirds of American children can't pass a basic physical; 40 percent of boys and 70 percent of girls ages six to seventeen can't manage more than one pull-up; and 40 percent of all kids show early signs of heart and circulation problems, according to a report by the President's Council on Physical Fitness and Sports.

To parents worried their kids might get hurt playing outside, Louv asks, "So where is the greatest danger? Outdoors, in the woods and fields? Or on the couch in front of the TV?"

One thing is certain. The more fun kids have outdoors, the more they'll be willing to play there. So ramp up the "fun factor" and banish NDD!

 thumbs up

One Green Hour Every Day

The National Wildlife Federation (NWF) encourages parents to give their kids a "green" hour every day to play freely and interact with the natural world. Whether in a garden, a backyard, or the park down the street, find a safe and accessible green space where children can reconnect with nature. NWF's website (www.green hour.org) is rich in family-friendly content and hosts a supportive virtual community where families can learn, explore, and share their outdoor experiences and backyard adventures.

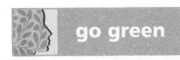

go green

Fun Things to Do with Kids

- **Watch wildlife.** In the spring watch nature come back to life as part of National Wildlife Federation's "Wildlife Watch" (www.nwf.org/naturequest/wildlife watch.cfm).

- **Take a hike.** Find a trail near you at American Hiking Society's Trail Finder website (www.americanhiking.org/trails/trailfinder.html). A two-week trial membership is free.

- **Go for a walk.** Many cities host urban wildlife jaunts. Ask your city Parks and Recreation department.

- **Bike a "Rail-Trail."** Check out the offerings at the Rails-to-Trails Conservancy's Trail Link website (www.traillink.com).

- **Count birds and butterflies.** Join the National Audubon Society's Great Backyard Bird Count (www.audubon.org/gbbc/index.shtml) or the annual census of the North American Butterfly Association (www.naba.org/ counts.html).

- **Go wild in your backyard.** Make it easy for birds, butterflies, and other wildlife to thrive in your backyard. The National Wildlife Federation shows you how (www.nwf.org/backyard).

- **Take a nature-oriented vacation.** Camp, kayak, canoe. Plan a visit to a national park at (www.nps.gov).

- **Scribble, draw, write.** Grab your kids, some paper, pens or colored pencils, and crayons, and plop down on your favorite park bench or under your favorite tree. Let your creative juices flow.

- **Make it easy.** Picnic in the nearest park, stroll through the botanic gardens, join the community garden.

- **Want more ideas?** Sign up for National Wildlife Federation's monthly e-newsletter of fun nature activities designed especially for parents and kids (www.nwf.org/kids).

Secrets to a Successful Hike with Kids

Having a hard time getting the kids to unplug long enough to take a hike?

- **Offer food.** Provide high-energy snacks along the way, plus a special treat for everyone who reaches the "summit" (whatever it is).
- **Take friends.** Kids are often more willing to do what they perceive to be a "chore" with playmates in tow.
- **Tell stories and sing songs.** Hiking won't seem like so much work if your son or daughter is engrossed in a story or belting out a tune.
- **Plan a "treasure" hunt.** Keep your children busy looking for special leaves, stones, paw prints, cloud formations, wildflowers, mosses, birds' nests, spiderwebs, and other natural "jewels."
- **Carry plenty of water or juice.** It's critical to avoid dehydration, especially on a long hike.
- **Find walking sticks.** Help your kids find sturdy "canes" they can use over and over again.
- **Dress the kids in layers.** Be prepared for changes in weather; most children can carry a light backpack and their own windbreaker or poncho.
- **Protect them from bug bites and poison ivy.** Stay on the trail to avoid itchy vines, and apply Deet-free insect repellent as needed.

 in my house

We started taking our kids camping when they were both still in diapers. They were used to playing outside anyway, so camping seemed normal, only better, since they got to sleep in a tent and roast marshmallows around a live fire. By the time they were five and seven, they could hike all day—as long as we included picnics, tree climbing, rock skipping, tag, and other games to keep them engaged and walking.

We also bicycled to local parks, visited horse stables, went to the zoo, and prowled the botanic garden. Going with friends whose kids were the same age as ours made it more fun for us all. During several spring breaks, we camped at Cinnamon Bay in the U.S. Virgin Islands. It's a wonderfully safe place where children can flit about wild as birds and find endless fascination in hermit crabs, land iguanas, bats, and the myriad fish they see when they snorkel. My son eventually joined the Boy Scouts. My daughter became more enthralled with the indoors as she entered her teen years, but we still made it a point to limit computer and TV time and go hiking as a family a few times a year. These days, though our children are almost adults, we continue to connect with nature as part of every family vacation. Not long ago, we spent a week white-water rafting, kayaking, rock climbing, and rappelling in West Virginia's New River Gorge. One night, my son built a roaring fire so we could make s'mores. My daughter threw a few logs on the coals, toasted her treat, then casually bid everyone a contented good night. When I checked on her a little while later, I found her snuggled up in her tent, a mischievous smile on her face. She was plugged into her iPod, watching the latest episode of *The OC*. That's okay. She was still under the stars . . . and doesn't a beach figure into *The OC* somewhere?

Control Consumption

Whether you have one child or more, you've probably already been dismayed by how much "stuff" they plow through on their road to adulthood. A middle-income family with a child born in 2000 can expect to spend about $165,630 ($233,530 when factoring in inflation) for food, shelter, and other "necessities" to raise that child over the next seventeen years, reported the U.S. Department of Agriculture in its 2005 Expenditures on Children by Families study. Still, even if you can afford all the extras that pile on as your family grows, you needn't feel like you have to buy them to be a good parent. Remember, wielding your Big Green Purse can be less about carrying it than leaving it at home.

How can you minimize what your kids use yet get the most eco-friendly products whatever you choose?

Before you buy:

- **Take stock of what you need.** It may be less than you think. Sure, you can pick from dozens of gorgeous strollers, swings, chairs, baby wraps, backpacks, clothes, toys, videos, games, and goodness knows what else. But if this is your first child, don't believe you "have to have it all." Learn from experienced parents what baby items are essential and which ones just add to the clutter. If you're having a second child, tally what you already have. "New" baby doesn't have to mean "new" stuff.

- **Shop at yard and garage sales.** Local sales are gold mines for recycled clothes, cribs, high chairs, baby swings, bassinets, changing tables, car seats, wagons, and more, all at prices a mere fraction of what you'd pay new. Check online newspaper ads for sale announcements, and keep an eye out for neighborhood posters announcing sale dates and times.
- **Buy at thrift stores.** Value Village, Salvation Army, Purple Heart, and local consignment shops offer many of the items you need to keep your baby or toddler happy. Since you may use these items for less than a year, it doesn't make sense to pay full price anyway.
- **Obtain gently worn items at a discount or even free via www.freecycle.com and www.craigslist.com.** Online bargains may lead you to perfectly good equipment while reducing the load at the landfill.

When your kids have outgrown or moved on from their clothes and gear:

- **Hold a yard sale.** Band together with neighbors for a block event to attract more customers. It's also a fun way to socialize and enjoy a day outdoors.
- **Sell clothes, toys, and equipment at a consignment shop.** It's convenient to pack everything up and sell it at one location.
- **Give your hand-me-downs to family or friends.** If friends don't want your discards, drive-by scavengers might. Leave filled bags and boxes marked "free" on your curb.
- **Donate.** Salvation Army and other charities may pick up at your convenience, and give you a receipt you can use to deduct the value of the donated goods from your taxes.

Keep Clothing in Check

Babies and toddlers bustle through one growth spurt after another. An infant at eight months is on average two and a half times larger than when she was born, and she just keeps on growing—and outgrowing whatever she was using only weeks before. Kids' clothes for their first year are sold in three- and six-month increments, but some babies don't even wear them that long. Talk about fast fashion!

- **Buy unisex.** Gender-neutral clothes are easier to share among siblings, neighbors, and friends. My daughter wore her brother's clothes, which we then gave to my niece, whose own two kids wore them before they were passed on to a local charity.
- **Buy slightly larger, stretchier clothes.** You'll get a few more months' wear out of them.
- **Check drawers.** Before you buy new, inventory what you still have that you can use for baby number two. Baby and toddler clothes never go out of style, so even if clothes are a couple of years old, they'll be fashionable (though honestly, baby won't care).
- **Set limits.** Work within a budget to keep purchases reasonable. Given the limited amount of time kids wear any one size, why spend a lot on clothes they may never get around to wearing?
- **Buy standards, rather than outfits.** Choose versatile pants, shorts, tops, and sweaters that you can mix and match. Kids may outgrow tops at a different rate than the bottoms, but you shouldn't have to dispose of both at the same time.
- **Make quick alterations.** Can you replace buttons to give a shirt a new look? Cut off pants to make them into shorts or capris?

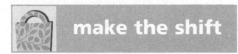

make the shift

Organic Cotton Clothing

From diapers and blankets to sweaters and shorts, kids' clothes are increasingly available in organic cotton. The choice is fortuitous, since more pesticides are applied on cotton than any other crop in the world. Only 1 percent of cotton is grown organically so far. Your purchases will not only swathe your children in healthy fabric, they'll also provide incentives to manufacturers to produce more cotton without toxic chemicals. Organic cotton clothing for children is available off the rack at Wal-Mart, REI, and Patagonia, and at dozens of online retailers. You can find a more complete listing in Chapter 8, as well as in the "Where to Shop" section at the end of this chapter.

The Diaper Dilemma

Your child could use between 5,000 and 8,000 diapers before she's toilet-trained. Should you choose cloth or disposables? If you choose cloth, should you wash the diapers at home, or get a diaper service? Or should you forgo diapers altogether (yes, you read that right)? And does it matter what kind of wipes you use?

Symbolic Moral Statement

Symbolically, using cloth diapers makes a great moral statement. I chose cloth when I had my kids because it seemed like "the right thing to do." I didn't want trees being ground down just so my kids could fill them up with poop. Nor did I care to have my kids wrapped in plastic 24/7. And I had no desire to contribute to the eighteen billion disposable diapers Americans are throwing away every year—a quantity, by the way, that's substantial enough to stretch to the moon and back seven times, according to one analysis.

For a while, I used a diaper service; then I washed the diapers myself. It was as easy as doing the rest of the laundry, and my kids never suffered from excessive diaper rash or inconvenience. They had child care at home, so we did not have to deal with day-care facilities that only accept disposables.

Environmental Analysis

It wasn't until long after my kids were out of diapers that a "life cycle" analysis was done on the environmental costs and benefits of disposable versus cloth diapers. I have to say, where once I had felt so virtuous about my diaper choices, this study left me feeling a bit disoriented.

It convincingly made the point that the diaper decision, like so many others, is all about trade-offs. The environmental consequences teeter between the amount of energy and water used to wash diapers and the amount of waste diapers create. According to the Institute for Lifecycle Environmental Assessment, disposable diapers produce substantially more solid waste, which includes: waste generated when the diaper is produced and processed, manufacture trimmings, and ash from electricity generation; the diaper itself; child waste; and packaging. Cloth diapers generate half as much solid waste. However, cloth diapers use more water and produce more waterborne waste.

The conclusion of this study, which was seconded by the Union of Concerned Scientists, was equivocal: If your community is concerned about water shortages, as is common in the West, it's best to use disposable diapers. If the area faces land-fill problems, a situation more common in densely populated urban areas on the eastern side of the country, it's best to use commercially laundered cloth diapers.

Notably, when this study was originally done in 1992, commercial laundry services were deemed more water and energy efficient than washing diapers at home. Today, appliances are significantly *more* efficient than they were in the nineties. If you are laundering diapers at home using a highly efficient washer and dryer, it's entirely possible you will save as much energy and water as a laundry service.

Health Considerations

Apart from the resource questions involved, many parents wonder what health issues diapers raise. Again, neither cloth nor disposables has the edge.

Bleaching the paper for most disposable diapers creates dioxin, a toxin that can persist in the environment and cause cancer and other health problems. But according to the Pesticide Action Network, cotton is the most insecticide-intensive crop in the world, so using cloth diapers made from conventionally grown cotton contributes to air, water, and chemical pollution. Organic cotton diapers and alternatively bleached disposable diapers are available in the marketplace, but both are quite expensive.

Because disposable diapers are superabsorbent, they keep infants drier longer. However, this phenomenon has a tendency to postpone a child's natural tendency to begin potty training by around a year. You may change more diapers in the short term if your babies wear cloth diapers, but they may transition out of diapers sooner, too.

Some parents worry that the ingredients used in the plastic and fragrances that make up disposable diapers could cause asthma or other illnesses in their children. To date, no specific diseases have been linked to the use of disposable diapers. You should probably wash cloth diapers in fragrance-free detergents and softeners anyway, for all of the environmental and health reasons explained at length in Chapter 3.

What to Do? It really comes down to what you value most.

You may prefer cloth diapers if the following are important to you:

- minimizing the amount of trash you create
- trying to live a "whole earth" lifestyle

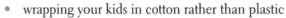

- wrapping your kids in cotton rather than plastic
- just feeling like "it's the right thing to do"

If you opt for a diaper service, find one that is already servicing your neighborhood, to reduce energy transportation costs associated with pickup and delivery. Explore your options at www.diapernet.org/locate.htm. Request fragrance-free detergents and water softeners.

You may prefer disposable diapers if the following are important to you:

- saving water
- convenience
- expressing your concern for the environment in other ways

If you opt for disposables, choose those made with nonchlorine-bleached, fragrance-free fiber.

What about early toileting, or even no diapers at all?

Billions of people around the world don't use diapers and still manage to raise healthy children. In this country, the no-diaper movement is gaining steam among parents who can devote time to recognizing their kids' cues for when they need to pee and poop. Children as young as fifteen months old have been potty-trained by parents who have learned to pick up on their babies' signals.

Check out Diaper Free! at (www.natural-wisdom.com/) for more information on this ancient but reviving child-care practice.

Baby Wipes

How you keep baby's bum clean is almost as controversial as what you wrap it with.

Throwaway wipes are usually made from a nonwoven fabric similar to the cotton/polyester/polypropylene blend used in diapers and dryer sheets. The sheets may be bleached with chlorine, which creates cancer-causing dioxin as a by-product. Cleansing power comes from water plus mild detergents mixed with moisturizing agents, fragrance, and preservatives. Many of the chemicals that infuse baby wipes are parabens (preservatives) and phthalates (in fragrances), which cause reproductive abnormalities among fish, frogs, and other aquatic wildlife. These same chemicals may have human health impacts, though no particular problems have been linked to baby wipes. Plus, disposables usually come in a nonrecyclable plastic tub that you have to toss in the trash once it's empty.

You can buy organic cotton cloth wipes. But they can be quite inconvenient if you have a mess to clean up and no easy access to rinse water.

If you choose disposables, look for the following baby- and earth-friendly features:

- no fragrance added
- refillable dispenser tub
- bleached with hydrogen peroxide or other nonchlorine bleach
- alcohol free
- plant-based oils and lotions (like aloe)

The Nurture Center's website (http://shop.nurturecenter.com/unniorrebawi.html) links to almost a dozen retailers that sell flannel, terry, and Egyptian cotton wipes and washcloths, as well as ecodisposables.

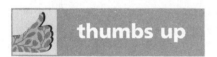

Tush Time

Find organic cotton diapers and wipes at:

- **Baby Bunz and Co.** (www.babybunz.com). Organic cotton and hemp diapers, diaper covers, swim diapers, and Fuzzi Bunz for naptime or nights.
- **Ecobaby Organics** (www.ecobaby.com.) Colorful assortment of diapers and diaper wraps, plus cloth "washies" instead of throwaway wipes.
- **Fuz Baby** (www.fuzbaby.com). Hand-dyed prints liven up the diapers outside; they're still organic cotton inside. Plus, wool diaper covers.
- **Little Beetle** (www.betterforbabies.com). Organic cotton fitted diapers and organic cotton velour "beetle boosters" for nighttime.
- **Tiny Tush** (www.tinytush.com). Fleece and terry cotton wipes, sold in packages of various quantities; one-size-fits-all organic cotton diapers may last

until your child reaches thirty-two pounds (though they may be a bit bulky on a newborn).

- **Under the Nile** (www.underthenile.com). Pure organic cotton terry knit in diaper liners, folded diapers, training pants, Velcro wraps, and baby wipes made with 100 percent organic Egyptian cotton.

These disposable nonchlorine-bleached diapers are plastic free to reduce their eco-impact:

- **gDiapers** (www.gdiapers.com) combine cloth and disposables. They consist of a conventional cotton cloth pant, nylon liner, and a superabsorbent pad that can be removed and flushed down the toilet. The cloth pant still requires laundering, and the pad is not completely bleach free, so it has some environmental costs. But the Natural Resources Defense Council says, "gDiapers seem to have the environmental edge over more conventional choices because they send no material to the landfill, use no elemental chlorine or plastics, and require much less washing (therefore, less water and energy usage) than regular cloth diapers."

- **Kushies Flushable Diaper Liners** (http://shop.nurturecenter.com/kuflbidili.html), the best of both worlds: wrap your baby in cloth diapers lined with a liner you can flush away.

- **Nature Boy and Girl** (http://shop.nurturecenter.com/naboygididib.html), a disposable diaper made from cornstarch-based material rather than plastic; it is not chlorine bleached and contains no perfume.

- **Seventh Generation** (www.seventhgeneration.com), a wood-pulp diaper that relies on absorbent polymer (gel) to keep babies dry and reduce diaper rash; baby wipes are disposable but fragrance free, and come with a reusable dispenser so all you need to do is replace the wipes, not the entire container. Training pants incorporate the same wood-pulp and polymer technology.

- **Tendercare** (www.tendercarediapers.com), Another wood-pulp diaper with a clothlike cover that's latex and perfume free.

- **Tushies** (www.tushies.com), made from wood pulp blended with cotton to increase absorbency; no gel, latex, perfume, or dye; wipes, which do not contain polluting parabens or propylene glycol, are either fragrance free or scented with aloe vera, chamomile, and vitamin E.

While we're on the topic . . .

Baby Bee Diaper Ointment (www.burtsbees.com), a Burt's Bees product, relies on chamomile, vitamins A and E, and almond oil to protect your baby from diaper rash.

Motherlove Diaper Rash and Thrush Cream (http://motherlove.com/product_diaper_rash_relief.php), a salve for diaper rash; also claims to be effective on yeast-infected nursing nipples. Ingredients include myrrh, Oregon grape root, calendula, yarrow, olive oil, and beeswax).

Keep Baby Clean—Not Sanitized

Chapter 3 extensively reviews the concerns that have been raised regarding exposing children as well as adults to the many unregulated chemicals that are often found in shampoo, soap, lotion, and other personal-care products. Children are particularly at risk because their immature organs and immune systems make them more susceptible to the accumulated impacts chemicals can have on development, learning, and, long term, cancer and other serious health issues.

This is one area where uniform and meaningful environmental standards would encourage manufacturers to meet the highest possible bar for producing safe products that will not endanger kids. But with no such standards on the horizon, your best bet is to take the following sensible precautions:

- **Limit the number of products you use on your kids.** Babies and toddlers do not need powder, body lotion, perfume, moisturizer, makeup of any kind, nail polish, body wash, or body spritzers—even if they are made from "natural" ingredients. Most very young children need only some gentle soap and water, possibly some shampoo, and some kind of ointment to help prevent diaper rash.
- **Choose personal-care products that have the fewest, and safest, ingredients.** See Chapter 3 for specific recommendations.
- **Limit or avoid products that contain fragrance, phthalates, parabens, and triclosan or other antibacterial agents.** Choose shampoo, soap, baby wipes, diapers, toothpaste, ointment, and skin cream with no fragrance or antibacterials added.
- **Prioritize your spending.** Shift money away from personal-care products kids don't need into organic cotton clothing, organic food, or other eco-items that benefit both baby and the planet.

You can find more safe personal-care product recommendations for children as well as adults at www.biggreenpurse.com (search: babies and kids).

Focus on Food

One of the main ways kids are exposed to pesticides is through the food they eat. According to the EPA's "Guidelines for Carcinogen Risk Assessment," children receive 50 percent of their lifetime cancer risks during the first two years of life. Since as many as four hundred chemicals can be used in conventional farming to control weeds and kill insects, it's not surprising that as much as half of conventionally grown produce contains measurable toxic residues. Kids ages two to four have higher pesticide residues concentrated in their blood if they eat conventionally farmed fruits and vegetables than do kids who eat organically, so diet clearly makes a difference, says organic food expert Lisa Barnes on her website (www.petitappetit.com). A University of Washington study of pesticide breakdown products (metabolites) in preschool-aged children found that those eating organic fruits and vegetables had concentrations of pesticide metabolites six times lower than children eating conventional produce. The findings reinforced the warning Consumers Union has issued to parents of small children, urging them to limit or avoid conventionally grown foods known to have high pesticide residues such as green beans, pears, strawberries, and tomatoes grown in Mexico.

What can you do?

- **Feed your kids organic produce and dairy products.** Chapter 6 lists fruits and vegetables that are most important to buy organically.
- **Grow your own organic produce.** Chapter 9 offers tips on how to cultivate a pesticide-free garden.
- **Make your own baby food from organic produce you grow or buy.** Get ideas from *The Petit Appetit Cookbook: Easy Organic Recipes to Nurture Your Baby and Toddler*, by Lisa Barnes (www.petitappetit.com).

Start with Breast Milk

Even though you've probably heard that breast milk contains harmful chemicals, pediatricians and health professionals agree that breast milk is best for a newborn baby and growing infant. Dr. Sandra Steingraber, Ph.D., biologist, mother, and author of *Having Faith: An Ecologist's Journey to Motherhood,* notes that "breast milk is not just food. It is also medicine. It swarms with antibodies and white blood cells drawn from your own body. By drinking it, your infant comes to share your immune system."

Your child also benefits mightily from it, says Dr. Steingraber. Breast-fed infants:

- have lower rates of hospitalization and death;
- develop fewer respiratory infections, gastrointestinal infections, urinary tract infections, ear infections, and meningitis;
- succumb less often to sudden infant death syndrome; and
- produce more antibodies in response to immunizations.

Studies also consistently show that children who are breast-fed as infants:

- suffer less from allergies, asthma, diabetes, colitis, and rheumatoid arthritis;
- have higher IQ scores; and
- are less likely to develop obesity and cancer.

Breast-feeding is good for you, too. If you nurse after giving birth, notes Dr. Steingraber, you will:

- bleed less after childbirth;
- lose less blood during the chaotic days of early motherhood, because breast-feeding suppresses menstruation;
- be at lower risk for hip fracture after menopause; and
- experience lower rates of ovarian and breast cancer.

I nursed my son for eight months, and my daughter for almost eleven. In both cases, apart from the wonderful bond I developed with my kids, breast-feeding made it remarkably easy to lose the extra weight I'd gained during both pregnancies.

That being said, I did worry about chemical contamination in my breast milk. As startling as it may seem, breast milk carries concentrations of organochlorine pollutants, like dioxin, PCBs, and DDT, that are ten to twenty times higher than those in cow's milk. Children who were breast-fed as babies have higher levels of chemical contaminants in their bodies than those who were formula-fed. DDT and PCBs remain the most widespread contaminants in human milk worldwide, notes Dr. Steingraber, but flame retardants, pesticides, wood preservatives, toilet deodorizers, and dry-cleaning fluids lurk there as well.

Given these risks and benefits, what can you do to provide your baby with the best nutrition possible?

- **Breast-feed.** Breast milk is still the most nutritious food for your baby.
- **Avoid home and garden pesticides** before, during, and after your pregnancy. These chemicals can easily find their way into your body when you breathe or through your skin. They can get into your milk while you are nursing.
- **Eat healthy.** Favor a low-fat, organic diet high in fruits, vegetables, and safe fish. (avoid tuna steaks, sea bass, oysters from the Gulf Coast, marlin, halibut, pike, walleye, white croaker, and largemouth bass). See Chapter 6 for more healthy eating suggestions.
- **Avoid cleaning chemicals and fumes.** That includes dry-cleaning fumes, solvents from paints and finishes, glues, and other building products.

 thumbs up

Making Our Milk Safe

To mobilize women to protect their breast milk from harmful chemicals, four friends founded Making Our Milk Safe—MOMS (www.safemilk.org). The California-based organization, which has more than three hundred members in twenty-eight states, works to educate new moms and pregnant women while trying to change corporate practices that expose women to dangerous toxins. "There should be nothing more basic than a mother's right to provide clean and healthy breast milk for her child," says cofounder Mary Brune. "Nobody wants their kids exposed to toxic chemicals. This is a human issue—something we all, as parents, are confronted with."

Organic Formulas

If you want or need to use formula, you have at least two organic options:

- **Earth's Best** (www.earthsbest.com/products/infant-formula.php) soy and dairy products are made without the use of growth hormones, steroids, antibiotics, pesticides, or chemical fertilizers.
- **Similac Organic Infant Formula** (abbottnutrition.com/products/products.aspx?pid=223) is an organic, milk-based, iron-fortified infant formula marketed as a supplement or alternative to breast-feeding.

Baby Bottles

Debate is growing about whether dangerous chemicals leach from plastic baby bottles into the breast milk or formula they contain. The State of California has banned toys and baby products containing more than trace amounts of plastic-softening phthalates. The Consumer Product Safety Commission has urged parents to make sure that the soft vinyl teethers and toys their babies chew or suck are not made from PVC plastic, which also contain the toxins. What else do you need to know about baby bottles to help keep your children safe?

Bisphenol A (BPA) is an industrial chemical used to make polycarbonate plastic, the key ingredient in clear, shiny baby bottles and many other plastic products. When heated or stressed, BPA can leach out of the bottle and into the breastmilk or formula it contains. Research indicates that at very low levels, BPA can disrupt normal hormone function, cause hyperactivity, impair learning, and affect the onset of puberty, among other health problems.

Research conducted by Case Western Reserve Medical School shows that very low doses of BPA can have measurable health effects. In its own study, *Consumer Reports* scientists bought six different bottles and heated plastic from each in simulated infant formula. The plastic from each of the bottles leached BPA into the test formula. Based on testing with an intact bottle, *Consumer Reports* calculated that babies who used the bottles they tested could be exposed to a BPA dose forty times higher than what is conservatively defined as safe.

The Children's Health Environmental Coalition recommends the following precautions:

- **Avoid polycarbonate plastic containers.** They are generally clear and rigid, and may have the recycling symbol 7 marked on the bottom.

- Select bottles made of tempered glass or nonleaching polyethylene or polypropylene (recycling symbols 1, 2, or 5).
- **Do not heat breast milk and infant formula in plastic.** Dangerous chemicals are more likely to leach when plastic is heated.
- **Discard scratched plastic bottles.** They may host unhealthy bacteria.
- **Avoid plastic bottles that are decorated on the inside.** The printing can leach into the formula when heated.
- **Discard cracked or chipped glass bottles.**
- **Avoid disposable nursers.** The plastic bags may leak or burst, and babies risk choking on the plastic tab inside.

 make the shift

Safe Baby Bottles

The following baby bottles do not contain BPA or PVC plastic:

Born Free Natural Baby Products (www.newbornfree.com/catalog.aspx), available at Whole Foods, Toys Я Us, and Babies Я Us, include safe plastic baby bottles in small and large sizes, sippy cups, and trainer cups.

EvenFlo (www.evenflo.com) makes glass bottles in varying sizes with latex nipples.

Baby Food

Even though you may want your baby to eat organic food, there's not a lot of choice at the grocery store. The two brands you're likely to see:

- **Earth's Best** (www.earthsbest.com/) offers cereals, single-ingredient fruits and vegetables, frozen foods, and organic teething biscuits.
- **Healthy Times** (www.healthytimes.com/hthome.htm) includes single ingredients, fruit and vegetable blends, dinners, and cereals.

Given the limited options as well as their premium price, you may decide to make your own:

- Steam the same organic fruits and vegetables you'd serve yourself: pumpkin, squash, peas, carrots, apples, plums, beans, and more.

- Use a blender or food mill to puree the food to the consistency your child can easily eat and digest.
- Refrigerate or freeze extra servings to save preparation time on future meals.

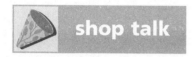

Baby Talk

To capitalize on consumers' growing interest in healthy, pesticide-free food, many stores are producing their own "natural" and organic brands. Urge your store manager to talk to headquarters about expanding the store's line to include baby food. Begin talking to the manager when you're pregnant and continue asking for organic options after your baby is born. If your store doesn't stock any organic infant food, suggest they order national brands, like Earth's Best and Healthy Times.

What's for Lunch?

Before you restock the food you pack in your child's lunch, you may want to replace the lunch box itself.

Research commissioned by the Center for Environmental Health (CEH) in Oakland, California, showed that the lining in some kids' lunch boxes contained high levels of lead, a toxin that hinders brain development and can cause behavioral and other developmental disorders. Children may be exposed to lead in lunch boxes if they eat food that's been carried in them or if they handle the boxes and then put their hands in their mouths.

Since you can't tell by looking whether a lunch box contains lead, the CEH recommends avoiding vinyl lunch boxes altogether. You can test any vinyl lunch boxes you already own using a handheld lead-testing kit. If your hardware store doesn't carry one, you can order one from LeadCheck (www.leadcheck.com).

If the box tests positive, contact the CEH toll-free at 800-652-0827. The organization will help you interpret the results and may also use your product as evidence in its campaign to get the lead out of kids' lunch boxes.

To date, CEH has only tested soft plastic lunch boxes. Brands that have tested high include Generation Sports, Frozn/Ingear, Roundhouse/Targus, Crayola, American Studio, Igloo, Sanford, Fast Forward, Arizona Jean Company, JCPenney, Lisa Frank, Animations/Accessory Network, Holiday Fair/Mischief

Makers, Extreme Gear/Romar, SubZero/Global Advantage, Chill, Big Dogs, Childress baby bottle carriers, Innovo, and East End Accessories/Worldwide Dreams. Not all lunch boxes with these brand names necessarily contain lead, so test to be sure.

 make the shift

Avoid the Lunch Box Blues

- Reusablebags.com (www.reusablebags.com) sells organic and regular cotton bags, "Lunchbugs" cloth lunch bags, Earthpak bags made from recycled soda bottles, and Cool Totes insulated lunch bags, among many other styles.
- World of Good (www.worldofgood.com) offers a handwoven reed lunch box and is committed to fair trade.
- Mimi the Sardine (www.mimithesardine.com/bags/) sports fun, vinyl-free waterproof Lunchbugs online and in Whole Foods stores in the Northwest and Southwest.
- Progressive Kid (www.progressivekid.com/shop) offers Earthpak bags made from "upcycled" two-liter plastic bottles.
- Laptop Lunches (www.laptoplunches.com) makes a bento box sectioned off to hold fruit, cookies, a sandwich, and a drink so you don't need to use plastic baggies or sandwich wraps, helping reduce the sixty pounds of trash a year that one child's lunches create.

Other Lunch Box Tips

Once you make the right lunch box choice, choose to minimize trash. Include:

- Cloth napkin and reusable utensils
- Reusable sandwich holders rather than throwaway wraps
- Whole fruits without packaging
- Reusable drink containers rather than juice boxes or water bottles
- Snacks purchased in bulk and divvied up in reusable containers

big green purse

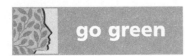

Snack Attack

Prepackaged organic snack food can be just as high in sugar and fat and create just as much trash as conventional snacks. When you're putting food together for the kids, consider these mindful munchies:

- Organic whole fruit
- Dried fruit (raisins, cranberries, apricots)
- Nuts (dry roasted, lightly salted)
- Nut butters made without sugar
- Whole-grain breads and crackers
- Pita bread and hummus
- Fresh vegetable slices dipped in hummus or yogurt lightly flavored with honey
- Fresh fruit slices dipped in vanilla yogurt
- Milk and soy yogurts mixed with fresh fruit and low-fat granolas and cereals
- Smoothies blended from vanilla yogurt, fresh fruit, and juice

Microwave Popcorn

These are sorry times for popcorn lovers. First, we were warned off microwave popcorn because the bag was contaminated with PFOA, the same chemical that makes Teflon pans slippery. Then diacetyl, which gives microwave popcorn its buttery taste, was blamed for causing bronchiolitis obliterans, or "popcorn lung." Several brands, including Orville Redenbacher, Act II, Pop Secret, and Jolly Time, are removing diacetyl from their manufacturing process, but the change is expected to take several months to a year. To be on the safe side:

- **Make popcorn the old-fashioned way:** put a little oil in a pot, cover the bottom with one layer of kernels, and heat until all the kernels have popped.
- **For a healthier alternative, use an air popper,** available online or at a local big-box store; it's inexpensive and safe for kids to use.

- **Make your own microwave popcorn.** Put one-quarter cup popping corn in a brown paper bag. Fold the bag over three times. Microwave on the popcorn setting.

Skip Canned Foods if You Can

It pains me to say this, because canned food has come to my rescue so many times. But it turns out that cans that serve up food also serve up unhealthy amounts of bisphenol A, the same ingredient that makes baby bottles unsafe. Pastas and soups contain the highest levels, though beverages (soft drinks, juices) have their fair share, too. When you have the choice, pick foods packaged in glass, or even in a box. Better yet, cook from scratch.

For more healthful food ideas, see Chapter 6.

Keep Toys Safe

Even before millions of Chinese-made toys were recalled because they were decorated with toxic lead paint, Environment California, a research and policy center, had released a report showing that products designed for babies and young children contain chemicals that have been linked to worrisome health problems. Those problems include the early onset of puberty, impaired learning development, reproductive defects, and cancer. One study tested soft plastic teethers, bath accessories, and other children's gear for phthalates (pronounced THA-LATES). Another tested changing pads, mattresses, and various sleep accessories for flame retardants. Toxic chemicals were found in most of the baby products examined.

Unfortunately, since manufacturers do not have to reveal whether their products contain dangerous ingredients, you have no way of knowing what poses a hidden hazard. Even if a toy or piece of equipment reveals it "contains phthalates" or is "treated with flame retardant," there is no "safe dose" for kids. Growing evidence indicates that low doses of many of these chemicals can cause ill effects. Ongoing exposure from multiple sources could become significant.

There is also the question of how toys are powered. Millions of kids' toys require batteries. While they may not pose an immediate health threat, batteries contain heavy metals like mercury, lead, cadmium, and nickel. The alkaline and button batteries used in most toys are the single largest source of mercury in our trash. If a child happens to swallow a button battery, she can become fatally ill.

Arts and crafts supplies can contain toxic substances that warrant vigilance, too. Dust, vapor, gas, and the aerosol from art supplies can easily infiltrate a young body if kids and parents aren't careful.

Despite these challenges, plenty of safe and healthy games, dolls, blocks, and figurines abound to entertain the children in your life. Here's a quick guide:

- **Look for PVC- and phthalate-free plastics,** like blocks from Brio, Ikea, and Lego.
- **Buy solid wood toys,** unfinished or finished with linseed, walnut, or other natural oil.
- **Use beeswax** instead of clays and colored doughs.
- **Purchase from local toy manufacturers** who can certify that they followed U.S. environmental, health, and safety regulations during toy manufacture.

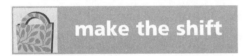

Toys You Can Trust

EcoMall (www.ecomall.com/biz/toys.htm) directs you to dozens of companies that sell a wide variety of toys and clothes for babies and toddlers made from organic cotton and untreated wood.

- **The Art & Creative Materials Institute** (www.acminet.org/) offers a catalog of arts and craft supplies that minimize indoor air pollution.
- **The Discovery Channel Store** (http://shopping.discovery.com) has toys, books, and a variety of nature-oriented amusements for kids and adults alike.
- **The Natural Baby Catalog** (http://naturalbaby.stores.yahoo.net/toys.html) features puzzles, pull toys, musical instruments, beeswax crayons and modeling clay, weaving looms, and wooden play sets.
- **Pristine Planet** (www.pristineplanet.com) sells wooden puzzles, solar-powered robots, and board books from the Golden Gate National Park Conservancy.

Toy Story

It's great to see a child enjoying a toy she loves. On the other hand, many kids have far more toys than they can play with during any reasonable period of time. The frenzy to fuel youngsters' desire for even more toys gets particularly intense around the Christmas holidays, when almost half of all kid-targeted novelties, games, and gadgets are sold. It's no accident that children through age fourteen influence $160 billion in spending in November and December, says James McNeal, author of *The Kids Market: Myths and Realities.* Companies like Mattel spend half their multimillion-dollar marketing budgets in the last three months of the year hyping toys they want tots to get their parents to buy.

How can you keep the lid on your kid's toy box?

- **Limit TV time.** Most child-targeted ads appear on NBC, ABC, CBS, Fox, CW, Nickelodeon, and Cartoon Network. Limit TV time from October 1 through December 31 (see "Connect with Nature," pages 283–84) to reduce pressure kids feel to demand toys they don't really need and probably don't really want.
- **Suggest alternatives.** Encourage friends and family to give nontoys: tickets to events, outings to special places, gift certificates to kid-friendly restaurants, savings bonds.
- **Donate what you have.** Before the holidays, have your kids clean out their toy chests and donate dolls, games, books, action figures, puzzles, and other playthings to charity.

Educate and Engage

Someday, when that little bundle of joy in your arms grows up, she may decide she wants to save the world. If she does, she'll have plenty of company, given the many student environmental organizations she can join.

High School Groups and Opportunities

Earth Day Network (www.earthday.net) coordinates worldwide Earth Day activities around the annual April 22 holiday, plus organizing other events and campaigns.

Ecology.com (www.ecology.com) provides links to global environmental issues, scientific research, school ecology clubs, environmentally related books, and other useful sites on the Web.

EcologyFund.com (www.ecologyfund.com/registry/ecology/res_student_links .html) provides links to student organizations, job listings, lesson plans for teachers, and student-oriented lifestyle tips.

Envirolink (www.envirolink.org) promotes a sustainable society by connecting individuals and organizations through new communications technologies. The site is a clearinghouse of environmental information, organizations, educational and government resources, publications, actions you can take, an environmental newsletter, and links to other environmental resources.

Environmentors (www.ncseonline.org/EnvironMentors), a project of the National Council for Science and the Environment, matches environmental professionals as mentors with high school students. The teams develop research projects. Students also participate in college prep courses, paid internships, and other environmental enrichment activities.

Free the Planet (www.freetheplanet.org) works to expand and strengthen the student environmental movement, provide resources for student activists, and work with students to win campaigns for strong environmental protections on such issues as forest protection, safe personal-care products, climate change, and sustainable college campuses.

Green Corps (www.greencorps.org) trains young people in grassroots environmental organizing and builds partnerships with environmental groups around conservation, corporate accountability, and public health issues.

National Wildlife Federation's Campus Ecology Program (www.nwf.org/campusecology/index.cfm) strives to help colleges and universities confront global warming through climate and wildlife-friendly practices that reduce their global footprint.

Oikos International, Students for Sustainable Economics and Management (www.oikosinternational.org) encourages business and economics students to gain an appreciation for environmental sustainability. While there are no local chapters in the United States, interested Americans can participate in the program when they travel abroad.

Public Interest Research Groups (PIRGs) (www.studentpirgs.org), independent state-based student organizations, work to solve public interest problems related to the environment, consumer protection, and government reform. The groups tackle global warming, mass transit, wetlands development, energy, and a wide variety of other local, state, and national environmental issues.

Sierra Student Coalition (www.ssc.org), the student arm of the Sierra Club, networks with high school and college students in 250 affiliated groups across the United States to protect the environment.

Sierra Youth Coalition (www.syc-cjs.org) is a Canadian environmental organization run by youth for youth, serving as the youth arm of the Sierra Club of Canada.

The Student Conservation Association (SCA) (www.sca-inc.org) offers conservation internships and summer trail crew opportunities to more than 3,000 people each year. The SCA focuses on developing conservation and community leaders while building hiking trails, protecting threatened habitats, and more.

Student Environmental Action Coalition (www.seac.org) includes hundreds of junior high school, high school, college, and community groups throughout the United States and Canada working on a wide variety of environmental campaigns.

SustainUS (www.sustainus.org), whose members range in age from fourteen to thirty, promotes sustainable development in schools and communities.

Teen Environmental Media Network (TEMN) (www.earthnewsradio.org) strives to train the next generation of environmental journalists through hands-on experience. Students select topics, research story ideas, and interview news sources.

College Curricula

If your child decides to study environmental affairs in college, she'll have plenty of wonderful programs to choose from:

Aquinas College (Michigan) offers business and environmental studies at the school's Center for Sustainability, and an undergraduate major in sustainable business.

Associated Colleges of the South Environmental Alliance (www.colleges.org/%7Enviro/alliances/sde_alliance.html) lists courses, majors and minors, and specific environmental programs on almost twenty college campuses based in the South.

California State University, Chico won the 2007 National Wildlife Federation's Chill Out competition for finding the most effective ways of all college campuses to fight global warming. The campus promotes environmental sustainability through education programs, while certifying buildings to meet green standards and installing rooftop solar collectors.

College of the Atlantic (Maine) offers one major, which focuses on human ecology. It was the first college in the United States to pledge to neutralize its carbon emissions, launching the American College & University Presidents Climate Commitment.

The Evergreen State College (Washington State) provides the produce for the campus food service from the school's organic farm; composts its organic waste; and purchases 100 percent of its power from green sources.

Green Mountain College (Vermont) bills itself as "Vermont's environmental liberal arts college," makes the environment a core part of its curriculum, and taps methane from local dairy farms to generate half the school's electricity.

Harvard University (Massachusetts) invests in energy conservation, uses green cleaning services, and provides organic and local produce in school cafeterias. Biodiesel is being made from kitchen oil for use in university buses, and almost two dozen building projects are going green.

Middlebury College (Vermont) is another carbon-neutral school where students host energy-saving contests in residence halls, promote use of public transportation, and turn down campus thermostats.

Oberlin College (Ohio) runs a car-sharing program on campus, has established a Center for Environmental Studies, maintains Ohio's largest solar panel array, and is aiming to use all earth-friendly cleaning products.

Stanford University (California) is where students can conduct climate and energy research, starting at the school's Global Ecology Research Center.

Tufts University (Massachusetts) was the first university to join the Chicago Climate Exchange and has won an award from the EPA for its climate initiatives.

University of Michigan, the School of Natural Resources and Environment, my alma mater, helped launch the environmental justice movement and continues to be a leader in environmental education and communication. The school's Center for Sustainable Systems weds engineering and environmental analysis to improve industrial processes for societal needs. The Environmental Justice Initiative addresses inequities arising from environmental, social, and political decision making. The Erb Institute for Global Sustainable Enterprise studies the environmental intersection of business, government, and nonprofit organizations and collaborates with students in a joint MS/MBA program. The Minority Environmental

Leadership Development Initiative works to increase the number of minorities hired in professional environmental positions. A master's degree in behavior, education, and communication can also be earned.

University of New Hampshire's thirty-acre organic dairy farm helps educate future sustainable farmers, while the institution's WildCAP program discounts student purchases of Energy Star computers and other energy-efficient items.

Yale University (Connecticut) intends to cut its greenhouse gas emissions 10 percent by the year 2020 by using renewable energy, buying carbon offsets, improving energy efficiency, and building greener buildings.

Other Don't-Miss Schools: University of California, Berkeley; Williams College; Dartmouth College; Illinois State University; University of California, Davis.

As for school gear, you can find earth-friendly ideas on backpacks and school supplies appropriate to kids of all ages at www.biggreenpurse; search "Back to School."

Where to Shop

Babies, toddlers, and kids have never had so much ecogear to choose from. These sites give you an idea of what's available.

Clothing

By law, fire-resistant and flame-retardant chemicals like PBDEs must be applied to infants' and children's sleepwear and mattresses. PBDEs have accumulated at alarmingly high levels in Americans' blood and breast milk. Health professionals are concerned that PBDEs may harm the developing fetus and breast-feeding infants and cause additional developmental disorders in young children. You should take precautions to ensure that your home is fire safe, such as installing fire alarms and fire extinguishers. You can also choose not to put your kids to bed in conventional pajamas that may have been treated with PBDEs.

All Natural Baby Clothes (http://allnaturalbaby.com/shop/natural-cleaning-product.asp) offers organic, cotton baby clothes and matching bedsheets made from cotton along with baby mattresses and a range of other nontoxic and practical items for the nursery or kitchen. Traditional styles.

Awakening Organics (www.awakeningorganics.com) specializes in a small, stylish line of organic cotton clothes in low-impact dyes for babies and young toddlers. Pants are either wide-leg, boot cut, or yoga style.

Baby Wit (www.babywit.com) sells organic cotton novelty clothes for babies and toddlers sporting punk, rock, political, and pop culture motifs designed to reflect their parents' taste and humor.

Bamboosa (www.bamboosa.com) sells soft, protective, natural bamboo clothing for women, men, and baby; includes tees, tank tops, long-sleeved jerseys, sleep slips, yoga pants, men's tees, and baby clothes.

Essere Organics (www.essereorganics.com) carries affordable organic baby clothes as well as bedding, towels, and other items for the whole family. Most of Essere's offerings are imported.

Green Babies (www.greenbabies.com) specializes in organic cotton clothing for newborns through age seven, as well as for boys and girls.

Hae Now (www.haenow.com) specializes in affordable, organic cotton tee shirts for infants, children, and adults. The cotton is grown in India without child labor under conditions that adhere to international standards of fair wages, work benefits, and environmental conditions. They are certified by Skal of Netherlands and only use nonchlorine bleaches and low-impact, azo-free reactive dyes for their vibrant colors.

Hanna Andersson (www.hannaandersson.com) sells cotton clothes for the whole family including a strong line of children's clothes. More than 50 percent of their Hanna products are now organic and carry the European certification Öko-Tex Standard 100.

Kidbean (www.kidbean.com) carries organic hemp or cotton infant and children's clothes up to size 12 as well as recycled and eco-friendly fleece outerwear; shirts; a broad range of diapers; and bedding (for adults as well), along with wooden play kitchens and a range of cooperative games and bath products.

Lapsaky Organic Cotton Baby and Children's Clothes (www.lapsaky.com) sells infant and toddler clothes (up to size 6X) online and through retail outlets that can be found through its website. Baby blankets and shopping bags are also offered.

Nature's Crib (www.naturescrib.com) features a range of organic cotton clothes for toddlers up to twenty-four months, as well as bedding, diapers, bibs, natural toys, wood furniture, and personal-care products for pregnant and nursing mothers.

Ohgeez Organic Clothing Co. (www.ohgeezorganic.com) offers American-made organic, versatile cotton clothing in sizes up to 8X. Clothes are practical and usually come in gray, brown, and other natural colors. Flannel sheet sets for children, receiving blankets, and washcloths are also available.

Patagonia (www.patagonia.com) retails outerwear and other casual and outdoor clothing for the whole family in organic and environmentally friendly fabrics including fleeces. In addition to purchasing items online, consumers can locate retailers on the website.

Sweetgrass Natural Fibers (www.sweetgrassfibers.com) offers hemp-based women's tops, pants, skirts, dresses; men's tops, pants; baby and kid clothes; and a bargain bin.

Susie Jane Organics, Inc. (SJO) (www.susiejane.com), is a boutique for clothes made from organic Peruvian pima, Egyptian cotton, and a few alpaca items. Some of the brands carried are speesees, Sckoon, Sweet Cottons, Oeuf, and Under the Nile—infant and toddler sizes only. Other products offered include wooden furniture, books, and games.

Bedding

You can buy PBDE-free mattresses that still satisfy fire-retardancy regulations (which require that a mattress resist both cigarette burns and an open flame). Look for organic cotton mattresses wrapped in flame-retardant wool whose labels say they meet the U.S. Consumer Product Safety Commission's (CPSC) and California's flammability-resistance standards.

The Clean Bedroom (www.thecleanbedroom.com) sells organic cotton sheets, bedding, mattresses, cribs, and beds for babies, young children, and adults, plus Hepa air cleaners and air filters.

Crib Organic Chemical-Free Mattresses (www.nontoxic.com/beds/crib.html) features organic cotton and organically grown wool mattresses, plus organic flannel, percale, or sateen sheets.

Ecobaby Bedding (http://ecobaby.com/cribmattresses.htm) includes organic cotton and wool crib mattresses with spring and rubber cores, plus mattress pads, comforters, sheets, and bumpers.

Kate Quinn Organics (www.katequinnorganics.com) offers fitted crib sheets, receiving and hooded blankets, and larger Sherpa blankets.

The Natural Baby Catalog (http://naturalbaby.stores.yahoo.net/bedding.html) markets receiving blankets, thermal baby blankets, flannel blankets, fitted cotton crib sheets, wool mattress pads, and cotton and wool pillows.

Furniture

Most conventional paints and finishes, even those used on baby furniture, contain toxic chemicals that your child could end up eating if she gnaws on the crib edge or inhaling as fumes from chemicals that "offgas" over time. When shopping, avoid cribs, bureaus, changing tables, and shelves made with laminated wood, pressed wood, chipboard, or particle board, any of which could emit formaldehyde and fumes from the glue and chemicals that hold the wood together. Instead, choose solid hardwood furniture protected with low-VOC paints or finishes, or buy unfinished hardwood furniture and treat it yourself with a safer, water-based polyurethane sealer.

American Solid Wood Crib (www.anaturalhome.com/product/A111 AMER/) is available in oak or ash with a tung-oil finish, comes with a matching changing table, and coordinates with a bookcase and dresser.

Argington (www.argington.com) inspires with safe but whimsical toy boxes, chairs, rockers, play tables, dressers, changing tables, and beds.

Celery Furniture (www.2modern.com/designer/Celery) features formaldehyde-free and bamboo cribs, changing tables, rocking chairs, and cradles.

Lilipadstudio (www.lilipadstudio.com) fabricates stools, tables, and chairs for toddlers from solid wood, then handpaints with nontoxic paints.

Natural Bassinet (www.ecobedroom.com/shop/bedding/baby.html) includes organic cotton and wool baby futons, liners, and covers, for babies up to twenty pounds.

Soaring Heart (www.soaringheart.com) offers for infants a handmade solid wood crib, and for older children, a "big bed" either as a solo bed, or with space to spare as designed by the versatile Four-in-One Sleep System.

Solid Pacific Coast Maple Crib (http://ecobaby.com/cribs.htm) comes in several designs, all finished with beeswax and tung oil.

Miscellaneous Accessories

Bibs

Look for organic cotton bibs at www.katequinnorganics.com, www.ourgreenhouse.com, and www.taraluna.com.

Strollers

Baby Planet (www.baby-planet.com) lets you recycle a stroller purchased there when you're finished with it; you can also donate any brand stroller to a family in need.

Teethers

Under the Nile (www.underthenile.com/underthenile/index.php) features 100 percent organic cotton teething rings, toys, and "teething veggies" for phthalate-free gum relief.

Toys

The following websites link to fun, nontoxic toys, games, stuffed animals, and arts and crafts.

Eco Fabulous (www.ecofabulous.com)
Great Green Baby (www.greatgreenbaby.com)
Honeysuckle Dreams (www.honeysuckledreams.com)
Maple Landmark Toys (www.maplelandmark.com)
Natural Pod (http://naturalpod.com)
Progressive Kid (www.progressivekid.com)
Sage Baby (www.sagebabynyc.com/SearchResults.asp?Cat=87&es=6)
Whittle Shortline Railroad (www.woodentrain.com)

Some specifics:

Baby Bunz (www.babybunz.com/shopping/category.php?mode=index& catid=9) has race cars, teething toys, rattles, dolls, rainbow cones, beads, and blocks made from nontoxic plastics and wood.

Green Toys (www.greentoys.com) includes tea sets, sand toys, cookware, and dining sets made from bioplastic, a corn and starch resin.

Holgate Toys (www.holgatetoy.com) sells color cones, lacing beads, Bingo bed, stools, and finger puppets.

Hugg-A-Planet (www.huggaplanet.com/index.html) has colorful cloth balls big enough to hug imprinted with the continents and other images.

ImagiPlay (www.imagiplay.com) features cardboard blocks, Noah's ark, African safari animals, and "Zoom to the Moon" portable rocket ship.

Natural Pod (http://naturalpod.com) has wooden bikes and toys, musical instruments, arts and crafts, children's jewelry, and "imaginative play" silks and shapes.

Nova Natural Toys & Crafts (www.novanatural.com) includes dollhouses, arts and crafts, wooden figures, castles and ramps, boats, chalk, and wooden kitchens.

NunoOrganic (www.nunoorganic.com) features organic cotton teddy bears, non-toxic crayons and paints, wooden cars, games, and jigsaw puzzles.

Peapods (www.peapods.com) has alphabet blocks, wooden cameras, art easels, and games.

Want to know more? Visit the toys page at www.biggreenpurse.com (search: toys).

If you still have Barbie, Batman, or Dora the Explorer, go to www.mattel.com/safety/us/ to make sure you've returned any toys that may pose a lead hazard to your child. You can buy a testing kit from leadcheck.com to test other toys and games. LeadCheck Swabs are nonhazardous and provide a rapid, sensitive, and specific test for leachable lead on toys. While you're at it, you can test wall paint, ceramics, vinyl lunch boxes, and miniblinds, too—all products that occasionally are contaminated with lead.

Kid Stuff Wrap-up

- **Simplify.** Set expectations for clothes, toys, and gear your child "needs" based on a realistic understanding of what she can actually use.
- **Redefine "new."** Meet needs for new items by sharing, swapping, and buying used from thrift shops, yard sales, www.freecycle.com, and www.craigslist.com.
- **Breast-feed your children.**
- **Be safe.** Switch to baby bottles, teethers, and toys free of PVC, pthalates, bisphenol A, and lead.
- **Skip canned food.** Choose fresh or frozen organic fruits and vegetables.
- **Dress your kids in organic cotton.** Look for hemp and recycled polyester, too.
- **Avoid PBDEs (fire retardants).** Use organic cotton sheets, and organic cotton and wool mattresses if possible.

And if you can do only one thing, keep your kids connected to nature. Picnic, walk, hike, bike, bird-watch, draw, stargaze, swim, or just sit and look up at the sky.

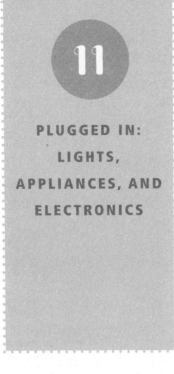

11

PLUGGED IN:
LIGHTS,
APPLIANCES, AND
ELECTRONICS

FROM THE MINUTE WE GET UP IN THE MORNING UNTIL THE MOMENT WE GO to bed, we depend on energy to maintain our busy schedules. Just flick a switch or push a button. Alarm clocks and coffeepots buzz to life. Toasters and TVs feed us body and (occasionally) brain. Hair dryers and dishwashers whir, computers and Cuisinarts stir.

It's so easy we probably aren't even aware that we're using energy, let alone how it affects the planet. Take electricity. Creating kilowatts is the leading cause of industrial air pollution in the United States. Most of our electricity comes from coal, and it leaves its mark not only on our well-lit households, but also in the smog, soot, acid rain, particulate matter, and other air pollutants that cause asthma and have been linked to increased heart disease among women. When we shift to power-saving strategies at home, we're standing up for cleaner air and our right to breathe it.

Abating electricity demand also helps moderate global warming. U.S. households produce 21 percent of the country's global-warming pollution. That's more than the entire heat-trapping output of the United Kingdom, according to Phillips Electronics and Environmental Defense. Eighty to 85 percent of the total energy

317

a building consumes—and the carbon dioxide it emits—comes from meeting our needs for heating, cooling, ventilation, and hot-water use, notes a study by the World Business Council for Sustainable Development.

You can reduce your emissions by up to two-thirds by taking advantage of the lifestyle suggestions and shopping options this chapter suggests. In fact, if every household in the United States made more energy-efficient choices, we could cut annual global-warming pollution by eight hundred million tons—more than the heat-trapping emissions generated by more than one hundred countries, another analysis from Environmental Defense and Phillips Electronics. That would go a long way toward stabilizing our climate and setting an example for the rest of the world.

But as important as lifestyle and shopping shifts are, they're not enough. We also need to transform the very sources of power we tap. To reverse climate change, clean up the air, and minimize pollution, solar, wind, and biomass need to play a bigger role in our energy future. It will be a challenge. Only 2 percent of U.S. electricity is currently fueled by renewable sources. If we want a cleaner world, renewable energy must play a bigger part.

The benefits will be tangible. According to the American Lung Association, the number of deaths in the United States associated with air pollution range from 50,000 to 100,000 per year. But an EPA study found that for every dollar we have spent on pollution controls since 1970, we have gained forty-five dollars in health and environmental benefits, thanks to fewer doctor visits, fewer work days lost, fewer hospitalizations, and fewer premature deaths. According to the Worldwatch Institute, implementary climate policies that will reduce air pollution could prevent at least eight million deaths in the next two decades.

One challenge we'll all have in common as we struggle with how to control our growing energy demands will revolve around electronics. During most of my youth, which was only one generation ago, my family—two parents and five siblings— shared one telephone, one television, three radios, and one phonograph. My kids have grown up in a house wired from top to bottom to accommodate three land phones, four cell phones, two PDAs (personal digital assistants), one fax machine, a minimum of one and sometimes two computer printers, two desktop computers, two laptop computers, a variety of CD and DVD players, a VCR, two iPods, one MP3 player, and six radios (though still no PlayStation or TiVo and only one TV).

Clearly, to make a dent in energy consumption, we have to curb our enthusiasm for electronics. In so doing, we'll reduce pollution, too, since e-waste is the fastest-growing component of trash. Between 1997 and 2004, more than 315 million computers became obsolete in the United States As of 2007, at least 750 million cell phones needed recycling in America. Another 150 million will be added this year and even more next year. Once in the waste stream, these devices may leak lead, mercury, cadmium, arsenic, and other toxic substances into the water supply. Municipalities that incinerate their waste instantly propel these toxins into the air, whereupon they return to earth in rainwater. And once in our air or water, this junk is almost impossible to remove.

Because women are usually the chief executive officers of our households, we already manage lifestyle and shopping decisions to keep our families on track and our budgets in line.

But we can be the "chief environmental officers," too, setting household guidelines that make saving energy and reducing e-waste a priority. When we do, we'll free up money we can shift to appliances and services that help us live a cleaner, greener life.

The Good News

Every chapter of this book has stressed the importance of the three Rs, and this one is no exception. Even though there is a technology fix for many of our energy problems, it won't do us any good unless we curtail the amount of energy we burn overall. This chapter starts with the first R by offering simple ways you can reduce the amount of energy you use to heat and light your home and run your appliances. If you follow these tips, you'll save money you can shift into other green purchases—or put in the bank for a sunny day.

You'll also find guidance on buying energy-saving compact fluorescent lightbulbs, the new LEDs, and a kilowatt-busting thermostat. The chapter reviews developments on energy-efficient appliances generally, though for specific product recommendations, check www.biggreenpurse.com (search "appliances"). With new models being introduced every season, the website is the best place to get up-to-date information.

Because it's important to tap into renewable energy whenever possible, you'll find a rundown on green power sources as well. Though federal and state investment dollars in alternative energy are disgracefully scarce, citizens can shift their own money into those sources when they're available locally. Fortunately, in at least six hundred communities, they are. If yours is one, take advantage of it.

As for electronics, these pages reveal why your computer is considered an energy "vampire," and where to recycle old electronics when you replace them with newer, more energy-efficient models.

Whether you plug in or unplug, you can save energy around the clock. All the better if that clock is solar-powered!

Use Your Big Green Purse

Your Big Green Purse can improve the outlook for energy in several ways. By saving energy you save money giving you the resources to shift your spending to technologies that may be more expensive but that are better for your household and the planet in the long run. By creating demand for wind, solar, and biomass you reduce the need for energy generated by more-polluting coal, oil, and nuclear power. By shopping for products and services produced by companies that also save energy or use renewable power sources, you provide an incentive to all manufacturers to become more energy-efficient.

How can you get started?

- Use energy more efficiently
- Replace lights, appliances and electronics with energy savers
- Shift to renewable green power
- Recycle electronics to reduce e-waste

Use Energy More Efficiently

The number of energy-sapping appliances we use is daunting, making energy efficiency a real priority.

WHAT DO YOU USE?

__ Television

__ Telephone

__ Cell phone

__ Personal digital assistant

__ Desktop computer (hard drive, monitor)

__ Laptop computer

__ Computer peripherals

__ Printer

__ Fax machine

__ Copy machine

__ Audio/stereo equipment

__ Television   __ Freezer   __ Crock-Pot

__ DVD player   __ Stove   __ Coffeemaker

__ VCR   __ Convection oven __ Water heater

__ Wireless devices __ Microwave oven __ Clothes dryer

__ Video game consoles __ Toaster oven __ Hair dryer

__ Portable DVD player __ Clothes washer __ Iron

__ Air conditioner __ Dishwasher   __ Steamer

__ Window fan   __ Blender   __ Batteries

__ Heating system __ Food processor

__ Refrigerator   __ Toaster

thumbs down

Environmental and Health Effects of Coal-Fired Electricity Generation

Acid rain   Mercury pollution   Soot

Global warming   Respiratory illness   Water pollution

Heart disease   Smog

The average home spends almost $1,900 on energy every year. You can reduce your bill 10 to 50 percent by making several energy-smart improvements.

Plug into a power strip. Any time an appliance is plugged into an electrical socket, it uses electricity, even when it's not turned on. In fact, 40 percent of the energy used to power consumer electronics is devoured when the devices are switched off. That's nearly 5 percent of the total electricity American homes consume. We spend about a billion dollars a year just to power TVs and VCRs that are "turned off."

You're not alone if you sometimes forget to shut down your computer or flick off the DVD player when you call it a night. Even if you had the best of intentions, many electronic devices don't have power switches at all, so the only way you can stop them from using energy is to unplug them. That's where power strips save the day. They let you plug several appliances or lots of office equipment into one larger outlet that you can turn off with minimal hassle. The Smart Strip model automatically cuts power to all devices that are plugged into it, so you only need to flip one switch rather than four or five. The Isole Power Strip works in tandem with a motion sensor that automatically turns devices on when you enter a room and turns them off when you exit. It's worth considering for computer workstations, entertainment centers, or any living space where you might want to automate lighting, music, or even the morning coffeepot.

You can buy Smart and Isole power ptrips at www.environmentalhome center.com.

Check www.amazon.com or your local hardware store for other options, like the Belkin 9-Outlet SurgeMaster or Craftsman Auto Switch.

And if you want to see what electricity you're using by the day, week, month or year, you can get a read from the Kill-a-Watt Electricity Usage Monitor Meter, also available on www.amazon.com and at some hardware stores.

 Get a star. When you buy a new appliance, light, or computer, remember: it has two price tags—what you pay to take it home, and what you pay for the energy it uses. Energy Star, a joint program of the U.S. Environmental Protection Agency and the U.S. Department of Energy, helps you save money and protect the environment by alerting you to the most energy-efficient products and services in the marketplace. Consumers who have chosen Energy Star have already made a big impact. Americans using qualified products saved enough energy in 2006 alone to avoid greenhouse gas emissions equivalent to those from 25 million cars—all while saving $14 billion on their utility bills. How does the program achieve such success? Energy Star appliances use 10 to 50 percent less energy and water than standard models. Over time, the money you save on your utility bills can easily make up for the cost of a more expensive but also more efficient Energy Star model. There are hundreds of Energy Star products to choose from, including computers, printers, fax machines, cameras, air conditioners, furnaces, dishwashers, refrigerators, clothes wash-

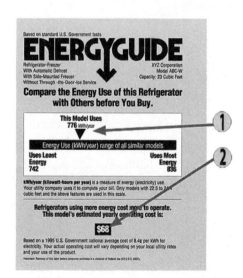

1) Estimates energy consumption on a scale showing a range for similar models.
2) Estimates yearly operating cost based on the national average cost of electricity.

How Do You Use Energy?

Heating and cooling—45%

Water heater—11%

Clothes washer and dryer—10%

Lighting—7%

Refrigerator—6%

Dishwasher—2%

Computer and monitor—2%

TV, DVD, electronics—2%

Other—15%

Source: Average Household Energy Estimates, Alliance to Save Energy.

ers and dryers, stoves, and many other home appliances. For a complete list and to locate stores where you can shop, go to www.energystar.gov.

Read the Label. The U.S. Department of Energy's Energy Guide label shows you how to compare different brands and models by providing an estimate of how much energy similar models use. The label also indicates what you can expect to pay every year to operate the appliance. Buy the most efficient model in your price range to meet your needs, remembering as you compare options that the model with the smallest kWh (kilowatts) consumption will use the least energy—and generate the least pollution.

Walk the walk. Once you buy an energy-saving appliance, make sure you take advantage of the savings it has to offer. Read the manual, visit product websites, or call the customer service hotline to answer any additional questions you have about conserving power.

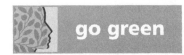

big green purse

Top Ten Ways to Save Energy (and Money) at Home

1. **Caulk or weather-strip windows and doors.** Materials for the average twelve-window, two-door house could cost about twenty-five dollars, but savings in annual energy costs might amount to more than 10 percent of your yearly heating bill. According to the Department of Energy, if every gas-heated home were properly caulked and weather-stripped, we'd save enough natural gas each year to heat almost four million more homes. Two sources of weather stripping online are M-D Building Products (www.mdteam.com) and Resource Conservation Technology (www.conservationtechnology.com). You can also find weather stripping at most hardware stores. To minimize indoor air pollution from the weather stripping materials you use, try Quick Shield VOC-Free Sealant (www.geocel usa.com).

2. **Install storm windows and doors.** Combination screen and storm windows and doors are the most convenient and energy efficient because they can be opened easily when there is no need to run heating or cooling equipment. Installing high-efficiency Energy Star windows can reduce heating and cooling costs by 15 percent annually; you can save from $125 to $340 a year when you replace single-pane windows with their Energy Star equivalents. If you don't want to buy new windows, cover existing windows with heavy-duty, clear plastic. You can buy a ready-made kit on Amazon.com. A third alternative? Thermal draperies, made with a thick, fiber-filled backing to fit snugly against the entire window frame, can reduce heat loss by as much as 50 percent and save you fifteen dollars per window each winter. Even simple heavy drapes can save about ten dollars per window annually.

3. **Insulate.** You can reduce your energy needs by as much as 20 to 30 percent and save about four months' worth of household energy by investing in insulation. Focus on your attic floor or top-floor ceiling, crawl space, exterior walls, basement ceilings and walls, and rooms over unheated spaces, like garages. The "Simply Insulate" website (www.simplyinsulate.com/savings/index.html), maintained by the North American Insulation Manufacturers Association, will tell you how much insulation you need. Consider cotton insulation made from recycled

cotton or denim scrap that has no impact on indoor air quality, unlike the formaldehyde ingredients in fiberglass insulation.

4. **Use a programmable thermostat.** This device allows you to predetermine temperatures for daytime and evening comfort as well as energy savings. It can save you as much as 20 percent if you opt to reduce temperatures by 5 degrees at night and 10 degrees during the day when most people are out of the house.

5. **Get an energy audit.** At low or no cost, your local utility may provide a specially trained auditor to examine your home and explain what inexpensive and free energy-conservation actions you can take to save money and energy immediately. The auditor may also take an infrared photograph of your home to help you pinpoint exactly where heat is being lost. You can do it yourself using the website http://hes.lbl.gov/ developed by the Lawrence Berkeley National Laboratory.

6. **Set your water heater to 120 degrees.** If you currently heat your water to 140 degrees, you may save as much as 10 percent annually on water-heating costs by cooling it slightly.

7. **Wrap your water heater in an insulating blanket.** This is one of the most cost-effective energy-saving steps you'll ever take. Insulating blankets or "jackets" cost only around ten dollars, but they can reduce the loss of heat through the walls of the tank by 25 to 40 percent, saving 4 to 9 percent on heating bills. Do it, and forget about it. The same goes for the hot water pipes that funnel hot water from the tank to your faucets.

8. **Use less hot water.** Wash laundry in cold water. Install low-flow showerheads and faucet aerators; you can find online retailers at www.biggreenpurse.com (search: water conservation). Fix leaky faucets. Wash full loads of laundry and dishes.

9. **Maintain your furnace.** If you heat with oil, have your furnace serviced at least once a year to use 10 percent less fuel (if you do this in summer, you'll get cheaper, off-season rates). Clean or replace the filters in your forced-air heating system each month. Dust or vacuum radiator surfaces frequently. When you replace your furnace, buy the most energy-efficient model you can afford. If you have a fireplace, keep the damper closed to avoid losing as much as 8 percent of your home's heated or cooled air.

10. **Upgrade your appliances.** When you replace your refrigerator, stove, dishwasher, or laundry appliances, choose Energy Star models, which use 10 to 50 percent less energy and water than the standard alternatives. If just one in ten homes used Energy Star–qualified appliances, the environmental benefit would be like planting 1.7 million new acres of trees.

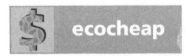

Tax Breaks and Mortgages

Federal Tax Credits help defray the cost of making energy-efficiency improvements or installing solar energy systems. Check the Energy Star website at www.energystar.gov/index.cfm?c=products.pr_tax_credits to see if you qualify.

Energy-efficient Mortgages (EEMs), along with Energy Improvement Mortgages (EIMs), can help you underwrite your mortgage by allowing you to pay to energyproof your home through the money you save on your utility bills. EEMs and EIMs may be offered by the Federal Housing Administration, the Department of Veterans Affairs, some state housing finance agencies, Freddie Mac, and Fannie Mae. You can get more information from the U.S. Department of Housing's Energy Efficient Mortgage Home Owner Guide, www.hud.gov/offices/hsg/sfh/eem/ eemhog96.cfm.

Replace Lights, Appliances, and Electronics with Energy Savers

Even before you think about buying light fixtures or bulbs you can take simple steps to reduce your lighting needs:

- **Use daylight as much as possible.** Remember—it's free. And it doesn't pollute.
- **Focus light on the task at hand.** Use dimmers for background lights.
- **Turn lights off when you leave a room.**
- **Replace fixtures that use two or more low-wattage bulbs with one that uses only a single bulb.** A single 100-watt bulb gives off 20 percent more light than two 60-watt bulbs and uses less power.
- **Keep light fixtures and bulbs clean** to take maximum advantage of their light.

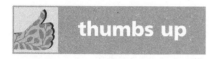

Occupancy Sensors

Occupancy sensors will turn your lights on and off automatically, saving energy every time you enter or leave a room. Check www.smarthome.com or www.amazon.com for occupancy sensors and motion detectors that can work in your home, office, and outdoors.

When you do decide to buy new lights, consider the facts:

- Lighting accounts for around 7 percent of the total energy you use in your home.
- It costs $50 to $150 a year in electricity to light the average home.
- It takes approximately 394 pounds of coal to keep a single 100-watt incandescent lightbulb burning for twelve hours each day for one year.
- Burning all that coal creates about 936 pounds of carbon dioxide—one of the biggest causes of global warming, climate change, and air pollution.
- An Energy Star compact fluorescent lightbulb (CFL) uses 66 percent less energy than a standard incandescent bulb and lasts up to ten times longer.
- A CFL can save more than $50 over the lifetime of the bulb. If you replaced five 75-watt bulbs with fluorescents, you'd save $250 over eight years.

How does a compact fluorescent lightbulb work? Here's how General Electric explains it:

Fluorescent lightbulbs (including compact fluorescents) are more energy-efficient than regular bulbs because of the different method they use to produce light. Regular bulbs (also known as incandescent bulbs) create light by heating a filament inside the bulb; the heat makes the filament white-hot, producing the light that you see. A lot of the energy used to create the heat that lights an incandescent bulb is wasted. A fluorescent bulb, on the other hand, contains a gas that produces invisible ultraviolet (UV) light when the gas is excited by electricity. The UV light hits the white coating inside the fluorescent bulb and the coating changes it into light you can see. Because fluorescent bulbs don't use heat to create light, they are far more energy-efficient than regular incandescent bulbs.

make the shift

Replace the Lights You Use the Most

To save the most energy and money, replace your highest-used fixtures or the light-bulbs in them with energy-efficient models. Typically, those include:

kitchen ceiling light
living room table and floor lamps
bathroom vanity
outdoor porch or post lamp

According to the EPA, if every American home replaced its five most frequently used light fixtures or the bulbs in them with ones that have earned the Energy Star, we would save close to $8 billion each year in energy costs and together prevent greenhouse gases equivalent to the emissions of 10 million cars.

Full Disclosure

* Some CFLs may take an extra second to warm up before they reach full brightness. Compact fluorescent bulbs are best used in fixtures that are left on for longer periods of time, rather than in fixtures that are turned on and off frequently.

INCANDESCENT VS. COMPACT FLUORESCENT LIGHTBULBS		
Bulb type	*100W Incandescent*	*23W Compact Fluorescent*
Purchase price	$0.75	$11.00
Life of the bulb	750 hours	10,000 hours
Number of hours burned/day	4 hours	4 hours
Number of bulbs needed	About 6 over 3 years	1 over 6.8 years
Total cost of bulbs	$4.50	$11.00
Total cost of electricity (8 cents/kilowatt-hour)	$35.04	$8.06
Total cost over three years	$39.54	$19.06
Total savings over three years with the Compact Fluorescent:		$20.49

Source: U.S. Department of Energy, Energy Information Administration.

big green purse

- CFLs may generally be used in enclosed fixtures as long as the fixture is not recessed. Totally enclosed recessed fixtures (for example, a ceiling can light with a cover over the bulb) create temperatures that are too high for compact fluorescent bulbs.

- Only CFLs designed to work with dimmers will do so. Read the label before you buy to get the right bulb for the fixture you have, and make sure you can return the bulb if it doesn't work to your satisfaction.

- Because CFLs contain minuscule amounts of mercury (significantly less than what is found in a fever thermometer), most municipalities prefer that you treat them as household hazardous waste. If you happen to break a CFL at home, don't inhale as you sweep the broken pieces into a plastic bag you can seal for later disposal. Keep in mind that the energy saved by using CFLs will actually cut more mercury pollution from coal-fired power plants than is added through manufacture of the bulbs, according to scientists at the Natural Resources Defense Council.

- The upfront cost of CFLs is somewhat higher than incandescents. But you'll save substantially more money on energy costs over the life of the bulb if you buy the CFL. You can use the Department of Energy online calculator (wwwl.eere.energy.gov/femp/procurement/eep_fluorescent_lamps_calc.html) to determine what you'll save over time if you make the CFL shift.

Want to buy an energy-saving bulb? Look here:

- Almost any local hardware store
- Home Depot's Eco Options label
- Wal-Mart; Sam's Clubs
- www.nolico.com/saveenergy/products.htm
- www.buylighting.com (for Neolite low-mercury bulbs)

thumbs up

Neolite bulbs (www.buylighting.com/NEOLITE-low-mercury-CFL-S-s/327.htm) contain only 1 mg of mercury (compared with the 4 mg in most CFLs).

To determine how many watts you need, check with:

- The EPA's Energy Star program on Compact Fluorescent Light Bulbs (www.energystar.gov/index.cfm?c=cfls.pr_cfls).

- Environmental Defense/Make the Switch campaign (www.environmental defense.org/page.cfm?tagID=632).

Should you turn the lights off or leave them on?

- Turn off incandescent bulbs whenever you leave the room. Only about 10 to 15 percent of the electricity that incandescent lights consume results in light—the rest is turned into heat. Turning the light(s) off will keep a room cooler and not greatly impact the light of the bulb.
- Turning a compact fluorescent on and off wears out the coating inside the fluorescent lamp, slightly reducing the life of the lamp. However, it is still more efficient to turn the light off if you will be gone for more than fifteen minutes. Programmable ballasts, the socket that holds the bulb, are also available to turn the light on gently.

 in my house

We started replacing our incandescent bulbs with compact fluorescents about twenty years ago. We liked the idea of using less energy and saving money on our light bill. All these years later, we still love how much time these bulbs save us. They last so long, we have only had to change most of them every eight years or so. Originally, the light from the bulbs was a little harsh, and it took us a while to get used to the few seconds a CFL needs to warm up before the light comes on. Today, bulbs offer soft light, bright light, white light, and many other hues. We don't even notice the slight pause before the light turns on.

LEDs

Compact fluorescent bulbs are the best energy-saving alternative right now, but bulbs that use light-emitting diodes, or LEDs, are gaining ground.

LEDs have been used in electronics for decades. They light up the panel on a VCR or cell phone, and they're common in flashlights. They also power Christmas lights, bicycle lights, and headlamps. Sylvania is selling an LED reading light and clap light.

What's the LEDs appeal? They're more efficient than compact fluorescents and, since they contain no mercury, offer a somewhat safer alternative. Though they're more expensive now, with consumer demand, the price will likely go down.

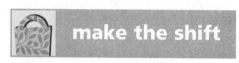

make the shift

LEDs for Your Lights

SuperBrightLeds.com (www.superbrightleds.com/led_prods.htm) has LED lighting available in a variety of consumer products, including track lights, truck lights, candelabra styles, and flashlights.

Led Light.com (www.theledlight.com) sells floodlights, LED controls, LED strips (some waterproof), ground and road lighting, motion-sensing security lights, under-cabinet lights, and rope lights.

The LED product Store (http://ledproductstore.com/ConsumerItems.htm) retails flashlights, key chain flashlights, light orbs and light washers, bicycle lights, wearable safety lights, and other clothing; also, novelty items such as jewelry, candles, sunglasses, and ice cubes.

During the holidays, check hardware and department stores for LED string lights.

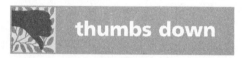

thumbs down

No Halo for Halogen Torchieres

These six-foot-tall lamps have been banned on most college campuses because they get so hot they've been known to set dormitories ablaze. According to urban legends, students were using the torchieres' 970 degrees to cook dinner in their rooms. If you like the torchiere style, get one that can take a CFL. You'll save an amount of carbon dioxide equivalent to driving a medium-size car 734 miles, calculates the Rocky Mountain Institute.

Appliances

Appliances—especially refrigerators, dishwashers, clothes washers and dryers, stoves, and ovens—account for about 20 percent of your household's energy consumption.

The good news? You can find any appliance you need in a model that will save you energy (and in the case of clothes and dishwashers, water, too). The bad news? You have so many choices!

make the shift

Energy-Efficient Appliances

When it's time to replace an appliance, buy the most energy-efficient model in your price range. Shift the money you'll save on energy to the cost of the new, more-efficient appliance. To find the right appliance for you, check these sources:

- **Consumer Reports Greener Choices** (www.greenerchoices.org) for ratings on the most efficient appliances.
- **U.S. Environmental Protection Agency Energy Star Program** (www.energy star.gov) for a list of all the appliances that qualify for the Energy Star.
- **American Council for an Energy Efficient Economy:** their *Consumer Guide to Home Energy Savings* describes energy-efficiency ratings for most appliances, along with recommendations that can help you find the most efficient model in your price range. Even though the guide was last updated in 2005, it is still helpful.

What to look for in individual appliances:

Refrigerators and Freezers
Energy Star refrigerators use at least 15 percent less energy than standard models. If you can only upgrade one appliance to an energy-efficient model, it should be your fridge (and freezer, if separate), since it runs all the time.

- Consider a refrigerator with freezer on top, as it is more efficient than one with a freezer on the side.
- Look for heavy door hinges that create a good door seal.
- Keep the refrigerator compartment set between 38 and 42 degrees F, the freezer about 0 degrees to 5 degrees.

- Periodically clean the condenser coils on the back of your refrigerator to improve overall efficiency.

Washing Machines

Energy Star clothes washers use 50 percent less energy than standard washers and sometimes as much as 50 percent less water.

- The Modified Energy Factor (MEF) measures the energy used during the washing process, including machine energy, water-heating energy, and dryer energy. The higher the MEF, the more efficient the clothes washer is.
- Most full-size Energy Star–qualified washers use eighteen to twenty-five gallons of water per load, compared to the forty gallons used by a standard machine. The water factor measures the gallons of water used per cycle per cubic foot (for example, a 3.0-cubic-foot washer using twenty-seven gallons per cycle has a water factor of 9.0). The lower the water factor, the less water the machine uses. The water factor is listed on the EPA's qualified product list.
- Most Energy Star washers extract more water from clothes during the spin cycle. This reduces the drying time and saves energy and wear and tear on your clothes.
- Energy Star–qualified clothes washers are available in both top-loading and front-loading designs. In horizontal-axis or front-loading machines the tub itself rotates, making the clothes tumble into the water. Redesigned vertical-axis (V-axis—top-loading) washers use sprayers to wet the clothes from above or a moving plate in the bottom of the tub to lift and bounce clothes through the wash water. After completing the rinse cycle, these washers spin clothes faster than conventional top-loading washers, so the remaining moisture content of the clothes is lower, reducing the energy required for clothes drying.

Note: If you buy a high-efficiency washing machine, you'll only need half as much laundry detergent. You can also buy "High E" or "HE" laundry detergent specially formulated for efficient washing machines.

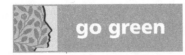

Extra Energy Savings

Even with an Energy Star model, you can save extra energy if you:

- Wash full loads—clothes washers are most efficient when operated with full loads.
- Wash clothes in cold water.

Clothes Dryers

Energy Star does not label clothes dryers because most dryers use similar amounts of energy.

To reduce the amount of energy your clothes dryer uses:

- Use the moisture-sensor option, which automatically shuts off the machine when the clothes are dry.
- Choose a high spin speed or extended-spin option to reduce the amount of remaining moisture, thus starting the drying process before you put your clothes in the dryer.
- Air-dry clothes if it's convenient.

Dishwashers

Energy Star dishwashers use at least 25 percent less energy than standard models. You can save around $100 over the life of the dishwasher if it's an Energy Star model.

- **Don't rinse your dishes before loading them.** If necessary, wipe them off with a wet sponge.
- **Run your dishwasher with a full load.** Most of the energy used by a dishwasher goes to heat water. Since you can't decrease the amount of water used per cycle, fill your dishwasher to get the most from the energy used to run it.
- **Avoid the heat-dry, rinse-hold, and prerinse features.** Instead use your dishwasher's air-dry option, or prop the door open after the final rinse to dry the dishes.

Hang It on the Line

Here's a simple, affordable "technology" that's making a comeback: the clothesline. It can save you as much as two hundred dollars a year in energy costs, creates no global warming gases or air pollution, and ensures that you get some exercise when you hang your laundry out to dry.

- **Vermont Clothesline Company** (www.smartdrying.com) offers three different clothesline styles.
- **Rawganique** (www.rawganique.com) sells an organic hemp rope you can string between two poles, two trees, or the laundry room walls.
- **Abundant Earth** (www.abundantearth.com.) makes drying racks you can use indoors or out.
- If you think your neighbors might object to seeing your sheets or nightgown drying in the breeze, get some moral support from **Project Laundry List** (www.laundrylist.org).

- **Install your dishwasher away from the refrigerator or freezer.** Dishwashers produce moisture and heat, which will make your refrigerator or freezer use more energy.

Gas Stoves, Electric Ranges

Electric stoves use less energy than those fueled by gas but usually cost more to operate due to the high cost of electricity. Stoves that rely on natural gas have an added benefit: natural gas emits only half the carbon of coal, none of the sulfur, and less nitrogen. Using a gas stove instead of one powered by coal-fired electricity does not add significantly to global warming.

Another option: induction cooktops. Induction cooking uses 90 percent of the energy produced compared to only 40 percent for a gas burner and 50 percent for traditional electric ranges. Induction cooking is based on magnetic fields: each "element" or induction coil generates a magnetic field that induces heat into the cookware placed on top of it. Induction cooktops offer the same instant control as gas and are the fastest of all cooktop types to heat and cook food. But be aware: you must use pots and pans that are either cast iron or the kind of stainless steel that supports a magnetic charge—if a magnet clings to your pot, it will be good to go on an induction cooktop.

Microwave Ovens, Toaster Ovens, Slow Cookers

Consider these additional energy-saving options, especially when cooking or reheating small- to medium-size meals and for defrosting. A microwave oven will use between one-fifth and one-half less energy than a conventional oven.

in my house

I use mostly gas appliances. That goes for my oven and range, clothes dryer, and the way I heat my house. When I replaced my clothes washer five years ago, I bought a water- and energy-saving front-loader. When I got a new oven, I chose one with a convection option. That saves me time and money, since it's quicker to cook with convection heat. Convection heat also seems to do a better job baking cookies.

One thing I should have done with my new appliances is bought extended war-

ENERGY COSTS OF VARIOUS COOKING METHODS				
Appliance	*Temp.*	*Time*	*Energy*	*Cost*
Electric oven	350° F	1 hr	2.0 kWh	16¢
Convection oven (elec)	325° F	45 min	1.39 kWh	11¢
Gas oven	350° F	1 hr	1.12 kWh	7¢
Frying pan	420° F	1 hr	.9 kWh	7¢
Toaster oven	425° F	50 min	.95 kWh	6¢
Slowcooker	200° F	7 hr	.7 kWh	6¢
Microwave oven	High	15 min	.36 kWh	3¢

Source: *Consumer Guide to Home Energy Savings,* American Council for an Energy Efficient Economy.

ranties on them. Their parts don't wear out that fast, but the computers running them seem to. This probably has less to do with their energy efficiency than with the state of developing technology. I've had the computer panel replaced on the washer twice, and the dryer needs it soon. As soon as I bought the appliances I should have purchased lifetime warranties to cover all repairs.

Repair, or Buy New?

Appliances are in a class by themselves when it comes to the idea of replacements. Because they use so much energy, it often makes more sense to buy new, energy-efficient models than to spend time and money repairing old power hogs. Here are a few rules of thumb, courtesy of *The Green Guide, Consumer Reports*, and Whirlpool Corporation.

- If the cost to repair a household appliance is more than half the price of a new product, buy the newer model and save money on your energy bill.
- Replace top-loading washing machines with high-efficiency front-loaders; you'll save both water and energy.
- If your broken dryer has a moisture sensor on it, you may be able to repair it and achieve gains similar to current models. Otherwise, replace with a new, energy-efficient model. Or think about a clothesline.
- Replace refrigerators purchased before 2001, when new energy standards were instituted, then contact earth911.com or your local utility to recycle the model you're replacing.
- Replace dishwashers with Energy Star models to save energy and water.
- Replace air conditioners and water heaters if they're more than ten years old. They're probably on their last leg, giving you the opportunity to upgrade to more efficient models.
- Repair computers as long as you can. Regular maintenance will extend their life; adding memory and other upgrades will keep your computer current as technology advances.
- Replace but recycle small appliances like coffeemakers, toaster ovens, food processors, blenders, and bread makers.
- Fill out the free warranties on every appliance you buy, and purchase extended warranties on all major appliances. Using inexpensive or free warranties, I've had printers, cell phones, iPods, my washing machine, and many other appliances repaired at no or low cost.

If you need help finding repair services, check with Point and Click Appliance Repair (www.pcappliancerepair.com).

You can find parts and do-it-yourself tips at Repair Clinic (www.repairclinic.com).

Shift to Renewable Green Power

If you've gotten tired of tilting at windmills, maybe it's time to put one up in your backyard. You won't be alone. Thousands of consumers are turning to wind, as well as solar and even corn pellets as a way to power their homes with renewable fuel.

Even if you don't want to build your own windmill, chances are you can buy wind power. About 75 million electricity customers in forty-two states have the option to buy green energy through their utility or an alternative power supplier, according to the government's National Renewable Energy Laboratory.

Where Does Green Power Come From?

Wind. Nonpolluting turbines rely on strong winds to generate electricity. Wind energy is most economical in places where average wind speed is at least seventeen miles per hour. Locations as diverse as Brooklyn, New York, southern California, and western Maryland all generate substantial power by tapping the wind.

Solar. The sun's energy produces electricity either using photovoltaic (PV) cells or by trapping sunlight in a thermal system. PVs convert sunlight directly into electricity. You may already be using them in landscape lighting, to charge batteries, or on your roof. Solar thermal systems harness the sun's energy to heat a fluid that produces steam, which then turns a turbine and generator.

Geothermal. Geothermal energy converts the hot water or steam lying deep below the earth's surface into electricity. Geothermal plants in the United States currently provide enough electricity to supply the homes of 3.5 million people. Known geothermal reserves and technology could supply the entire country with electricity for thirty years, reports Environmental Defense.

Biomass. Vegetation or animal waste can be converted into energy for electricity and fuel to heat homes and other buildings, including factories and to power vehicles. Individuals are adapting their oil-burning furnaces to biodiesel and their wood-burning stoves to run on corn. Wood pellets—small plugs of compressed sawdust and wood shavings left over by lumber mills—are being used to heat more than 600,000 homes in New England.

big green purse

To find green power in your area, visit the Department of Energy's "Green Power" page (www.eere.energy.gov/greenpower/buying/buying_power.shtml).

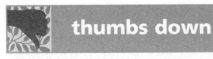

thumbs down

House Power the "Old Way"

Most of the energy that powers our homes comes from conventional sources that are neither efficient nor clean.

- **Coal** generates more than 50 percent of the electricity in the United States, but it also accounts for about one-third of the country's carbon dioxide emissions, making it a major source of global warming. Emissions from coal-fired power plants also contain mercury, which pollutes our lakes and oceans and contaminates the fish we eat.
- **Nuclear** is exorbitantly expensive. Plus, there's still no solution for safely storing the radioactive waste generated by nuclear power plants.
- **Natural gas** is more abundant than coal or oil, but prices are going up as demand increases and supplies shrink.
- **Oil** spews large amounts of carbon dioxide when it's burned, and given dwindling supplies, it is not a fuel we can count on long-term for either electricity or heating.
- **Large-scale hydropower dams** destroy ecosystems and interfere with fish migrations. It is unlikely additional hydropower facilities will be built.

By shifting your spending to green power, you support renewable energy industries that are working to clean up the air and water, reduce climate change, and make clean energy more affordable.

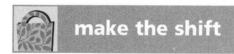

make the shift

How to Buy Green Power

- **Purchase green power directly.** Around six hundred utilities now offer wind power and green power (a combination of wind, solar, and biomass) to their customers, at comparable or marginally more expensive rates. (I pay slightly more than an extra penny a kilowatt hour for 100 percent wind power from my Maryland utility.)
- **Buy Renewable Energy Certificates (RECs) or Green Tags.** RECs and Green tags help subsidize the construction of power plants powered by renewable energy sources. While you may not receive any green power directly, your investment helps offset the environmental impact caused by generating electricity from coal, oil, natural gas, or nuclear power. Learn more at www.green-e.org or www.green tagsusa.org.
- **Patronize businesses that buy green power.** If you can't buy it yourself, support companies that do. You'll know who they are by the Green-e label that verifies they're purchasing or generating certified renewable energy. For more information, see www.green-e.org/gogreene.shtml.

You can also generate your own clean energy.

- **Windpower.** According to the U.S. Census Bureau, reports Josh Dorfman in *The Lazy Environmentalist*, approximately 17 million U.S. households are capable of capturing wind energy. You'll need at least half an acre of unobstructed land and average wind speeds of at least 10 mph, plus local zoning that permits construction of a windmill at least forty-two feet tall, the optimum height. Check with your utility to set up an interconnection agreement so you can use power lines and feed excess electricity back into the grid. One Skystream (www.sky stream.com) 3.7 windmill can meet half the annual energy consumption needs of a typical home. Buy two and you can get off the grid completely.
- **Solar power.** Some solar systems are so effective at reducing equivalent air pollution and global warming emissions it's like planting eight acres of trees or offsetting 114,000 miles driven by the average car. Ready Solar (www.ready solar.com) helps you capitalize on any available tax credits, financing packages,

rebates, and other options to make purchasing solar panels for your home affordable. Real Goods (www.realgoods.com) sells ready-made solar electric kits for rooftops and other applications. Evergreen Solar (www.evergreensolar.com) manufactures thin solar panels that require less silicon than conventional models; the panels help reduce roof construction costs and integrate solar panels into the roof's structure. Home Depot has teamed with BP Solar to offer BP Solar Home Solutions, a solar design and installation program that takes advantage of state and utility incentives to "make solar power more affordable than ever."

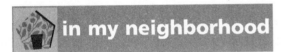

in my neighborhood

Where I live, in Montgomery County, Maryland, just outside Washington, D.C., people are fueling their homes in many clean and empowering ways:

- We buy 100 percent of our electricity from the wind turbines that supply our local utility.
- The family up the street replaced their oil-burning furnace with one that runs entirely on biodiesel.
- Two blocks away, neighbors have installed solar collectors on their roof and occasionally feed power back to the utility.
- The parents of my daughter's closest neighborhood pal have retrofitted their fireplace with a stove that burns low-polluting corn pellets.
- Friends intent on using less coal-fired electricity use solar batteries to power fans, reading lights, and other small appliances.

A Word About Batteries

Batteries' small size belies the impact their portable power has on the planet. Americans purchase two to three billion dry-cell batteries every year to power radios, toys, cell phones, watches, laptop computers, and portable power tools. An additional ninety-nine million lead-acid car batteries juice automobiles, boats, or motorcycles. What's the problem?

- Batteries contain heavy metals like mercury, lead, cadmium, and nickel.
- Household batteries, especially alkaline and button batteries, are the single-largest source of mercury in our trash.
- Mercury is highly toxic. Long-term exposure can permanently damage the brain and kidneys and the fetus in pregnant women.

Fortunately, the three Rs can come to the rescue once again. Reducing the number of new batteries used, recharging batteries to extend their reuse, and recycling batteries at the end of their life helps keep heavy metals out of landfills and the air while saving resources that would otherwise be used to make new batteries.

go green

Battery Basics

- **Buy fewer toys, appliances, and electronics that rely only on batteries for power.** As often as possible, choose products that can be powered electrically or by hand to avoid batteries altogether. You can find links to battery-free toys at www.big greenpurse.com (search: battery-free time).

- **Turn off battery-powered appliances when you're not using them to extend the life of the battery.** Remove the batteries if you're not going to use the appliance for a long period of time.

- **Choose rechargeables so you use fewer batteries overall.** But remember: rechargeables still contain heavy metals like nickel and cadmium.

- **When you've used up any battery, don't toss it in the trash.** Save it for a hazardous-waste pickup in your community, or take it to your local hazardous-waste-management facility (check with your city or county government for the nearest location).

- **Recycle batteries.** The Rechargeable Battery Recycling Corporation (www.rbrc.org/call2recycle/dropoff/index.php) will help you find the nearest drop-off point; to recycle throwaways, check with http://earth911.org/recycling/batteryrecycling.

 More than three hundred manufacturers encourage rechargeable battery recycling by placing the Battery Recycling Seal on rechargeable batteries and portable electronic products. When you see it, you know the battery can be recycled.

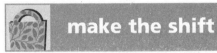

Buy rechargeable batteries

- **Battery Solutions Inc.** (www.batteryrecycling.com/household.html) provides downloadable instructions so you can recycle batteries in cell phones, laptop computers, flashlights, cameras, watches, hearing aids, toys, two-way radios, electric tools, clocks, and other electronic devices.
- **Green Batteries** (www.greenbatteries.com) offers many different types of rechargeable batteries, rechargers, and other accessories.
- **Solar Battery Saver SE 2** (www.batterystuff.com) charges a car battery via the cigarette lighter.
- **Solio** (www.solio.com/v2/) recharges batteries using power from the sun.
- **Sundance Solar** (www.sundancesolar.com) sells rechargeable alkaline, nickel-cadmium (Ni-Cd), and nickel-metal hydride (Ni-Mh) batteries.
- **USB Cell** (www.usbcell.com/products) makes AAA batteries that recharge by plugging into your computer.
- **Voltaic Pouch** (www.voltaicsystems.com) does double duty as a daypack whose solar panels charge cell phones, PDAs, MP3 players, and cameras.

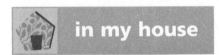

We've pretty much given up on throwaway batteries in our house. Happily, all of our electronics have batteries that can now be electrically recharged, and we rarely buy anything that requires throwaways. Our city picks up batteries a couple of times a year, so I keep a box in a bottom drawer in the kitchen where I put worn-out batteries until pick-up day. Meanwhile, my son got a hand-cranked radio for Christmas and it works like a charm. No batteries, no electricity. Try it.

Electronics

The key message behind *Big Green Purse* is to use your consumer clout to make a difference. When it comes to electronics, your pull is substantial. In fact, here's a number that may surprise you: women buy more electronic gear than men do. According to the Consumer Electronics Association, women are influencing 88 percent of household consumer electronics purchases, initiating spending amounting to at least $65 billion in purchases every year.

This impact has captured the attention of most electronics companies, who've redesigned several products to meet women's desires for sleeker, lighter, more colorful cell phones, PDAs, laptop computers, and even televisions. Sharp refashioned its flat-panel TVs, calling the product line Aquos "to connote fluidity and a softer touch," reported CNN. It promoted the product beyond sports and prime-time slots to Lifetime, the Food Network, and The Learning Channel. On Mother's Day, a Circuit City ad featured an Aquos in a kitchen.

Women's spending power in the electronics marketplace is being felt throughout the industry. Radio Shack's customers shifted from 20 percent female in 1997 to 40 percent female in 2004. In an effort to capture more of the female dollar, Sony developed its LIV line, sold exclusively at Target stores, to include CD players for the kitchen and shower radios in colors from stainless steel to lime.

All of this speaks volumes for the clout women could have if we used our purses to favor technology that was not only sleek and snazzy but also energy efficient, nontoxic, and recyclable.

You face three critical decisions when buying new e-ware. What is the most energy-efficient technology you can buy? What products are made from the cleanest, greenest materials possible? Where can you recycle your electronics when the time comes?

Buy Energy-Efficient Electronics

Buying the most energy-efficient electronics will save you money on operating costs and reduce the amount of energy you use—which will also reduce the amount of air pollution and greenhouse gas you produce. Follow these general guidelines when shopping for electronics.

- **Buy a laptop rather than a PC, which consumes five times as much energy.**
- **Switch to an LCD monitor.** The typical old-style 20-inch CRT monitor consumes about 150 watts of power, while a new 20-inch flat-panel LCD uses about 30 watts; the difference in energy expense amounts to about twenty dollars a year for a typical American user.
- **Choose highly efficient power supply units.** Look for the "80 Plus" label, which indicates the power supply is at least 80 percent efficient.

- **Buy Energy Star equipment.** Over its lifetime, Energy Star–qualified equipment in a single home office (e.g., computer, monitor, printer, and fax) can save enough electricity to light an entire home for more than four years.

make the shift

Energy Star Computers

When you're ready to purchase new electronics, check out your options at the Energy Star website (www.energystar.gov/index.cfm?fuseaction=find_a_product.showProduct Group&pgw_code=CO).

go green

Energy-Saving Tips

Personal computers use about the same amount of energy to reboot as they use when they are on for about two seconds, says the U.S. Department of Energy in its *Consumer's Guide to Energy Efficiency and Renewable Energy*. To conserve power:

- **Turn off the monitor if you're taking a break of twenty minutes or more.**
- **Turn off both the CPU and monitor if you're not going to use your PC for more than two hours.** (Remember, plugging your computer, printer, and fax machine into the same power strip will make it easier to turn all your office equipment on and off.)
- **Activate the power-down or *sleep mode* feature for the CPU and monitor.** Energy Star computers power down to a sleep mode that consumes 15 watts or less power, which is around 70 percent less electricity than a computer without power-management features. Energy Star monitors feature two successive "sleep" modes, one that reduces power consumption to less than or equal to 15 watts, and another that cuts power consumption to 8 watts, which is less than 10 percent of the energy it normally uses.
- **Skip the screen saver.** Using a screen saver may consume more kilowatts than not,

and the power-down feature may not work if your screen saver is activated. Modern color monitors do not need screen savers at all.

Recycle Electronics to Reduce E-Waste

Buy "Green" Electronics

E-waste is the fastest-growing part of the waste stream. There are 500 million obsolete computers in the United States alone, notes the Silicon Valley Toxics Coalition (SVTC), a grassroots organization working to promote human health and environmental justice in the high-tech industry. More than 130 million cell phones are thrown out each year; 20 to 24 million TVs and computers are stored annually in homes and offices. Despite this mounting electronic mess, little recycling occurs. Only 10 percent of unwanted or obsolete computers are refurbished or reclaimed.

Keeping electronics out of the trash protects the environment and your health, too. Manufacturing computers, cell phones, PDAs, printers, fax machines, and other high-tech gadgets typically involves thousands of toxic chemicals, including solvents, gases, heavy metals, and acids. Lead, cadmium, and brominated flame retardants dot circuit boards. Lead oxide and barium fill cathode ray tube monitors. Mercury infiltrates switches and flat-screen monitors. Polyvinyl chloride (PVC) lines electronic cables and wires.

If electronics are simply tossed in a landfill, these chemicals can escape into the air and water, eventually adding to the toxic body burden we already carry. Of greater concern is the fact that so much e-waste is shipped to developing countries, where electronics are dismantled by unskilled, unprotected workers. Even in the United States, reclaiming tech trash may be done by untrained prison help who face toxic threats from the chemicals these electronics contain.

Both Greenpeace and the SVTC, working with the Computer TakeBack Campaign (CTBC), rate electronics companies on the progress they make in reducing their use of toxic substances and increasing electronics recycling. You can use these report cards to choose the most socially and environmentally responsible company in the marketplace.

The Silicon Valley Toxics Coalition. The most recent computer report card issued by the SVTC ranks HP and Dell at the top of the list for their efforts to reduce e-waste, increase recycling, and eliminate some of the toxic chemicals in their products. You can see the complete report card at www.svtc.etoxics.org/site/PageServer? pagename=svtc_computer_report_card.

Greenpeace. In 2006 Nokia and Dell shared the top spots in the Greenpeace ranking, thanks to their belief that producers should bear individual responsibility for taking back and reusing or recycling their own-brand discarded products. Since the end of 2005, all new Nokia cell phones have been free of cancer-causing polyvinyl chloride and the company promised that all new components would be free of harmful brominated flame retardants (BFRs) beginning in 2007. Dell has also set ambitious targets for eliminating these same harmful substances from their products. In 2007 Lenovo, which bought IBM's consumer electronics division in 2005, scored top marks on its e-waste policies and practice. The company offers take-back and recycling in all the countries where its products are sold. Plus, Lenovo reports the amount of e-waste it recycles as a percentage of its sales. However, the company has yet to put products free of the worst chemicals on the market. For more information, visit www.greenpeace.org (search: "Guide to Greener Electronics").

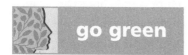

E-Trash Tips

- **Use a smartphone.** Combine an MP3 player, digital camera, digital video recorder, GPS navigation instrument, and laptop computer in a single device rather than many you'll have to throw away.
- **Consider an energy-saving all-in-one home computer system.** Combine television, TiVo, music system, and home computer.
- **Resist the urge to buy a new machine.** Marketers may be in the business of selling new products every year, but you don't need to be in the business of buying them. Upgrade existing equipment first, using software, adding RAM, a new video card, and other options.
- **Upgrade vicariously.** Visit computer showrooms, surf technology websites, read digital newspaper and magazine columns. Understand that whatever you buy will be out of date the minute you bring it home. Since there's no way to keep up, keep the right perspective instead.
- **Recycle.** More on that below.

The Electronic Product Environmental Assessment Tool (EPEAT) helps the public and private sectors evaluate, compare, and select desktop computers, notebooks, and monitors based on their performance in eight categories, such as energy conservation, packaging, and reduction of toxic materials. The program has identified more than two hundred desktop computers, laptops, and monitors that meet its standards. Products in the online EPEAT registry include computer monitors made partly out of plant-based materials. You can find a complete listing of EPEAT registered merchandise, which also meets Energy Star criteria, at www.epeat.net.

Recycle ALL Electronic Gear

Cell phones, computers, printers, monitors, fax machines, and copiers are loaded with toxic metals and chemicals that pollute groundwater and contaminate the air. They can also poison workers who dismantle the machines if they're not properly trained—and in developing countries, where most of the world's e-trash is shipped, it is often women and children who do this deadly work. Make a difference by recycling all the electronic gear you discard.

- **RIPMobile (Recycle Inactive Phones;** www.ripmobile.com) Once you tell RIPMobile what old phones (and some PDAs) you have, they'll calculate what your booty is worth and pay you in RIP mobile points (a point is worth a dollar). You send the phone and accessories to RIP for inspection. If they measure up, you'll receive a gift certificate to redeem at a vendor like Circuit City or Starbucks. You can also donate your points to a charity through the company's sister site, www.CollectiveGood.com.
- **AT&T and Cingular Reuse & Recycle.** Both companies recycle used wireless phones, accessories, and batteries.
- **FedEx Kinko's.** Drop-off boxes in their outlets accept cell phones.
- **eBay** (http://ebay.eztradein.com/ebay/) If your electronics still work reasonably well, trade them in on eBay's EZ Trade In site. Print a mailing label, send your items to the company, and receive payment back via PayPal. eBay accepts PC and Apple desktop and notebook computers, SLR and point & shoot cameras,

servers, home projectors, multimedia projectors, cell phones, computer monitors, PDAs, game systems, camcorders, and iPods.

- **Swaptree** (www.swaptree.com). This online community trades CDs, DVDs, and video games. There's no money back, but it's an easy way to recycle.
- **Staples.** This retailer accepts cell phones, printer toner cartridges, computers, computer printers, monitors, fax machines, and other e-waste, though not televisions.
- **www.earth911.com.** For information to help you recycle televisions and other electronics, plug in your zip code here.
- **Storefronts.** Many companies, including Dell and Apple, will recycle your old computer for free when you buy a new one from them. HP offers trade-in discounts on new hardware if you recycle your computer there. Most companies have some kind of recycling policy in the works; check before you buy. **Note:** Remember to erase the memory of your cell phone or computer hard drive before you recycle it.
- **Charities.** If a local school or charity can't use your computer, contact Computer Aid International (www.computer-aid.org), a nonprofit that refurbishes electronic gear and distributes it to educational, health, and charitable organizations in developing countries.

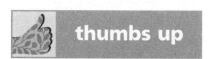

Your Home Videos

Got unwanted laser discs and VHS tapes? Send them to GreenDisk (www.greendisk.com). The company will erase the contents and resell the tapes to cities and police departments to use in day-to-day operations; your discs will be shredded and sold for plastics reuse.

Appliances, Lighting, and Electronics Wrap-Up

- **Insulate and weatherize your home.** Use a programmable thermostat to regulate temperatures automatically.
- **Use a compact fluorescent** each time you need to replace a lightbulb.
- **Plug office equipment—computer, printer, fax machine, phone—into a power strip.** You'll find it easier to stop wasting energy.
- **Replace appliances with Energy Star models.** Start with the refrigerator and freezer, which run constantly.
- **Buy "green" home energy.** Choose wind or solar power.
- **When buying new electronics, purchase the "greenest" model available.** Check with Greenpeace and the Silicon Valley Toxics Coalition for up-to-date ratings.
- **Resist the urge to upgrade every year.** That goes especially for appliances, cell phones, PDAs, and computers.
- **Recycle all electronics.** Contact www.earth911.com to find nearby locations to recycle cell phones, fax machines, PDAs, printers, and more.

If you can do only one thing, replace kitchen, bathroom, porch, living room table, and living room floor lamps with compact fluorescent lights. You'll conserve energy, clean up the air, reduce global warming, and save money.

big green purse

HOME, GREEN HOME: FURNITURE, PAINT, FLOORING, AND FABRICS

IF YOU'VE EVER RUN TO THROW OPEN THE WINDOWS SO YOU COULD CATCH your breath in a newly painted room, if you've ever had to hold your nose while applying a powerful epoxy, then you already know that paints and finishes release volatile organic compounds, or VOCs, which cause headaches, muscle achiness, and, on occasion, asthma and other respiratory disorders. You may have felt similar discomfort from a new piece of furniture, since it's not uncommon for tables, chairs, bureaus, and cabinets to be glued together with products containing formaldehyde, a cancer-causing chemical that seeps into the air from the resin used to cement plywood, particleboard, and medium-density fiberboard. Adhesives in carpeting and flooring and the finishes used to protect them make many people uncomfortable, too, as they also contribute to the indoor air pollution that plagues so many homes today.

In addition, the manufacture of home furnishings—including the resources used, their transformation into a useful product, their transportation to the retailer where you buy them, and their ultimate disposal—racks up "life cycle" costs that threaten the outdoor environment. Rain forests may be ravaged to supply trees for our coffee tables, dining room floors, and bed frames. Pesticides used to grow cotton for our draperies, upholstery, and bed linens run off into groundwater. Global warming inevitably figures into the tableau, since converting any raw material to a useful product takes energy, which releases climate-changing carbon dioxide into the atmosphere. Designing women we may be, but these are not the decor results we had in mind.

The Good News

Before you feel as if your only recourse is to live in a tree, take heart: new manufacturing standards sought by consumers and created by pioneers in the home and commercial-furnishings industry are generating interior-design options pure enough to adorn Mother Nature's own abode.

The Institute for Market Transformation to Sustainability's comprehensive SMART standard (http://mts.sustainableproducts.com) gives you one idea of what to choose. The SMART standard promotes a particularly green way of manufacturing that:

- Reduces waste and eliminates emissions
- Uses renewable energy like wind and solar power
- Closes the loop on manufacturing, making new products out of old ones to save energy and use resources wisely
- Seeks efficiencies in transporting raw materials as well as finished products to save energy and reduce air pollution
- Ensures that workers are treated fairly
- Creates policies and market incentives that reward sustainability
- Takes a product's entire life cycle into account, encouraging environmental responsibility from the moment resources are tapped, through their manufacture into merchandise, to the time they're either recycled into a new product or disposed of.

Such "sustainable" standards motivate manufacturers to minimize their environmental impact on almost every measurable scale. Just as important, they provide a filter you can use to separate proven "green" products from those whose manufacturers attempt to "greenwash" their attributes with unsubstantiated claims.

Those "green" products offer tangible benefits neither you nor the planet will want to miss. Furniture made from recycled materials like steel and soda bottles helps protect the environment by saving energy, water, and many natural resources. Desks, tables, and flooring crafted of wood that has been grown sustainably or reclaimed from warehouses, abandoned buildings, and riverbed floors help keep forests intact. Favoring organically grown cotton and hemp for draperies, furniture covers, towels, and sheets significantly reduces the amount of pesticides applied to the land. By painting with no- or low-VOC paint, you keep the air in your house sweeter, and that makes you sweeter, too.

But even before you buy, you'll want to consider what you're going to put where. That's why the chapter begins by focusing on basic eco-design principles. In keeping with the overriding Big Green Purse "Less is more" message, these pages also encourage you to look for salvaged and recycled furnishings before you buy new, and to renovate before you build. Of course, the way you actually construct your house is key, but that subject is too big for this book. This chapter touches instead on a few of the basics. You can find links to topics like framing, roofing, insulation, and renewable building materials, and other nitty-gritty home construction concerns in the Little Black Book at the end of this book and at www.biggreenpurse.com (search: home).

When you are ready to choose paint, furniture, fabrics, or flooring, you'll find suggestions for sustainable products like those certified by the SMART initiative, as well as others that are making an honest effort to minimize their environmental impact.

By the time you finish reading, hopefully you and your home will both feel SMART.

Use Your Big Green Purse

There are more "green" home furnishings on the market than ever before (though you'll have to do most of your shopping online). Start here to decorate with eco-friendly flair.

- Design to minimize
- Use salvaged and reclaimed materials
- Build and decorate with locally made products
- Recycle or donate excess materials
- Favor sustainable furnishings

Design to Minimize

"Eco" shouldn't be an afterthought. Beginning with the design process, identify ways you can make your home more earth-friendly. Minimize use of synthetic, nonrenewable, nonrecyclable resources while maximizing design with nontoxic, high-quality materials and objects. Consider whether you can renovate a room rather than build a completely new structure. Whether building new, renovating, or just giving your space a touch-up, aim for styles that are simple and relaxing. Recommends Kimberly Rider, author of *The Healthy Home Workbook: Easy Steps for Eco-Friendly Living*:

- Use as much natural light as possible.
- Be inspired by and connected to the rhythms of nature.
- Respect the earth and use resources wisely.
- Integrate layers of natural materials, rich textures, and inspiring colors.
- Strive for furnishings and design that are comfortable, practical, functional, and efficient.
- Be unique; choose a style and objects that mean something to you.
- Create surroundings that promote physical, mental, and spiritual health.
- Be flexible; let your design and furnishings evolve and change as your household needs change.

How to Get Started

- **Building a new house?** Before you do, visit www.usgbc.org, the website of the U.S. Green Building Council; www.greenhomebuilding.com; or read the "Minnesota Green Affordable Housing Guide" (www.greenhousing.umn.edu) for excellent overviews of earth-friendly options, particularly in cold climates. The American Lung Association's "HealthHouse" (www.healthhouse.org/index.asp) includes a list of builders and ways to create a more comfortable indoor environment.
- **Remodeling?** "Green Home Remodeling Guides" from the city of Seattle will help (www.seattle.gov/dpd/GreenBuilding/SingleFamilyResidential/Resources/RemodelingGuides/default.asp). You'll learn how to hire design and building professionals, use salvaged materials when you renovate, and choose paint that won't give you a headache.
- **Need energy-efficient designers and builders, as well as appliances?** Check in with the U.S. EPA Energy Star program (www.energystar.gov) or Green Building Blocks (www.greenbuildingblocks.com). Then hustle on over to the

Department of Housing and Urban Development's "Energy-Efficient Rehab Advisor" (http://rehabadvisor.pathnet.org); in about five seconds this online calculator will tell you how much money you'll save by incorporating energy-efficiency measures into room-by-room renovations.

- **Want information on other aspects of green living?** Drop by www.biggreen purse.com (search: LiveGreen).

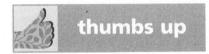

Your Spirit of Place

Architect Travis Price III says, "Nature's beat—even the simple rhythm of night and day—impacts the use of [a] building, its temperatures and light, its aging process,

Be a "LEED"er

Whether you're renovating a room or building a home from the nails up, the "Leadership in Energy and Environmental Design (LEED) Green Building Rating System" can guide you in creating a space you'll be proud to call "green." An initiative of the U.S. Green Building Council, LEED promotes sustainability by recognizing performance in five key areas that affect human and environmental health:

- sustainable site development
- water savings
- energy efficiency
- materials selection
- indoor environmental quality

To learn how you can be a LEEDer, visit www.usgbc.org.

its views. Yet working with what is natural has a deeper level, too. It is about embracing the environment: the daily and seasonal cycles, the rhythms of life. . . ." See how Price applies his sustainable-design philosophy in *The Archaeology of Tomorrow: Architecture & the Spirit of Place.*

Use Salvaged and Reclaimed Materials

There is probably nothing you want to furnish your home with that you can't find through salvage, and generally at less than half the price. Furniture, fabric, cabinets, flooring, accents, draperies, and appliances are yours for the picking, and they'll help you create a unique and beautiful home.

Do an Internet search of "salvage furniture" plus the name of your town or city to find nearby warehouses you can browse. Or you can check with businesses like the Loading Dock (www.loadingdock.org), a nonprofit materials reuse center in Baltimore, Maryland, whose motto is "Don't Dump. Donate!" The organization's inventory includes:

- Adhesives
- Banisters
- Bathtubs
- Bifold doors
- Carpet
- Caulk
- Cinder blocks
- Countertops
- Doors
- Door sweeps

- Electric lights
- Floor covering
- Gas stoves
- Hardware
- Insulation
- Kitchen cabinets
- Lumber
- Marble
- Paint
- Plumbing fixtures

- Roof shingles
- Shelving
- Sinks
- Stairs
- Tile, ceramic
- Toilets
- Vinyl flooring
- Wallpaper

Similar facilities exist as part of the Reuse Development Organization, including Urban Ore, in Berkeley, California; Materials for the Arts, in New York City; and Barnraisers in Albany, New York.

If you do buy used goods, you'll save money. The Loading Dock calculates that its 5,000 members save $2.3 million every year shopping in its warehouses as opposed to traditional big-box stores or online. Salvage shopping benefits the environment, too. The Loading Dock has rescued more than 33,000 tons of building materials from landfills since it opened its doors in 1984. Plus, the group diverts 24,000 gallons of paint and other toxic materials from landfills annually.

Build and Decorate with Locally Made Products

You'll reduce the environmental impacts of long-distance transportation, help support your local economy, and create a market for materials that are more likely to meet U.S. standards for environmental protection and human health and safety if you shop closer to home. Items likely to be available locally or even regionally include:

- straw bales and other construction materials
- wood flooring
- kitchen and bath cabinets made by local craftspeople
- handcrafted living room, bedroom, and dining room furniture
- glasswork, pottery
- throw rugs, area rugs
- photography, painting

For a list of craft shows and art fairs by zip code, visit www.festivalnet.com; weekend sections of newspapers and online community calendars provide directories, as well.

What about making it yourself? Yes, it will take more time, and the result is somewhat unpredictable (I speak from experience!). On the other hand, it can be extremely satisfying to do the work, and making accents, curtains, throws, and collages for your home will result in decor that's yours and yours alone.

- With a sewing machine, finish the edge on fabric to make a window treatment or pillow.
- Embroider fabric with designs you create, or follow a pattern.
- Reupholster simple seat cushions, or get ambitious and tackle more-complicated pieces of furniture.

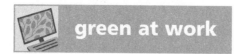

Offices Can Be Green, Too

Use the same earth-friendly flair at work that you use at home.

- Decorate your office with personal items rather than stock kitsch.
- If the company is repainting, suggest nontoxic materials that will minimize indoor air pollution.
- Recommend carpeting made from recycled fibers.
- Choose furniture made from sustainable wood or recycled sources. Companies to consider include Herman Miller (www.hermanmiller.com), the Knoll Group (www.knoll.com), Steelcase (www.steelcase.com), and Guilford of Maine (www.guilfordofmaine.com).

Recycle or Donate Excess Materials

To minimize how much you trash, recycle or donate excess building materials.

- When we replaced our wall-to-wall carpeting with wood (see "In My House," page 359), the floor installer wanted to charge us a fee to dump the carpeting and padding at the local landfill. Instead, we carted the waste to a nearby recycler who took it off our hands for free.
- Contact www.earth911.org to find the nearest place to donate leftover paint, fabric, wood, and other building materials.
- Remember the maxim, "One woman's junk is another woman's treasure." If you're renovating your home, donate unwanted items to charities like the Loading Dock.
- Habitat for Humanity's ReStores accept a wide variety of household items; so does your local Salvation Army, and they'll pick up at no charge.

When my neighbors redid their kitchen, a nonprofit organization removed the old cabinets intact, as well as the still-working appliances, and carted them off to a family in need.

Before you think about giving your furniture or cabinets away, ask yourself if you can put them to use somewhere else. When we renovated our kitchen, we transferred a couple of the cabinets to the basement bathroom. It saved us a few hundred dollars and reduced what we tossed in the trash.

Favor Sustainable Furnishings

Designs made from recycled and renewable products serve two mistresses: the aesthetic, who's looking for visual, spiritual, and emotional satisfaction; and the practical, who wants to achieve function and flexibility. As you read the following listings, you may want to circle or check the options that sound particularly appealing for your next redo.

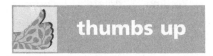

Buying or Selling

When you are ready to buy, www.GreenerBuilding.org makes it easy to identify the right building products, and to locate local dealers and helpful programs that sell reliable, certified environmental materials for your home.

For an explanation of the benefits of green building and renovating, log on to www.builditgreen.com.

And when you're ready to sell, list your home on www.greenhomesforsale.com.

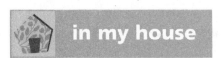

As 2006 was drawing to a close, I had to face the facts: my home had gotten dingy. The wall-to-wall carpeting, originally a nice soft gray to complement the peach walls, had gone almost white in the places where we'd scrubbed to remove proof that someone had spilled his juice or ground a chocolate chip under her heel. The twenty-year-old furniture sagged and sighed every time we sat down. Even our artwork was looking a little artless, never mind the fact that we didn't have quite enough to cover the many nicks the walls had sustained from kids, pets, parties, and day-to-day living. It was time for a makeover. Though we weren't going to tear down walls or build new rooms, the work we did turned out to be pretty major:

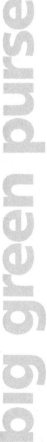

- We replaced our wall-to-wall carpet with Forest Stewardship Council (FSC)–approved Brazilian cherrywood bought at a local green supplier (www.amicus green.com). We coated it with a clear, water-based sealant that created almost no perceptible indoor air pollution.

- We had the entire house repainted in Pittsburgh Paint's Pure Performance Paint. There are many new no- and low-VOC options these days. I chose Pure Performance because it was no-VOC; I work at home and would not have been able to tolerate the minor indoor air pollution even a low-VOC paint generates.

- Even though our furniture was twenty years old, since it was structurally sound, we decided to reupholster rather than replace it. I was not able to find any organic or earth-friendly fabrics locally and ran out of the time necessary to shop intelligently for recycled or organic fabric online. Ultimately, I chose a cotton/polyester blend that is supposed to be durable enough to last another twenty years.

- I repainted some furniture, polished some, and donated what I couldn't use—chairs, lamps, an ottoman—to the Salvation Army. Having them pick it up was easier than having a yard sale, and I got a tax deduction for giving my items to a charity.

- For home accessories, I "shopped" locally—in my attic. I browsed around and found interesting "new" items that have sentimental as well as artistic appeal, like knickknacks from past family vacations and crafts I'd picked up at local art fairs. Rather than buy knockoff prints by famous artists that meant nothing to me, I framed family photographs to give our house a more personal touch. I'm also acquiring artwork made by friends and shopping at local art galleries and seasonal crafts fairs that feature designs made by regional artists.

Replacing the floor and repainting the entire house were the most expensive parts of the project, and doing them in an eco-friendly way made them slightly more so: the FSC-certified floor cost about $1,500 more than its conventionally produced counterpart, while the no-VOC paint added $600 to the cost of the job. On the other hand, I lost absolutely no time due to health or discomfort from the paint or the chemicals used to treat the floor. More important, my family was able to live in the house during the entire renovation.

Furniture

Unleash your ingenuity as well as your green spirit when it comes to furnishing your home in an eco-friendly way. The Sustainable Furniture Council (www.sustainable furniturecouncil.org) offers these tips:

- **Fashion furniture from interesting existing materials,** like wheel frames, grapevines, and door frames (all of which make creative table bases).
- **Use lumber reclaimed** from fencing, flooring, and structural supports and paneling.
- **Choose fast-growing wood** varieties or species from sustainably managed forests, such as mango and bamboo.
- **Avoid species known to be threatened,** like new teak and mahogany and woods from fragile tropical or subtropical regions, such as the Philippines, Indonesia, and South America.
- **Apply water-based finishes** rather than common varnishes, lacquers, and shellacs, which can contain toxic petroleum- or synthetic-based solvents.
- **Choose upholstery made from organic cotton,** durable hemp, or fabrics woven from recycled cotton and polyester blends.

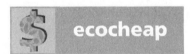

To be honest, furnishings made from recycled, organic, or sustainable materials can be more expensive than mass-produced department store models—they're more often priced comparably to higher-end options. But remember, your purchase now can make a difference in the long run by helping bring the price down: every time any of us chooses a green option, those choices become more affordable for all of us eventually.

- **Consider antiques,** which rack up nothing in additional energy, water, and other manufacturing costs. They reduce the amount of trash entering landfills because that "old" furniture is not thrown away. Plus, many antiques add character and charm to your living space.
- **Buy online.** Check eBay, www.freecycle.com, www.craigslist.com, and other on-line communities for quality items at reduced prices.
- **Sell online.** Use the proceeds to purchase (more-expensive) ecofurnishings. Using my neighborhood Listserv, I sold two chairs for half of what I paid for them, then

used the proceeds to buy a beautiful photograph produced by a local artist. Meanwhile, my neighbor got a great deal on the chairs.

• **Shop at crafts fairs.** Local artisans make exquisite but affordable furniture out of wood and materials they salvage in their community; weavers create beautiful pillows, cushions, throw rugs, and blankets from organic wool and cotton. Many merchants will customize their crafts to meet your specific needs.

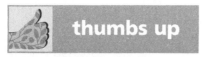

Have a Healthy House as Well as a Green One

• **The Healthy House Institute** (www.healthyhouseinstitute.com) offers dozens of useful links, articles, tips, and product reviews.
• **GreenGuard** (www.greenguard.org) will help you find products that emit no or low chemicals, benefiting indoor air quality.

Flooring

There are so many green flooring options these days, it should be relatively easy to find one that appeals to both your aesthetic eye and your pocketbook.

Carpet. The most earth-friendly carpeting uses recycled fibers. Manufacturers like Forbo and Interface are aggressively recapturing used carpet, grinding it up, and recycling it into new products. You can be even more eco-friendly by installing carpet squares rather than wall-to-wall broadloom. In the event the dog diddles, your child piddles, or soda water just won't remove that stubborn red wine stain, you don't have to replace the entire carpet. Just pull out the offensive square and install a new one. Nontoxic glues and low-VOC padding also add to the increased appeal of green carpeting.

Carpet Woes

• Most carpet is made from synthetic oil-based materials backed with PVC that outgas harmful chemicals long after the carpet has been installed.

- Adhesives used to glue carpet to the floor typically contain volatile organic compounds (VOCs) that also pollute indoor air long after the carpet is installed.
- Most carpet is not recycled. In fact, the amount of carpet that is discarded and sent to landfills every year covers an area greater than New York City.

If you opt for carpet, choose wool or recycled fibers, natural padding, and a product that meets environmental standards that will protect your indoor air quality.

Wood. Salvaged wood is being reclaimed from old bars, abandoned factories and warehouses, the bottom of lakes and rivers that once served as shipping channels for logging operations, and old boats. Once the nails are removed, the wood is stripped, sanded, and readied for installation or remanufacture into a new product.

Hardwood from sustainably managed American plantations should bear the FSC logo, which signifies that the wood was grown without the use of poisonous chemicals or other practices that would wreck the land. Woods from sustainably managed tropical plantations may also bear the FSC logo. But since the standards are often difficult to enforce in extremely remote regions of the world, there is less certainty that the wood lives up to standards. On the other hand, buying FSC-certified tropical wood is better than buying wood from tropical rain forests that bears no standards. The FSC standard matters most when applied to teak, mahogany, rosewood, ebony, and cherry, all of which are grown in tropical regions where logging is still out of control.

Also look for flooring and furniture made from "secondary species"—sweet gum, madrone, California oak—which take pressure off more-endangered trees like mahogany and teak. You might even consider products made from so-called "lower" grades of wood—specimens that may feature knots or streaks. These lower grades are just as functional as other woods, often have more character, and, again, help reduce demand for higher-grade lumber.

Cork. Strong and versatile, cork is harvested from the bark of trees that grow in the Mediterranean, primarily Portugal. The bark is gently peeled from the trees every nine years or so; the trees are not cut down, since they're needed to regenerate the bark. Cork can be fine-grained or marbleized in appearance and comes in many shades and hues, from the color of light honey to dark walnut. Cork is easy to maintain, durable, resilient, and flame retardant.

Bamboo. A fast-growing and long-lived plant, bamboo can grow to a height of forty feet and a diameter exceeding six inches in five or six years. Because bamboo is a grass, it does not require replanting when harvested. Its extensive root system will continue to send up new shoots for decades. "Eco-bamboo" is grown in managed forests and harvested by hand with minimal impact to the local environment. It can be used in its natural color or stained. *Beware*, though: Most bamboo flooring comes from China, which by now is notorious for unreliable factory conditions, use of toxic chemicals, and general lack of environmental standards. This makes it essential that you buy bamboo only from a reliable supplier whose product carries the FSC label and who can vouch for the environmental quality of its products.

Linoleum. Natural linoleum is a durable flooring choice made from linseed oil, pine resin, wood flour, cork powder, limestone dust, natural pigments, and jute. It can be used anywhere you need a resilient floor, as well as for counters and desktops. You can buy natural linoleum in tiles, sheets, and panels that click into place and require no adhesives. You can also use natural linoleum to replace vinyl flooring.

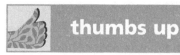 **thumbs up**

Floor Covering You Can Count On

C&A, a Tandus Group company, is one operation that really deserves to be called "eco." C&A purchases used vinyl-backed carpet, regardless of manufacturer, and processes it into 100 percent recycled-content backing for new C&A carpeting, closing the recycling loop by using the old product to make a new one. Because of the California Sustainable Carpet Standards the company adheres to:

- C&A has recycled more than 35 million pounds of carpet and manufacturing waste.
- The company has reduced both energy use and greenhouse gas emissions from its operations by 28 percent per square yard.
- The average face weight of their products is 20 percent below the industry average, but the carpet lasts up to three times longer than conventional carpeting.

Forbo, manufacturers of Marmoleum natural linoleum, has achieved SMART sustainable certification by creating a nature-friendly floor covering that's easy to clean, made from readily renewable natural ingredients, and based on life-cycle assessment to reduce environmental impact.

Milliken Carpet, another SMART-certified carpet company, has reduced energy and water consumption by 50 percent since 1995 while reusing rather than wasting used carpet through its Earth Square recycling program. Chances are, some of the Milliken carpet tiles you buy will consist of recycled fibers from other Milliken products.

Paint

Paint contains many volatile organic compounds, or VOCs, that "outgas" after they are applied. Indoors, these VOCs cause headaches, nausea, achy bones, and general discomfort. Outdoors, they contribute to smog and air pollution. Whether for indoors or out, your best bet is to buy low- or no-VOC paint. It's now available from almost a dozen companies in thousands of colors and in standard eggshell, glossy, and semigloss finishes. You can also select no-VOC water-based paint, stains, finishes, and paint stripper.

Paint How-tos

To get the most out of the paint you use:

- **Buy only what you need.** Measure carefully. It's better to go back for more than to be stuck with too much leftover paint you can't use.
- **Prevent paint from drying out.** Cover the paint can with plastic wrap, hammer the lid securely back into place, and store the paint upside down.
- **Use up stored paint.** Apply it for touch-up jobs or smaller projects. Blend similar colors for larger jobs; use as a primer.
- **Donate leftover paint.** Schools, churches, community groups, and kids' clubs may be looking for a free way to give their buildings a face-lift, and you can take a tax deduction when you make the gift.
- **Don't pour paint down the drain.** You can rinse latex paint off brushes, but otherwise leave leftover paint you can't use in open cans in a protected outdoor shed. When the paint air-dries, you can throw it away.
- **Circulate air.** Keep windows open and fans blowing to move air—and paint fumes—out of the house. Avoid as much indoor air pollution as possible.

Lead alert: If your home was painted prior to 1978, the paint probably contains lead. Lead dust is extremely toxic, especially to children and pets. Before you paint, take the precautions recommended on the Environmental Protection Agency's Web page "Lead in Paint, Dust and Soil" (www.epa.gov/lead). In short, never sand lead paint. Call on a professional certified in lead-paint abatement, whether the paint is indoors or outside where pets and wildlife can be exposed.

---

thumbs down

Unprotected Painters

Many homeowners hire immigrant workers to paint their homes, refinish their floors, and handle other messy jobs that potentially expose laborers to hazardous substances. Workers have shown up at my home to scrape, sand, paint, and caulk dressed only in T-shirts and blue jeans, not the protective goggles, face masks, and impervious long-sleeved work suits they need to prevent toxic dust from settling on their skin. If you are hiring work crews to refurbish your home, help keep them safe. Insist that they wear proper protection. If necessary, provide it. Alternatively, find a crew that is licensed under OSHA (Occupational Safety and Health Administration) standards to perform the tasks at hand.

Fabric

Consider two factors when you evaluate fabric for furniture or draperies: the cloth itself and how it's been colored. Cloth options stretch across the eco-spectrum, beginning with the rich and elegant and ending with the practical and serviceable. (You can read a more extensive discussion of the environmental costs incurred in creating fabric in Chapter 8.) They include:

- Organic silk (produced without killing the worms that spin the silk)
- Organic cotton
- Recycled polyester
- Hemp
- Hemp/silk or hemp/cottonblends
- Cotton twills and brushed twills made without chemical finishes or sizing
- Linen

Color options are equally varied. Conventional dyeing processes can wreak environmental havoc. Cotton is often bleached white first with chlorine or hydrogen peroxide, a process that produces dioxin, a carcinogen and potential hormone disrupter. Fabric dyes likely include toxic heavy metals such as chrome, copper, and zinc; even natural dyes may use heavy metals in the mordant, or dye-fixing, agent. Because cotton naturally resists dye, some of the chemicals used during coloring may be discarded, polluting rivers and land. "Low-impact" or "natural" dyes help, but it would be better to set a standard for growing and dyeing cotton that encourages the safest production possible. Hemp and cotton can be grown naturally in different hues, but that's only a partial solution. Not everyone wants to live in the same shades of gray, taupe, green, cream, and white.

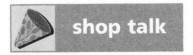

Ask for Eco

It's difficult to find organic or hemp fabrics on the shelves of most retail outlets, though you can usually special-order through catalogs and magazines. To get an idea of what to look for, peruse the pages of http://organicclothing.blogs.com, a comprehensive website devoted to natural and sustainable fibers and ecofashion. Green Sage (www.greensage.com/fabricstore) also showcases a beautiful array of sustainable fabrics you can restyle into upholstery, draperies, and accessories that can be ordered online or at specialty shops. *Natural Home Magazine* (on newsstands or at www.naturalhomemagazine.com) bursts with green home makeovers, new product links, and eco-design tips that often include organic and recycled fabrics.

Where to Shop

The following online and neighborhood retailers will help you find the most earth-friendly furnishings for your home.

Furniture

ABC Home and Carpet (www.abchome.com/end_splash.htm) is a major New York City–based retailer of imports, furniture, and rugs. The company is committed to retailing and sourcing sustainable products manufactured by fair labor practices.

Asiantique (www.asiantiqueweb.com) specializes in antiques and handcrafted reproductions made from teakwood reclaimed from old buildings and ships.

Baltix (www.baltix.com) features office furniture made from sustainable natural materials that contain no harmful adhesives, formaldehydes, or VOCs.

From the Mountain Sources LLC (www.fromthemountain.com) helps manufacturers, importers, and consumers source the sustainable manufacture of home furnishings that are handmade, unique, storied, fair-trade manufactured, and affiliated with green industries. The site lists where some handmade products answering these criteria may be purchased (www.fromthemountain.com/interior_pages/where_to_buy.htm).

Getknu.com (www.getknu.com) is an environmentally committed manufacturer of contemporary office furniture. Proprietary hardware is custom manufactured from 40 percent recycled steel that is 100 percent recyclable. Wood components are produced from FSC-certified multi-ply birch whenever possible, engineered veneers are Scientific Certification Systems (SCS)–certified sustainable, and even the pencil drawers are recyclable plastic. No contact adhesives are used in the manufacturing of Knú products. Recycling is an important priority and the company practices carbon offsetting.

Groovy Stuff (www.groovystuff.com) sells reclaimed teakwood furniture refashioned from plantation teak and farm implements from a bygone era into contemporary and organic furnishings.

Industrial Woodworking Corporation (www.industrialwoodworking.com) manufactures high-end, contemporary nonupholstered furniture, ready-to-assemble home-office solutions, and cabinets, as well as seating and case goods–related furnishings. Many supplies (including particleboard) are certified to meet environmental sustainability standards. Manufacturing occurs without contact adhesives and utilizes only HAPS (hazardous air pollutant)-compliant (very-low-VOC) finishes, or waterborne finishes for wet coat (wood-finishing) operations. The company practices carbon offsetting.

Natural As Sleep (www.naturalassleep.com) offers 100 percent certified organic and fair trade bedding: mattresses are made with organic wool, cotton, and latex and use the Sonoid adjustable sleep system.

Organo (www.organonatural.com) designs use wheatboard, aluminum, steel, and sustainably harvested woods, plus low- and no-VOC finishes, to create tables, mirrors, frames, and accessories.

Restoration Hardware (www.restorationhardware.com/rh/index.jsp) carries the

Providence Collection of sustainably harvested teak indoor-outdoor furniture but does not prominently feature other ecologically friendly products.

Southcone (www.southcone.com) offers traditional and lush contemporary furniture manufactured from sustainably managed woods (with FSC certification when possible) and, often, with organic finishes. Attention is given to promoting sustainable economic prosperity for Indians in the Peruvian Amazon.

Tassajara Designs (www.tassajaradesigns.com) features one-of-a-kind pieces made in the U.S.A., with a local, legal workforce, using sustainable or alternative products whenever possible. Nonpolluting/nontoxic finishes and adhesives are standard. Nakashima-influenced slab furniture is a specialty.

Urban Woods (www.urbanwoods.net) describes its classic, contemporary furniture as "beyond sustainable." It is manufactured exclusively from reclaimed woods, organic cottons, and water-based finishes.

Viridian (www.viridiandesign.org/products/furniture.htm) has compiled a great list of manufacturers that create a wide variety of environmentally comfortable sofas, chairs, desks, and stools. Get a cup of tea, put on your favorite music, and go ahead and browse.

VivaTerra (www.vivaterra.com) sells furniture made from recycled or sustainable wood, as well as a variety of other sustainable luxury products.

Vivavi (www.vivavi.com) offers upscale, eco-friendly furniture for homes. The company is powered by 100 percent clean wind energy and is also a member of 1% for the Planet, an alliance of socially and environmentally responsible businesses that donate 1 percent of all sales to environmental organizations. Vivavi selects furniture made from renewable materials that replenish quickly, like bamboo, and sources wood products that are certified to have been responsibly harvested by groups like the Forest Stewardship Council (FSC). The company also strives to ensure that the products it features are created by workers who earn a fair wage for their labor.

Fabric

Peruse the listings of these ecofabric designers for cloth and upholstery to meet your green decorating needs.

Ambatalia Fabrics (www.ambataliafabrics.com) sells hemp, organic plant-dyed wool, vintage lace, custom sewing services, plant-dyed indigo, and buttons.

Anna Sova (www.annasova.com) offers ecosafe silk and organic cotton draperies.

Aurora Silk (www.aurorasilk.com) retails organic silk, yarns, and threads, and provides tutorials if you want to raise your own silkworms.

Clothworks (www.cameronclothworks.com/) and **Furnature** (www.furnature.com/fabrics.html) sell organic cotton upholstery as well as upholstery fabric. Furnature's SafeWash removes unpleasant fabric finish and dye odors from almost any fabric.

Do-it-yourself Organics at Heart of Vermont (www.heartofvermont.com) retails twills and flannels, as well as organic cotton and pure wool pillow kits and organic cotton futon covers.

Green Sage (www.greensage.com) features organic textiles for reupholstering furniture or sewing draperies or cushions.

Hemp Traders (www.hemptraders.com) looks like a good place to get upholstery-quality hemp, a strong, long-lasting fabric that's easy to launder, as well as knits, muslin, and linen.

Interface Fabrics (www.interfacefabricsgroup.com/home.html) markets Terratex, a fabric made from recycled polyester, corn-based "PLA" fibers, and sustainable wool.

Loop Fabric (www.loopfabric.co.uk/index.html) features an exclusive range of textiles derived entirely from sustainable, biodegradable, and/or certified organic fibers, including muslin, linen, hemp, silk, corduroy, canvas, and knits.

Maharam (www.maharam.com) designs upholstery fabric and curtain material in beautiful colors, and offers designs made from "post-industrial polyester."

Twill Textiles (www.twilltextiles.com/climatex.html) features pesticide residue–free wool and organically grown ramie dyed and processed with nontoxic chemicals; the manufacturer claims the product is 100 percent biodegradable and can be returned to the earth as mulch or ground cover.

Mattresses, Bedding, and Linens

Given how much time we spend (or should spend) sleeping, the furniture and fabrics we use in our bedroom deserve some special attention. Several organizations and health groups encourage consumers to consider "eco" mattresses when they shop. Why? Most mattresses are filled with polyurethane foam and other materials that have been treated with flame retardants as well as water-, stain- and wrinkle-resistant chemicals. At the least, these chemicals, which include PBDEs, can pollute the air inside your home. If you're particularly sensitive, they could make you sick. According to the Children's Health Environmental Coalition (CHEC), there is some evidence that PBDEs can interfere with thyroid hormone, which is critical to the developing fetus. According to some studies, women in the United States have the highest levels of PBDEs in their bodies in the world. Mattresses and mattress pads are also being treated with water and stain repellents to guard against damage to these products. One such repellent is Teflon, the same product used as a nonstick coating on pans. Recently, Teflon has come under attack because its main ingredient, perfluorooctanoic acid (PFOA), is so widespread in the environment and in people.

The solution? Untreated organic cotton and wool mattresses for cribs as well as adult-size beds. CHEC cautions that, if you choose an untreated option, make sure you have working smoke detectors near the bedrooms and do not allow candles, matches, lighters, and cigarettes in bedrooms. If you're worried about the mattress collecting dust, mold, or mildew, you can encase it in a full-mattress cover.

Many bed linens, meanwhile, may be treated with fabric finishes to repel stains or wrinkles. These chemicals may be released over time into the air we breathe. They may also irritate the skin. Organic cotton sheets, pillowcases, and comforters can help solve the problem.

EcoBedroom (www.ecobedroom.com) sells baby bedding, duvets, comforters, shams, bamboo and organic wool blankets, mattress pads, and softeners.

Heart of Vermont (www.heartofvermont.com) specializes in sateen, wool, and cotton sheets, pillowcases, comforters, fitted crib sheets, and futons for cots and chairs.

Natural As Sleep (www.naturalassleep.com) specializes in 100 percent certified organic and fair trade bedding: mattresses made with organic wool, cotton, and latex.

A Natural Home (www.anaturalhome.com) offers chenille organic cotton blankets, natural latex rubber pillows, organic cotton quilts, organic cotton percale sheets, and handwoven cotton rag rugs.

Nirvana (www.nontoxic.com/cbedding/index.html) sells nontoxic, organic cotton sheets, cotton blankets, and wool comforters.

Organic Mattresses (www.organicmattresses.com) features organic mattresses in any size or firmness using only natural latex or innerspring cores and naturally safer® organic wool and certified organic cotton, plus sheets, blankets and "puddle pads."

Rawganique (www.rawgamoqie.com) features towels, curtains, and bath mats made from organic cotton, hemp and linen.

Carpet

"Green" carpets don't have to be green—they come in many colors and designs. The best options, like those listed below, meet either SMART, SCS Sustainable Choice, or the equivalent California Gold, Platinum, or Silver standards for sustainability. They contain a high level of post-consumer or recycled content, have no or minimal impact on indoor air quality, can be recycled, avoid PBDE flame retardants, and have completed a life-cycle analysis.

Bentley Prince Street (www.bentleyprincestreet.com) sells several product lines that have been certified to meet the California Gold standard, including High Performance PC broadloom carpet, Prestige PlusRC broadloom carpet, and EncoreRC Carpet Tile.

FLOR (www.florcatalog.com), a modular carpet company, says it stands for "Mission Zero." Inspired by its parent company, environmental leader Interface, Inc., Flor seeks to eliminate any negative impact on the environment by 2020. Since 1995, Flor has reduced manufacturing waste sent to landfills by 63 percent and absolute greenhouse gas emissions by 56 percent worldwide. FLOR's R&R program (Return-Recycle) makes it easy for customers to ship used carpet tiles back to the mill, where the old tiles are recycled into new product.

InterfaceFLOR Commercial (www.interfaceflor.com) includes many sustainable product lines in a wide variety of colors, styles, and applications.

Milliken Carpet (www.millikencarpet.com) patterned carpet tiles have achieved platinum and gold certification.

The Mohawk Group (www.themohawkgroup.com) features product lines achieving gold, silver, or platinum certification, among them, Durkan, Lees, and Mohawk Commercial Colorstrand.

Shaw Contract Group (www.shawcontractgroup.com). The company's EcoWorx line has achieved California Gold standard.

Wood

Eco Timber (www.ecotimber.com) offers FSC-certified and reclaimed wood flooring. The company's HealthyBond adhesive is virtually VOC free (7 grams per liter), and many of the products are formaldehyde free. Prefinished floors are UV-cured at the factory to further decrease VOCs.

Salvaged Wood

North Coast Timber (www.northcoasttimber.com/products.html) sells western red cedar, Alaskan yellow cedar, Sitka spruce, and Douglas fir.

Timeless Timber (www.timelesstimber.com) salvages logs from underwater, recovering and processing two million board feet of lumber each year without sawing down one single tree. In addition to flooring, Timeless Timber wood is used for countertops and paneling.

Other Flooring Options

Bamboo Plyboo (www.plyboo.com). Sustainably produced bamboo is used for flooring as well as countertops, cupboards, and furniture.

DuroDesign (www.duro-design.com). Bamboo, cork, oak and eucalyptus flooring with low-VOC finishes.

Edipo cork flooring (www.duro-design.com). Bamboo, cork, oak, and eucalyptus flooring finished with low-VOC sealants.

EnviroPLANK terrazzo plank flooring (www.enviroglasproducts.com). Ecological flooring tiles combine 100% recycled glass and porcelain terrazzo. EnviroGLAS combines lightweight epoxy resin with multicolored glass chips from discarded bottles, mirrors, and plate windows, and porcelain chips from discarded toilets, sinks, and tubs to achieve a surface harder than traditional marble terrazzo.

Marmoleum (www.themarmoleumstore.com). Made from linseed oil, wood flour, rosin, jute, and limestone to have no indoor air-quality impact. Available in a comprehensive range of design elements.

Natural Cork and More (www.naturalcork.com) offers a wide variety of colors in classic and earth designs, and in parquet squares.

Paint and Wall Coverings

American Clay (www.americanclay.com) makes a natural-clay plaster alternative to cement, gypsum, acrylic, and lime; manufactured in the United States, American Clay's products use natural clays, recycled and reclaimed aggregates, and vibrant natural pigments available domestically.

AnnaSova (www.annasova.com) wall finishes contain 99.9 percent food-grade ingredients that the company claims are so safe, leftovers can be "thrown in the garden." Products include paint, stucco, and "texture."

Auro Paint (www.aurousa.com) manufactures mineral- and plant oil–based paints that utilize rosemary, eucalyptus, castor, and linseed.

Green Seal (www.greenseal.org/findaproduct/index.cfm#paints) has certified dozens of other no- or low-VOC paints worth considering.

The PPG Architectural Finishes Pure Performance line (www.pittsburgh paints.com) sells no-VOC paints in hundreds of colors in eggshell, semigloss, and glossy finish.

Safecoat (www.safecoatpaint.com) makes an all-purpose paint that eliminates solvents, heavy metals, chemical residuals, formaldehyde, and other harmful preservatives; seals surfaces (from wood to metal to concrete, carpets, and much more), reducing "outgassing," the emission of toxins into the environment.

Sherwin Williams' GreenSure line (www.sherwin.com/do_it_ yourself/ sherwin_williams_products/greensmart.jsp), in fourteen hundred colors, comes in low- and no-VOC options.

Home, Green Home Wrap-up

- **Don't make "eco" an afterthought.** Whether renovating or building new, make your home more earth-friendly right from the start.
- **Simplify.** Reuse before you renovate, and renovate before you build.
- **Be a "LEEDer."** Build and decorate based on sustainable U.S. Green Building Council principles that save energy and water and conserve materials.
- **Buy local.** Build and decorate using locally made materials.
- **Protect indoor air quality.** Choose formaldehyde-free furniture, organic cotton and hemp fabrics, and no- or low-VOC paints and finishes.
- **Save forests.** Choose FSC wood furniture, flooring, and cabinetry.

And if you can do only one thing, purchase furnishings that meet sustainable standards from the beginning of their production phase to the end. You'll get the most environmental benefit for your buck while encouraging other manufacturers to achieve sustainable standards, too.

ACKNOWLEDGMENTS

Writing this book would have been a solitary task if not for the grandstand of supporters cheering me on every step of the way. Gail Ross, my loyal agent and friend, offered many suggestions that improved on the original idea, providing the kind of strategic guidance that showed yet again why she is the best in her field. Howard Yoon's insights strengthened the concept and broadened its appeal. The proposal never would have gotten out the door without the devotion of the talented staff at the Gail Ross Literary Agency. Many thanks.

From the beginning, the team at Avery has embraced my vision as their own. Every writer should be blessed with a publisher as stalwart as Megan Newman, an editor as sure as Lucia Watson, and a publicist as relentless as Anne Kosmoski. Miriam Rich, Jessica Lee, Molly Brouillette, Kate Stark, and Amanda Tobier made up the rest of the Avery dream team, spoiling this author forever. Avery's copy editors, proofreaders, and page designers played a critical role, too, working to meet deadlines that would have flummoxed others less competent or committed. Thank you, all.

There is no way I can ever express my gratitude to Mandy Katz, Chris Intagliata, Susan Katz Miller, Colleen Cordes, Susan Orlins, and Robyn Jackson—the members of Calliope, my writers' group—for their generous spirit, perceptive editorial comments, and unfailing encouragement. If *Big Green Purse* "sings," it is because I often heard their voices in my ear when I was writing. Marika Partridge, who gave me my first big green purse, was there at the beginning, too: I am happily in their debt.

Research assistants Elizabeth Higgins Null and Carey Ciochina both did a terrific job ferreting out information, often under pressure of last-minute deadlines. Genna Duberstein helped extend *Big Green Purse* to social networking communities on the Internet. Thank you.

Mary Hunt, a sharp analyst of the power of the purse in her own right as well as an accomplished author and blogger, provided invaluable insights, direction, and assistance that have helped give the *Big Green Purse* message both depth and breadth.

I will never cease to appreciate the support of my friends, especially Selma Jaskowski, Bruce Hathaway, and Karen Sagstetter; Annie Prutzman and "Chicken"; Donna Scarboro and Ralph Steinhardt; Wolfgang and Gertrud Mergner; Anthony Garrett, Christopher Palmer, and Roger DiSilvestro. The Alaska Wilderness League, on whose board I serve, could not have been more gracious during the leave of absence I have had to take while writing this book. Thanks especially to executive director Cindy Shogan and board chair Tom Campion. I also appreciate the early brainstorming I did with my former colleagues at Vanguard Communications under the magnanimous direction of Maria Rodriguez.

I am particularly grateful to Peter Barnes, Luke Newton, and the Common Counsel Foundation for the opportunity to spend two weeks researching and writing at the incomparable Mesa Refuge writers' center. Thanks, too, to my fellow "refugees," Rebecca Clarren and Jamie Kitman, for their good humor, lively conversation, and that delicious last supper.

I am indebted to the hundreds of nonprofit organizations that are working locally, nationally, and internationally to protect the environment. Mike Italiano and the Institute for Market Transformation to Sustainability were especially helpful in explaining the important role standards play in motivating companies to reduce greenhouse gases and meet other important environmental goals. I am also grateful to Rebecca Graham of Scientific Certification Systems, James Simpson of the Marine Stewardship Council, Katie Miller of the U.S. Forest Stewardship Council, Cassie Hayes of the Chlorine Free Products Association, Vicki Katrinak of the Coalition for Consumer Information on Cosmetics, Linda Chipperfield of Green Seal, Inc., Jennifer Rudolf of TransFair USA, Ellen Hunt of Humane Farm Animal Care, and Taryn Holowka at the U.S. Green Building Council for their cooperation in the use of their labels to help consumers avoid greenwashing. Ginny Miller and New Society Publishers were extremely generous in providing review copies of many excellent books that helped illuminate my thinking on environmental issues and the way consumers can use their clout to protect the environment. Thanks to Robert Engelman of Worldwatch Institute for providing key insights into the relationship between population and environmental degradation. In the important intersection between women's health and the environment, I was particularly informed by Environmental Working Group, the Campaign for Safe Cosmetics, the excellent reports published by Women's Voices for the Earth, and the proceedings of the Women's Health and the Environment Conference series sponsored by the Heinz Foundation. I am particularly grateful to Ben Dappen, the Big Green Purse webmaster, who has helped maintain and update www.biggreenpurse.com no matter how vague my suggestions or how tight the deadlines.

By and large, writing this book demanded a punishing schedule of twelve- to fifteen-hour days almost every day for six months. My body would look like the chair I've been sitting in if not for my mutt, Heaven, who nuzzled me away from my computer every three or four hours and insisted I stretch my legs by taking her for a walk. Good dog.

My sisters, Jean Mehi and Laureen MacEachern, have been staunch supporters of this book from its onset; their love and encouragement have been invaluable. My brothers, Hugh and John, and my father, Angus Hugh, will also be proud, even if they don't carry a purse.

I could not have written a single word without the support of my husband, Dick Munson, who rejoiced equally at the completion of a paragraph as at a page. His flexibility in accommodating my writing priorities made it possible for me to meet my deadlines. Our children, Dana and Daniel, were as patient as teenagers can be during the many hours I was holed up in my office. I owe them a lot of homemade cookies.

Finally, I would like to acknowledge the constant good cheer and encouragement of my mother, Ann MacEachern. Her appreciation for my work, but especially her excitement for the ideas expressed in *Big Green Purse*, helped assure me that I was on the right track.

THE BIG GREEN
PURSE "LITTLE
BLACK BOOK"

Want to learn more about the topics discussed in Big Green Purse? These books, reports, and websites are in my Little Black Book. You're welcome to add them to yours.

Environmental Background

State of the World 2004; Special Focus: The Consumer Society, A Worldwatch Institute Report on Progress Toward a Sustainable Society, Linda Starke, ed., W .W. Norton & Company, 2004.
U.S. Environmental Protection Agency (www.epa.gov)
The Green Guide (www.thegreenguide.com)
Natural Resources Defense Council (www.nrdc.org)
Earth Share (www.earthshare.org)
Alaska Wilderness League (www.alaskawild.org)

Women's Health and the Environment

"What We Know: New Science Linking Our Health and the Environment," by Heather Sarantis, The Collaborative on Health and the Environment, 2007.
Women's Health and the Environment (www.womenshealthandenvironment.org)
Women's Voices for the Earth (www.womenandenvironment.org)
Environmental Health Perspectives (www.ehponline.org)
Environmental Risks and Breast Cancer, Vassar College (http://erbc.vassar.edu)
Center for Environmental Oncology of the University of Pittsburgh Cancer Institute (www .environmentaloncology.org/ec.htm)
State of the Evidence: What Is the Connection Between the Environment and Breast Cancer? edited by Nancy Evans, Breast Cancer Fund/Breast Cancer Action, 2006.
Making Our Milk Safe (www.safemilk.org)
"Are We Living in a Chemical Stew?" by Dr. Sandra Steingraber, 9th Annual Conference on Women's Health and the Environment, Keynote Address, October 24, 2005.

Global Warming

An Inconvenient Truth: The Planetary Emergency of Global Warming and What We Can Do About It, by Al Gore, Rodale Books, 2006.

Intergovernmental Panel on Climate Change (www.ipcc.ch), a joint initiative of the World Meteorological Organization (WMO) and the United Nations Environment Programme (UNEP) to understand the risks of human-induced climate change, its potential impacts, and options for adaptation and mitigation.

Field Notes from a Catastrophe: Man, Nature, and Climate Change, by Elizabeth Kolbert, Bloomsbury, USA, 2006.

www.stopglobalwarming.org

Climate Change website of the U.S. Environmental Protection Agency (www.epa.gov/climate change)

Marketplace Impacts

Institute for Market Transformation to Sustainability (www.mts.sustainable products.com)

Cradle to Cradle: Remaking the Way We Make Things, by William McDonough and Michael Braungart, North Point Press, 2002.

Consumers Union Guide to Environmental Labels (www.eco-labels.org)

In Women We Trust (www.inwomenwetrust.com)

Center for a New American Dream (www.newdream.org)

Branded! How the "Certification Revolution" Is Transforming Global Corporations, by Michael E. Conroy, New Society, 2007.

Ecoaction and Lifestyle Changes

Big Green Purse (www.biggreenpurse.com)

Earth 911 (www.earth911.org)

The Consumer's Guide to Effective Environmental Choices: Practical Advice from the Union of Concerned Scientists, by Michael Brower, Ph.D., and Warren Leon, Ph.D., Three Rivers Press, 1999.

Consumer Reports Greener Choices (www.greenerchoices.org)

The Lazy Environmentalist: Your Guide to Easy, Stylish, Green Living, by Josh Dorfman, Stewart, Tabori and Chang, 2007.

The Live Earth Global Warming Survival Handbook: 77 Essential Skills to Stop Climate Change, by David de Rothschild, Rodale Books, 2007.

Personal-Care Products

Third National Report on Human Exposure to Toxic Chemicals, Department of Health and Human Services Centers for Disease Control and Prevention, July 2005.

Environmental Working Group (www.ewg.org)

U.S. Food and Drug Administration: Cosmetics (www.cfsanifda.gov/~dms/cos=toc.html)

Campaign for Safe Cosmetics (www.safecosmetics.org)

Women's Voices for the Earth (www.womenandenvironment.org)

Exposed: The Toxic Chemistry of Everyday Products and What's at Stake for American Power, by Mark Schapiro, Chelsea Green, 2007.

Driving and Transportation

Divorce Your Car! Ending the Love Affair with the Automobile, by Katie Alvord, New Society Publishers, 2000.

Plug-in Hybrids: The Cars that Will Recharge America, by Sherry Boschert, New Society, 2006.

Forward Drive: The Race to Build "Clean" Cars for the Future, by Jim Motavalli, Sierra Club Books, 2001.

Beat High Gas Prices Now! The Fastest, Easiest Ways to Save $20–$50 Every Month on Gasoline, by Diane MacEachern, Andrews-McMeel, 2005.

Green Streets Initiative (www.gogreenstreets.org)

U.S. Environmental Protection Agency: Green Vehicle Guide (www.epa.gov/greenvehicle/about.htm) and Fuel Economy Guide (www.fueleconomy.gov)

Coffee, Tea, Cocoa, and Chocolate

Global Exchange (www.globalexchange.org/economy/coffee)

Rainforest Alliance (www.rainforestalliance.org)

Smithsonian Migratory Bird Center (www.natzoo.si.edu/smbc/Research/Coffee/coffee.htm)

The Songbird Foundation (www.songbird.org/sunvsshade.htm)

TransFair USA (www.transfairusa.org)

The Cocoa Tree (www.cocoatree.org)

Food

A Field Guide to Buying Organic, by Luddene Perry and Dan Schultz, Bantam Dell, 2005.

Six Arguments for a Greener Diet: How a Plant-based Diet Could Save Your Health and the Environment, by Michael F. Jacobson, Ph.D., Center for Science in the Public Interest, 2006.

"Still Waters—The Global Fish Crisis," by Fen Montaigne, Kennedy Warne, and Chris Carroll, National Geographic, April 2007.

Environmental Defense's Oceans Alive list of smart seafood choices (www.oceansalive.org/home.cfm)

Monterey Bay Aquarium's Seafood Watch (www.mbayaq.org/cr/seafoodwatch.asp)

Environmental Working Group's Shopper's Guide to Pesticides in Produce (www.foodnews.org/walletguide.php)

Food Routes Buy Local Network (www.foodroutes.org)

Green Cleaners

Consumer Reports' online Greener Choices consumer guide to cleaners (www.greenerchoices.org/products.cfm?product=greencleaning&page=RightChoices)

Household Hazards: Potential Hazards of Home Cleaning Products, by Alexandra Gorman, Women's Voices for the Earth, 2007.

Green Clean: The Environmentally Sound Guide to Cleaning Your Home, by Linda Mason Hunter and Mikki Halpin, Melcher Media, 2005.

Green This! Volume One: Greening Your Cleaning, by Deirdre Imus, Simon & Schuster, 2007.

Nontoxic & Natural: How to Avoid Dangerous Everyday Products and Buy or Make Safe Ones, by Debra Lynn Dodd, Jeremy P. Tarcher, 1984.

Clothing, Accessories, and Jewelry

Sustainable Cotton Project (www.sustainablecotton.org)

Organic Exchange cotton network (www.organicexchange.org)

"Nanotechnology's Invisible Threat: Small Science, Big Consequences" (www.nrdc.org/health/science/nano/fnano.pdf)

Project on Emerging Nanotechnologies, Woodrow Wilson Center for International Scholars (www.wilsoncenter.org/index.cfm?fuseaction=topics.home&topic_id=166192)

Textiles page of the Environmental Protection Agency's municipal solid waste website (www.epa.gov/epaoswer/non-hw/muncpl/textile.htm)

No Dirty Gold jewelry campaign (www.nodirtygold.org)

Global Witness campaign to stop blood diamonds (www.globalwitness.org/campaigns/diamonds)

Lawn, Garden, and Patio

Rodale's Chemical-Free Yard & Garden: The Ultimate Authority on Successful Organic Gardening, by Anna Carr.

The Landscaping Revolution: Garden with Mother Nature, Not Against Her, by Andy Wasowski and Sally Wasowski, Contemporary Books, 2000.

Native Plant Information Network (www.wildflower.org/plants)

Armitage's Native Plants for North American Gardens, by Allan M. Armitage, Timber Press, 2006.

The Natural Habitat Garden, by Ken Druse, Timber Press, 2004.

Plant Native (www.plantnative.org)

"Healthy Lawn Healthy Environment," Environmental Protection Agency (www.epa.gov/pesticides/controlling/garden.htm)

Lawns (Rodale's Organic Gardening Basics), Rodale Books, 2000.

Redesigning the American Lawn: A Search for Environmental Harmony, 2nd ed., by F. Bormann, Yale University Press, 2001.

The Chemical-Free Lawn, by Warren Schultz, Rodale Press, 1989.

National Coalition for Pesticide-Free Lawns (www.beyondpesticides.org/pesticidefreelawns/index.htm)

Pesticide Information Resources

Northeast Organic Farming Association Organic Land Care (www.organicland care.net)

The National Pesticide Information Center (www.npic.orst.edu)

U.S. Environmental Protection Agency, Office of Pesticide Programs (www.epa.gov/pesticides)

Pesticide Action Network (www.panna.org)

Bio-Integral Resource Center (www.birc.org)

Northwest Coalition for Alternatives to Pesticides (www.pesticide.org)

Babies and Kids

Institute for Children's Environmental Health (www.iceh.org)

Children's Environmental Health Network/Mt. Sinai Center for Children's Environmental Health and Disease Prevention Research (www.cehn.org/cehn/resourceguide/mscfcer.html)

The Learning and Developmental Disabilities Initiative (LDDI), a working group of the Collaborative on Health and the Environment (www.healthandenvironment.org)

Healthy Child Healthy World (www.healthychild.org) (Formerly known as CHEC—Children's Health Environmental Coalition)

Raising Healthy Children in a Toxic World: 101 Smart Solutions for Every Family, by Philip J. Landrigan, M.D., Herbert Needleman, M.D., and Mary Landrigan, MPA, Rodale Press, 2002.

Mothers & Others for a Livable Planet Guide to Natural Baby Care: Nontoxic and Environmentally Friendly Ways to Take Care of Your New Child, by Mindy Pennypacker and Aisha Ikramuddin, John Wiley & Sons, 1999.

Having Faith: An Ecologist's Journey to Motherhood, by Sandra Steingraber, Ph.D., Perseus Books, 2001.

Our Children's Toxic Legacy: How Science and Law Fail to Protect Us from Pesticides, 2nd ed., by John Wargo, Ph.D., Yale University Press, 1998.

"Keeping Kids Safe: A Guide for Safe Food Handling and Sanitation," United States Department of Agriculture (www.fns.usda.gov/TN/Resources/appendj.pdf)

Appliances, Lights, and Electronics

A Consumer's Guide to Energy Efficiency and Renewable Energy, U.S. Department of Energy (www.eere.energy.gov/consumer/your_home)

Consumer Reports Greener Choices Appliance report (www.greenerchoices.org/pcategories .cfm?pcat=appliances)

U.S. Environmental Protection Agency Energy Star Program (www.energystar.gov)

Consumer Guide to Home Energy Savings by the American Council for an Energy-Efficient Economy (www.aceee.org/consumerguide/#about)

EPA's Energy Star program on Compact Fluorescent Light Bulbs (www.energystar.gov/index .cfm?c=cfls.pr_cfls)

Environmental Defense "Make the Switch" campaign (www.environmentaldefense.org)

Alliance to Save Energy (www.ase.org/section/_audience/consumers/homecheckup)

American Solar Energy Society (ASES) (www.ases.org)

American Wind Energy Association (AWEA) (www.awea.org)

Electronics: A New Opportunity for Waste Prevention, Reuse, and Recycling (www.epa.gov/osw/ elec_fs.pdf)

WasteWise Update: Electronics Reuse and Recycling (www.epa.gov/wastewise/pubs/wwupda14 .txt)

eCycling: Basic Information (www.epa.gov/e-Cycling/basic.htm)

Silicon Valley Toxics Coalition (http://svtc.etoxics.org)

Furniture, Paint, Flooring, and Fabrics

Your Green Home: A Guide to Planning a Healthy, Environmentally Friendly New Home, by Alex Wilson, New Society Publishers, 2006.

The EPA's EnergyStar Web page on energy-efficient doors, windows, and skylights (www.energy star.gov/index.cfm?c=windows_doors.prwindows)

Green Remodeling: Changing the World One Room at a Time, by David Johnston and Kim Master, New Society Publishers, 2004.

Build It Green (www.builditgreen.org)

U.S. Green Building Council (USGBC) (www.usgbc.org)

Alliance to Save Energy (www.ase.org)

A Primer on Sustainable Buildings, by Dianna L. Barnett and William D. Browning, Rocky Mountain Institute, 1995.

The Healthy Home Workbook: Easy Steps for Eco-Friendly Living, by Kimberly Rider and Thayer Allyson Gowdy, Chronicle Books, 2006.

NOTES

Introduction

"Women spend eighty-five cents of every dollar in the marketplace." Marti Barletta, CEO and founder, TrendSight Group, "Primetime Women" e-newsletter, April 2, 2007.

Data on weekly household grocery expenses was gleaned from the Food Marketing Institute, as reported in *Frozen Food Digest*, October 2006.

"Fifty percent of purchasing agents for companies now are women." Marti Barletta, CEO and founder, TrendSight Group, and author, from online excerpt of *PrimeTime Women: How to Win the Hearts, Minds, and Business of Boomer Big Spenders*, Kaplan Business, 2007.

The rain forest facts, such as the statement that tropical rain forests are disappearing at the rate of six soccer fields a minute, came from "The Gasping Forest," by Alex Shoumatoff, *Vanity Fair*, May 2007.

The statements on the impact of the environment on the health of women and children reflect research being done by the Collaborative on Health and the Environment as reported at www.womensenvironmentalhealth.org; the Center for Environmental Oncology at the University of Pittsburgh Cancer Institute; Environmental Working Group; Women's Voices for the Earth; and the Children's Environmental Health Network/Mount Sinai Center for Children's Environmental Health and Disease Prevention Research.

The impact of phthalates on pregnant women came from "Exposure to Phthalates Commonplace in Pregnant Women; May Shorten Duration of Pregnancy by One Week." *Environmental Health Perspectives*, November 4, 2003.

The impact of phthalates on young girls is documented in "Phthalates Overview," *Environment California*, www.environmentcalifornia.org/environmental-health/stop-toxic-toys/phthalates-overview.

"Nearly 88,000 hybrid-electric vehicles were sold nationwide during 2004," reported J.D. Power and Associates, a marketing information and research firm based in Agoura Hills, California (www.bankrate.com/brm/news/auto/20030507a1.asp). The company also reported that "the market is still on track to sell 345,000 hybrids in 2007" in a press release, "Hybrid Vehicle Sales on Pace to Reach Record Sales in 2007."

Bruce MacKay of Del Laboratories, the maker of Sally Hansen nail polish, was originally quoted in the story "Looking good could be hazardous; Makeup, perfume and moisturizer may contain harmful chemicals," by Beth Greer, *San Francisco Chronicle*, September 27, 2006.

The details of Unilever's commitment to convert its tea brands to sustainable practices are detailed in the report "Unilever Commits to Rainforest Alliance Certification" on the Rainforest Alliance Farm to Market Web page (www.rainforest-alliance.org/agriculture/newsletter/fm_07_summer.html).

The Harry Potter facts and figures came from analysis by the Canadian group Markets Initiative and the article "Next thing you know, even Voldemort will be hugging trees," by Kate Sheppard, www.grist.org, July 18, 2007.

Chapter 1. If It Can Happen to an Alligator, Can It Happen to Your Son? Why Your Big Green Purse Matters

Information on the impact of pesticides on reproductive organs of alligators and other wildlife was gleaned from several articles, including "PCBs Diminish Penis Size," Rachel's Hazardous Waste News #372, January 13, 1994, and Janet Raloff, "The Gender Benders," *Science News*, Vol. 145 (January 8, 1994), pp. 24–27.

The findings on the 148 chemicals found in human blood or urine were reported in the *Third National Report on Human Exposure to Environmental Chemicals*, The Centers for Disease Control and Prevention (Atlanta): CDC, 2005.

Environmental Working Group's research on chemicals found in breast milk, cord blood, and urine and their link to cancer was reported in, "We're Exposed to 126 Chemicals Every Day: Common Chemicals: Breast Cancer Link?" by Colette Bouchez, WebMD Feature (www.webmd.com/breast-cancer/features/common-chemicals-breast-cancer-link).

Understanding of the impact of the environment on women's health, a topic addressed throughout the chapter, was derived from "What We Know: New Science Linking Our Health and the Environment," by the Collaborative on Health and the Environment (www.womenshealthandenvironment.org); the "Vallombrosa Consensus Statement on Environmental Contaminants and Human Fertility Compromise," October 2005; and *Exposed: The Toxic Chemistry of Everyday Products and What's at Stake for American Power*, by Mark Schapiro, Chelsea Green, 2007. "Declines in Sex Ratio at Birth and Fetal Deaths in Japan and U.S. Whites but not in Africa-Americans," by Devra Lee Davis, et al., *Environmental Health Perspectives*, April 2007, further explains how men exposed to dibromochloropropane, certain pesticides, alcohol, lead, and solvents, as well as those employed in sawmills and the aluminum industry, father fewer sons than expected. As reported in these same findings, men exposed to unusually high levels of dioxin fathered only daughters.

Information on contamination of breast milk by environmental toxins was found at Natural Resources Defense Council, "Healthy Milk, Healthy Baby," (www.nrdc.org/breastmilk/envpoll.asp).

Documentation on the impact of climate change on the Mendenhall Glacier was compiled in the report "Effects of Climate Change on Marine and Terrestrial Ecosystems in the Area of Juneau, Southeast Alaska," by Ashley Kelly, et al. (http:seagrant.naf.edu/nosb/papers/2005/juneau-stellar.html).

Background on climate change was drawn from the U.S. Environmental Protection Agency (www.epa.gov/climatechange/basicinfo.html), the Intergovernmental Panel on Climate Change (www.ipcc.ch), and *An Inconvenient Truth*, by Al Gore, Rodale Books, 2007.

The news about the impact of climate change on poison ivy was drawn from "Climate Changes Are Making Poison Ivy More Potent," by Tara Parker-Pope, *The Wall Street Journal*, June 26, 2007; p. D1.

Insights on the potential impact of global warming on asthma and allergy were gained from "Global Warming May be Spurring Allergy, Asthma," by Gautam Naik, *The Wall Street Journal*, May 3, 2007, p. 1.

Understanding of the impact of climate change on women came from IUCN—The World Conservation Union, "Climate Change and Disaster Mitigation" (www.iucn.org/themes/pbia/about/news.htm).

The consequences to business of climate change were reported in "Climate Change Futures: Health, Ecological and Economic Dimensions," Harvard Medical School, November 1, 2005.

Understanding of threats to our water supply came from www.abc.net.au/news/newsitems/200704/s1891582.html, "Water on Tap: What You Need to Know," U.S. EPA; the Environmental Protection Agency's website on safe water (www.epa.gov/safewater/mcl.html); "The Rise of Big Water," by Charles C. Mann, *Vanity Fair*, May 2007; "Arsenic in Drinking Water," National Academy 2001 Update, National Research Council Press Committee on Toxicology 2001; "Emerging Water Shortages Threaten Food Supplies, Regional Peace," Worldwatch Institute Press Release, July 17, 1999.

Information on chemicals in the Chesapeake Bay and Potomac River was drawn from "Water Worries," by Greg Peterson, *E Magazine*, July/August 2007, pp. 16–20.

Details on the impact of climate change on mangroves appeared in *State of the World 2006*, the Worldwatch Institute, W. W. Norton & Company, Danielle Nierenberg, project director, Linda Starke, editor.

Chapter 2. Cutting Through the Confusion: The Big Green Purse Principles

The statistics about how much we throw away came from the Environmental Protection Agency Office of Solid Waste and the Green Home newsletter (www.greenhome.com).

I got many useful ideas for ways shoppers could choose less packaging from "Consumer Choices Can Reduce Packaging Waste," by Kenneth R. Berger, University of Florida IFAS Extension Service, Institute of Food and Agricultural Services (http://edis.ifas.ufl.edu/AE226#FOOT NOTE_1) and *The Consumer's Handbook for Reducing Solid Waste*, by the U.S. Environmental Protection Agency (www.epa.gov/epaoswer/non-hw/reduce/catbook/index.htm).

The phrase "Less stuff, more fun" was coined by the Center for a New American Dream (www.newdream.org).

Details on how much time people spend shopping (six hours) as opposed to playing with children (forty minutes) were provided by the New Road Map Foundation (www.ecofuture.org/pk/pkar9506.html) in the report "All-Consuming Passion: Waking Up From the American Dream." The same report noted that about 53 percent of grocery and 47 percent of hardware store purchases are spur of the moment; the percentage of shoppers surveyed across the country who were shopping for a specific item is only 25 percent.

Information about polystyrene came from the U.S. Department of Health and Human Services (www.atsdr.cdc.gov/tfacts53.html), Agency for Toxic Substances and Disease Registry.

"The Consumers Union Guide to Environmental Labels" (www.eco-labels.org) was an invaluable source of information on the various eco-labels I reference in this chapter.

The origin of the meaning of the word "hypoallergenic" is explained in "Hypoallergenic: What's in a Word?" October 3, 2000, CBC News: Marketplace Microscope (www.cbc.ca/consumers/market/microscope/micro_2000/hypoallergenic.html). The word was invented by advertisers who used it in a cosmetics campaign in 1953. The U.S. Food and Drug Administration says, "There are no federal standards or definitions that govern the use of the term hypoallergenic. The term hypoallergenic means whatever a particular company wants it to mean."

Information about the energy required to transport food came from "Home Grown," a paper published by the Worldwatch Institute in 2002.

The statistics on the impacts of bottled water on the environment came from "Tapped Out: The True Cost of Bottled Water," by Solvie Karlstrom, *Green Guide* 121, July/August 2007.

My reports on women and their objections to packaging are based on intercept research I conducted between 2004 and 2006.

Rolling Hills Wildlife Adventure Museum and Zoo (www.rollinghillswildlife.com/get_involved/recycle.html) reported that each year, people in the United States produce 154 million tons of garbage, enough to fill the Louisiana Superdome from top to bottom, twice a day, every day.

The statistic revealing that Americans produce enough trash to fill sixty-three thousand garbage trucks each day came from Trash Trivia (www.cqc.com/~ccswmd/trivia.htm).

Chapter 3. Beauty . . . or the Beast? Cosmetics and Personal-Care Products

Information about cosmetics-labeling requirements came from the *Cosmetic Labeling Manual*, U.S. Food and Drug Administration, Center for Food Safety and Applied Nutrition, Office of Cosmetics and Colors (www.cfsan.fda.gov/~dms/cos-labl.html).

"Common Chemicals: Breast Cancer Link?" by Colette Bouchez, WebMDFeature, Nov 6, 2006, was the source of the quotes by Prof. Janet Gray of Vassar College and Dr. Julia Smith, Director of Breast Cancer Screening and Prevention at the Lynne Cohen Breast Cancer Preventive Care Program at NYU Cancer Institute and Bellevue Medical Center in New York City.

"New Site Gives Consumers Brand-by-Brand Safety Ratings for Over 14,000 Personal Care Products—Finds Few Popular Health and Beauty Brand Ingredients Are Industry-Screened for Safety" (www.ewg.org/reports/skindeep2/newsrelease.php).

Product-use survey results were originally reported in "Exposures Add Up—Survey Results" (www.ewg.org/reports/skindeep2/findings/index.php?content=exposure_survey#begin).

Facts about fragrances and their source as the most common cause of skin problems came from the National Women's Health Information Center—Office on Women's Health, U.S. Department of Health and Human Services (www.4woman.gov/faq/cosmetics.htm#l).

The connection between fragrances and asthma, headaches, and migraines was reported in "Fragrance: emerging health and environmental concerns," by Betty Bridges, *Flavour and Fragrance Journal*, Volume 17, Issue 5, 2002, pp. 361–371. Published online April 16, 2002.

The link between phthalates and male genital irregularities was reported in "Decrease in Anogenital Distance among Male Infants with Prenatal Phthalate Exposure," Shanna H. Swan, et al., *Environmental Health Perspectives*, May 2005, Volume 113, Number 8.

Preservatives are the second-most common cause of skin problems, according to research reported in "A Whiff of Danger: Synthetic Musks May Encourage Toxic Bioaccumulation," *Environmental Health Perspectives*, January 2005 volume 113, Number 1 (www.ehponline.org/docs/2004/7301/abstract.html).

Links between breast cancer and parabens were reported in a news release from the University of Reading (www.extra.rdg.ac.uk/news/details.asp?ID=304).

The importance of protecting the body's immune system was reported in "Antibacterial Household Products: Cause for Concern," by Dr. Stuart Levy, director, Center for Adaptation Genetics and Drug Resistance, professor of molecular biology and microbiology, and of medicine, Tufts University School of Medicine, Boston. Presentation from the International Conference on Emerging Infectious Diseases 2000 in Atlanta, Georgia, sponsored by the Centers for Disease Control National Center for Infectious Diseases (www.cdc.gov/ncidod/eid/vol7no3_supp/levy.htm).

Dr. Fran Cook-Bolden and Dr. Sarah Boyce Sawyer were originally interviewed on the topic of cosmetics and personal-care products by Natasha Singer in *The New York Times*, January 4, 2007.

Additional background on the impact of chemicals on the environment and human health was taken from "Household Pollutants Disrupting Fish Genes," *National Geographic News*, July 29, 2002 (www.news.nationalgeographic.com/news/2002/07/0729_020729_fishhormones.html); and "Common Industrial Chemicals in Tiny Doses Raise Health Issue," by Peter Waldman, *The Wall Street Journal*, July 25, 2005. "Chemicals from underarm deodorants and other cosmetics can build up inside the body, according to a study," BBC News, 11/01/04 (http://news.bbc.co.uk/2.hi/health/3383393.stm). "Antibacterial soaps presenting new kind of hygiene problems," by Pamela Roberts, Silicon Valley/*San Jose Business Journal*, March 30, 2001 (www.bizjournals.com/sanjose/stories/2001/04/02/focus2.html).

Birth control information was sourced at www.4women.gov/FAQ/ birthcont.htm, "Birth Control Methods" (www.womenshealth.gov), the Federal Government Source for Women's Health Information.

Douche information came from the Federal Government Source for Women's Health Information (www.4women.gov/FAQ/douching.htm).

Chapter 4. Car Talk . . . and More: Driving and Transportation

Numbers that report on women's driving patterns were culled from "What Women Want: 82% of Women Find Environmentally Friendly Vehicles 'Extremely Important' or 'Somewhat Important.' " Good Housekeeping Institute/J.D. Power and Associates study, 2004.

U.S. women have slowly and steadily increased their participation in the labor force from 46 percent of all women (age 16+) in 1974 to almost 60 percent in 2004. Oregon Labor Market Information System, "Women in the Labor Force," by Pamela Ferrara, March 22, 2007.

Information on the air pollution caused by driving came principally from "Clean Cars—Clean Air—A Consumer Guide to Auto Emission Inspection and Maintenance Programs," U.S. Environmental Protection Agency (www.epa.gov/otaq/cfa-air.htm), and "Automobiles and Carbon Monoxide" U.S. Environmental Protection Agency, Office of Mobile Sources, EPAA-400-F-005.

The statement that cars, trucks, and other mobile sources account for almost a third of the total air pollution in the United States came from the U.S. Department of Energy—Energy Efficiency and Renewable Energy Biomass Program "National Energy Security" (wwwl.eere.energy.gov/biomass/printable_versions/national_energy_security.html).

Data concerning the benefits of public transportation and lack of mass transit options in rural communities were sourced from "Public Transportation: Benefits for the 21st Century," by the American Public Transportation Association, July 2007.

"A two-adult household that also relies on mass transit can save as much as $6,251 every year compared to an equivalent household with two cars and no access to mass transportation," according to "Public Transportation and Petroleum Savings in the U.S.: Reducing Dependence on Oil," Linda Bailey, ICF International, January 2007.

The statement "The good news is, for every additional mile you get to the gallon, you keep one ton of CO_2 out of the atmosphere in a year" is based on data that appeared in "An Eco-System of One's Own," by Alex Shoumatoff, *Vanity Fair*, May 2007.

The original analogy comparing "the amount of carbon an average gas-powered car generates to tossing a five-pound bag of charcoal briquettes out my window every twenty miles or so," was made by John Ryan, writing in *In Over Our Heads: A Local Look at Global Climate*, as referenced by Jim Motavalli in his book *Forward Drive: The Race to Build "Clean" Cars for the Future*, Sierra Club Books, 2001.

Data noting that the ten years between 1995 and 2005 marked the hottest decade on record were provided by the National Climatic Data Center, NOAA Satellite and Information Service, "State of the Climate in 2005," *Bulletin of the American Meteorological Society*, June 2006 Volume 87.

"Right now, our cars and light trucks depend on oil for 95 percent of their fuel." Energy Information Agency, Energy Outlook 2002.

Oil spill data, including the reference to the two hundred confirmed releases each week since 2000, came from www.fueleconomy.gov/feg/oilspills.shtml.

"Almost 60 percent of the oil we use right now is imported." Energy Information Agency (www.eia.doe.gov/kids/energyfacts/sources/non-renewable/oil.html#Howused).

The original conjecture that NOx emissions are powerful enough to dissolve a twenty-pound steel cannonball was made by Jim Motavalli in *Forward Drive: The Race to Build "Clean" Cars for the Future*, Sierra Club Books, 2001.

Commuting distances are taking 10 percent more time, given how much traffic there is, according to the National Household Travel Survey conducted by the Center for Transportation Analysis at Oak Ridge National Laboratory and MacroSys Research and Technology (http://nhts.ornl.gov/2001/pub/STT.pdf).

"Meanwhile, every year, the average U.S. household spends more than a sixth of its budget on cars, more than on food and second only to housing; poor households spend twice that proportion," according to *Divorce Your Car!*, by Katie Alvord, New Society Publishers, 2000.

"The hidden cost of the automobile to the average American taxpayer is $1.19 per mile," according to "The True Cost of Driving," Santa Cruz County Regional Transportation Commission, Commute Solutions Program (www.commutesolutions.org and www.sccrtc.org/pdf/TCODBro.pdf).

"A person who commutes to work by transit rather than driving alone saves two hundred gallons of gasoline per year," per the Virginia Transit Association (www.vatransit.com/benefits/environment.htm).

Public transportation saves more than 855 million gallons of gasoline a year, or forty-five million barrels of oil. These savings equal about one month's oil imports from Saudi Arabia, according to the American Public Transit Association (www.apta.com/research/info/online/how_transit_benefits.cfm#t).

"Transportation is the second-largest expenditure for U.S. households; it accounts for 18 percent of all annual spending, behind housing at 33 percent, according to the Bureau of Labor Statistics." Sourced from "High prices forcing many to drive less, downsize, take mass transit," by Larry Copeland, *USA Today*, May 18, 2007.

SUVs were originally designed to allow for off-road travel. But fewer than 10 percent of all sport-utility vehicles ever drive off road, according to a CarPoint survey, cited in *Business Wire*, September 4, 1998.

"Top 10 Ways to Use Less Gas" originally appeared in *Beat High Gas Prices Now! The Fastest, Easiest Ways to Save $20–$50 Every Month on Gasoline*, by Diane MacEachern, Andrews-McMeel, 2005.

Data on the safety of sport-utility vehicles were taken from "SUVs Not Safe Enough," a report from the National Highway Transportation and Safety Administration, as reported by CNN on January 15, 2003, http://money.cnn.com/2003/01/15/news/suvs/index.htm?cnn=yes.

My understanding of the differences between ethanol and gasoline were informed by "E85 Vs. Gasoline Comparison Test," by Dan Edmunds, director of vehicle testing, and Philip Reed, senior consumer advice editor, General Motors (www.gm.com/company/onlygm/energy/flexfuel.html), June 5, 2007.

Information concerning the impact of the ethanol industry on food prices came from "Food Prices Going Up? Blame Ethanol," *National Post*, July 10, 2007, http://communities.canada.com/nationalpost/blogs/posted/archive/2007/07/10/food-prices-going-up-blame-ethanol.aspx; "Blame your bill on corn, weather; Shoppers already dealing with high gasoline prices face surging costs for groceries driven partly by demand for biofuels," by Janet Rausa Fuller, June 6, 2007; "Ethanol Demand Threatens Food Prices," by Brittany Sauser, www.technologyreview.com/Energy/18173/ February 13, 2007; "A Culinary and Cultural Staple in Crisis: Mexico Grapples With Soaring Prices for Corn—and Tortillas," by Manuel Roig-Franzia, *Washington Post* Foreign Service, January 27, 2007, p. A1, and "Science A Go Go: U.S. Throws Away Half Its Food" (www.scienceagogo.com/news/20041024002637data_trunc_sys.shtml11/24/04).

Chapter 5. Hot Stuff: Coffee, Tea, Cocoa . . . and the Skinny on Chocolate

Facts about how much coffee Americans consume annually were drawn from E-Imports: Specialty Coffee Statistics (www.e-importz.com/Support/specialty_coffee.htm) and "Cut Out the Jive in Your Java," *The Green Guide* (www.thegreenguide.com/doc/int/coffee).

My understanding of the impact growing coffee has on the environment came in part from *World Agriculture and the Environment* by Jason Clay, Island Press, as cited on the World Wildlife Fund Web page on agriculture and the environment.

Information on the impacts of coffee on birds was drawn from "Coffee and Conservation" (www.coffeehabitat.com/2006/02/birds_and_coffee.html); "Sun vs. Shade," the Songbird

Foundation (www.songbird.org/sunvsshade.htm); and Smithsonian Migratory Bird Center (www.natzoo.si.edu/smbc/Research/Coffee/coffee.htm).

The threats to children from the production of cocoa and chocolate were illuminated in the Global Witness report "Hot Chocolate—How Cocoa Fuelled the Conflict in Côte d'Ivoire") (www.globalwitness.org/media_library_detail.php/553/en/global_witness_report_calls_on_chocolate_industry_); the Global Witness Ivory Coast Web page, "Natural Resources in Conflict." (www.globalwitness.org/pages/en/cote_divoire.html); "Blood Cocoa: Cocoa is Ingredient Spurring Ivory Coast Civil War," by Johnnie Paradies, Associated Content, June 20, 2007 (www.associatedcontent.com/article/280296/blood_cocoa_cocoa_is_ingredient_spurring.html?page=2); "Ivory Coast: Cocoa Fueled Civil War," by Lydia Polgreen, *The New York Times,* June 9, 2007 (www.nytimes.com/2007/06/09/world/africa/09briefs-cocoa.html?ex=1339041600&en=3679b4e9bc8a1d05&ei=5090&partner=rssuserland&emc=rss).

Much of the background information about tea came from ChinaMist, www.chinamist.com, Quintessential Tea, www.qleaftea.com, and Choice Tea, www.choicetea.com.

Data on the $400 million in electricity that coffeepots use annually came from the blog Ideal Bite.

Chapter 6. We Are What We Eat: Fruits, Veggies, Dairy, Meat, Poultry, and Seafood

Plastic bag information came from "Plastic Left Holding the Bag as Environmental Plague," by Joan Lowy, *Seattle Post Intelligencer,* July 21, 2004, and Worldwatch Institute, "Plastic Bags: A Necessary Eyesore" (www.worldwatch.org/node/1499); "Reusable Bags: Paper Bags Are Better Than Plastic, Right?" (www.reusablebags.com/facts.php?id=7); "When It Pays to Buy Organic," *Consumer Reports,* February 2006 (www.consumerreports.org/cro/food/diet-nutrition/organic-products/organic-products-206/overview/index.htm).

"When it Comes to Pesticides, Birds Are Sitting Ducks," by Mary Deinlein, Smithsonian Migratory Bird Center (www.nationalzoo.si.edu/ConservationAndScience/MigratoryBirds/Fact_Sheets/default.cfm?fxsht=8)

Much important information on the impact of pesticides, fertilizers, and animal wastes on ground and surface water was taken from *A Field Guide to Buying Organic,* by Luddene Perry and Dan Schultz, Bantam Books, 2005.

"It has been estimated that only 0.1 percent of applied pesticides reach the target pests, leaving the bulk of the pesticides (99.9 percent) to impact the environment." David Pimentel, "Environmental and Socio-Economic Costs of Pesticide Use," *Techniques for Reducing Pesticide Use,* John Wiley & Sons, 1997, p. 71.

"In the U.S., where meat is cheap, we consume more than a hundred billion pounds of animal products per year."*A Field Guide to Buying Organic,* by Luddene Perry and Dan Schultz, Bantam Books, 2005, p. 215.

A "dead zone" as big as the state of New Jersey spreads through the Gulf of Mexico every year as millions of tons of pesticides and fertilizers applied to Midwest farms are carried into the Gulf via the Mississippi River. *Six Arguments for a Greener Diet,* by Michael F. Jacobson, Ph.D., p. 97.

U.S. coastal ecosystems are receiving 100 to 400 percent more nitrogen than natural systems would experience, as reported in the testimony of the Honorable Eileen Claussen, member, Pew Oceans Commission, before the Subcommittee on Fisheries Conservation, Wildlife and Oceans, House Committee on Resources, May 24, 2001.

"Hogging It! Estimates of Antimicrobial Abuse in Livestock," by Margaret Mellon, Charles Benbrook, and Karen Lutz Benbrook, Union of Concerned Scientists, January 2001 (report available at www.ucsusa.org) provided details on the impacts antibiotics have on the meat we eat.

"Pesticides and Food: Why Children May Be Especially Sensitive to Pesticides," U.S. Environmental Protection Agency (www.epa.gov/pesticides/food/pest.htm) and Environmental Working Group's "Shopper's Guide" (www.foodnews.org/reduce.php) helped me understand that we don't know what impact multiple exposures to pesticides will have on healthy adults. The U.S. Environmental Protection Agency believes that infants and children may be especially sensitive to health risks posed by pesticides because their internal organs are still developing and maturing. Plus, in relation to their body weight, infants and children eat and drink more than adults, possibly increasing their exposure to pesticides in food and water.

Information on the need to eat a variety of fruits and vegetables came from *A Field Guide to Buying Organic*, by Luddene Perry and Dan Schultz, Bantam Books, 2005, p. 114.

"For most retailers, organic beef represents only 1 percent or 2 percent of overall beef sales because of limited supply," was originally reported in "American Consumers Hungry for Organic Beef," by Christopher Doering, Organic Consumers Association, June 30, 2004.

Information on growth hormones in milk and meat came from the Center for Food Safety (www.centerforfoodsafety.org/rbgh_hormo.cfm).

Data concerning the increased nutritional value of organic over conventional food came from "New research proves organic milk is higher in vitamins and antioxidants than nonorganic milk," Soil Association (www.soilassociation.org/web/sa/saweb.nsf/848d689047c6466780256a6b0029 8980/b1ab478889d5OpenDocument), March 2, 2005, and "Elevating Antioxidant Levels in Food through Organic Farming and Processing, by Charles M. Benbrook, Ph.D., The Organic Center for Education and Promotion, January 2005.

Impacts of agricultural pesticides on human health came from several sources: U.S. Environmental Protection Agency: "Pesticides and Food: Why Children May be Especially Sensitive to Pesticides" (www.epa.gov/pesticides/food/pest.htm).

"Although acute poisonings in the United States rarely result in death, the EPA estimates that three hundred thousand farm workers suffer acute pesticide poisoning each year" came from *A Field Guide to Buying Organic*, p. 81.

"U.S. consumers can experience up to seventy daily exposures to residues from persistent organic pollutants (POPs) present on food and dairy products raised the conventional way" came from "Nowhere to Hide: Persistent Toxic Chemicals in the U.S. Food Supply," by Kristin Schafer, Pesticide Action Network North America, 2000 (www.panna.org).

"More than 1 million children between the ages of 1 and 5 ingest at least 15 pesticides every day from fruits and vegetables. More than 600,000 of these children eat a dose of organophosphate insecticides that the federal government considers unsafe, and 61,000 eat doses that exceed benchmark levels by a factor of 10 or more" came from "Food for Thought: The Case for Reforming Farm Programs to Preserve the Environment and Help Family Farmers, Ranchers and Foresters," pp. 12–13, found at www.environmentaldefense.org/pubs/Reports. Original source: Environmental Working Group, *Overexposed: Organophosphate Insecticides in Children's Food*, 1998, pp. 1–3.

Several sources provided statistics on the amount of energy organic agriculture uses compared with conventional crops. Key among them was "Legume-based Cropping Systems Have Reduced

Carbon and Nitrogen Losses," by Lori Drinkwater, *Nature* magazine, November 18, 1998, pp. 262–265. The fifteen-year Farming Systems Trial conducted by the Rodale Institute in Pennsylvania showed that organic agriculture can reduce greenhouse gas emissions by effectively locking more carbon into the soil rather than releasing it into the atmosphere, as happens in conventional agriculture. According to the research, organic farming uses 50% less energy overall than conventional farming methods.

"Top Ten Reasons to Buy Organic Food" was adapted from an article by Sylvia Tawse, marketing coordinator for Alfalfa's Markets, an organic food marketplace in Boulder and Denver, Colorado (www.abbeysvegetarianrecipes.com/organic-foods.html).

"The reason to buy meat without antibiotics is not because the antibiotics in the meat are transferred to the person, but because of how the antibiotics increase the number of antibiotic-resistant bacteria," said Dr. Stuart Levy, director of the Center of Adaptation Genetics and Drug Resistance at Tufts University Medical School in a January 17, 2001, *New York Times* article by Marion Burros.

Additional information on the impact of livestock on the environment came from "Livestock a major threat to environment; Remedies urgently needed," November 29, 2006, Food and Agriculture Organization of the United Nations, FAO Newsroom.

"Exposure to pesticides can cause a range of ill effects in humans, from relatively mild effects such as headaches, fatigue, and nausea, to more serious effects such as cancer and neurological disorders. In 1999, EPA estimated that nationwide there were at least 10,000 to 20,000 physician-diagnosed pesticide illnesses and injuries per year in farm work. Environmental effects are evident in the findings of the U.S. Geological Survey, which reported in 1999 that more than 90 percent of water and fish samples from streams and about 50 percent of all sampled wells contained one or more pesticides. The concern about pesticides in water is especially acute in agricultural areas, where most pesticides are used." "Agricultural Pesticides: Management Improvements Needed to Further Promote Integrated Pest Management," U.S. Government Accountability Office [GAO-01-815, Page 4, August 2001].

The impact of pesticides on farmworkers, wildlife, and wells was reported by Donella H. Meadows, "Our Food, Our Future," *Organic Gardening*, September/October 2000. "In the past fifty years, more than 500 insect pests, 230 crop diseases, and 220 weeds have become resistant to pesticides and herbicides."

"High levels of pesticides, such as DDT, chlordane, and toxaphene, are present in beluga whales from the Arctic, where they were never used. Scientists June-Soo Park, Steve Sweet, and Terry Wade reported that DDT, for instance, can volatilize into the gaseous state and be transported in the air over long distances fairly rapidly," according to "Atmospheric Deposition of PAH, PCB, and Organochlorine Pesticides to Corpus Christi Bay," cited in *Science Daily Magazine*, September 21, 2001.

Information on the state of the world's fisheries came from "World Fisheries: Declines, Potential and Human Reliance," January 2006, University of Michigan, Global Change Course; Data showing that more than 75 percent of the world's fisheries are either fully fished or overfished came from the Monterey Bay Aquarium, "Frequently Asked Questions," Seafood Watch Program.

Marine Stewardship Council's Principles and Criteria for Fisheries (www.msc.org/assets/docs/fishery_certification/MSCPrinciples&Criteria.doc) describe the three main principles for a fishery to be deemed certified by the MSC; the principles strive to protect existing ecosystems while encouraging the sustainability of the habitat as well as the fish species.

Data on availability of safe and unsafe seafood came from the Monterey Bay Aquarium's Seafood Watch website (www.mbayaq.org/cr/cr_seafoodwatch/sfw_resources.asp#sss).

Information concerning the safety to consumers of eating fish contaminated with methylmercury came from the Food and Drug Administration and the Environmental Protection Agency. "FDA and EPA Announce the Revised Consumer Advisory on Methylmercury in Fish," March 19, 2004.

Chapter 7. Clean and Green: Cleansers, Scrubs, Polishes, and Fresheners

The green cleaning suggestions in this chapter are pulled from the cleansers page of www.big-green purse; the University of Missouri Extension Service's excellent online Household Hazardous Products Guide (http://extension.missouri.edu/xplor/wasteman/wm6003.htm); *Consumer Reports'* online Greener Choices consumer guide product ratings and analysis (www.greenerchoices.org/products.cfm?product=greencleaning&page=RightChoices); The "Green Guide Product Report on Laundry Supplies" (www.thegreenguide.com/reports/product.mhtml?id=78&sec-2; and "Hazards of Cleaning Chemicals," by the University of Colorado Health Services Center, Health and Safety Division, Guidance Note, January 2002. The statements "In 1985, a study by the National Toxicology Program, a unit of the U.S. Department of Health and Human Services, found that methylene chloride caused tumors at a statistically significant rate in at least two animal species. That is the definition of a carcinogen applied by government agencies. The Consumer Product Safety Commission says the chemical poses 'one of the highest cancer risks ever calculated for a consumer product.' Stripping one piece of furniture per year can put a person in the high-risk category, according to CPSC" were sourced from *The Healthy Home: An Attic-to-Basement Guide to Toxin-Free Living*, by Linda Mason Hunter, Pocket Books, 1989, p. 106.

Several home-cleaning recipes originally appeared in "EPA Office of Solid Waste Home Cleaning Recipes" (www.epa.gov/epaoswer/non-hw/reduce/catbook/alt.htm). *Greener ChoicesHome>Home & Garden>Cleaners: Buying guide 7/07 (www.greenerchoices.org/ratings.cfm?product=green cleaning) *Consumer Reports*, 2005 Annual Report of the American Association of Poison Control Centers National Poisoning and Exposure Database, Melisa M. Wai, M.D., et al. (www.aapcc.org/2005.htm).

A fifteen-year study in Oregon found a 54 percent higher death rate from cancer in women who stayed home than those who worked elsewhere, according to a presentation given at the National Center for Health Statistics conference. "Use with Caution," by Jessica A. Knoblauch, *EJ Magazine*, Fall 2006.

Information on reducing hazardous products in the home was sourced form the Family and Consumer Sciences website published by the North Carolina State University Cooperative Extension Service (www.ces.ncsu.edu/depts/fcs/housing/pubs/fcs3682r.html).

Background information on "the ridiculous number of sprays, powders, liquids, and pastes we're using to polish, disinfect, deodorize, unclog, and otherwise 'clean' our homes and apartments," came from Linda Mason Hunter, *The Healthy Home: An Attic-to-Basement Guide to Toxin-Free Living*, Pocket Books, 1989.

I discussed the impact on women's health of various cleaning products, such as phthalates, air sanitizers, aerosol sprays, laundry detergents, toilet bowl cleansers, glass cleaners, and other products, based on the report "Household Hazards: Potential Hazards of Home Cleaning Products" by Alexandra Gorman, Women's Voices for the Earth, 2007; various excellent reports on cleansers in *The Green Guide*; and recommendations of Green Seal and Scientific Certified Systems (SCS).

Information about indoor air pollution levels created by household hazardous products came in part from the Center for Health, Environment and Justice (www.besafenet.com/pvc/newsreleases/target-suds_news_release.htm). Additional background was gleaned from the EPA's Indoor Air Quality website (www.epa.gov/iaq).

Chapter 8. Eco Chic: Clothing, Accessories, and Jewelry

The data on cotton's impact on the environment comes from the Sustainable Cotton Project; the Organic Exchange; the Organic Trade Association; REI, Inc.'s Web page on Eco-Sensitive Materials, "The Truth About Cotton" (www.greenfeet.com); "The Secret Life of Clothing" (www.sierraclub.org/sierra/200407/hidden.asp); the Organic Clothing blog (http://organic clothing.blogs.com/my_weblog/2007/05/global_warming_.html); "What Should My Clothes Be Made Of?" by Lucy Siegle, *The Observer* magazine (http://observer.guardian.co.uk/magazine/story/0,,1715437,00.html), February 26, 2006; and "Waste Couture: Environmental Impact of the Clothing Industry" by Luz Claudio, *Environmental Health Perspectives*, September 2007, Volume 115, Number 9. Specific statements—that less than 1 percent of cotton is grown organically; approximately 25 percent of all insecticides and more than 10 percent of the pesticides used in the world are used to grow cotton; it takes one-third pound of pesticides and fertilizers to produce enough cotton to make just one T-shirt; most synthetic fibers, including polyester and nylon, come from petroleum products—come from "Organic Cotton Facts," Organic Trade Association (www.ota.com/organic/mt/organic_cotton.html).

My explanation of the cost of organic fiber was particularly informed by "Why Is Organic Clothing Worth the Extra Money?" (http://organicclothing.blogs.com/my_weblog/2006/12/the_high_cost_o.html).

Information on the impact that textiles have on the solid waste stream came from the "Textiles" page of the EPA's Municipal Solid Waste website (www.epa.gov/epaoswer/non-hw/muncpl/textile.htm) and Retex Frequently Asked Questions regarding clothes recycling (www.retexnorthwest.com/faq.htm).

The figure, "Of the 9 million tons of clothes thrown out every year in the U.S. only 2 million tons are recycled," came from Gaia Movement Trust (www.gaia-movement.org/TextPage.asp?TxtID=135&SubMenuItemID=103&MenuItemID=47). The growing popularity of organic clothing among parents was documented in "Popularity of chemical-free products has boomed as parents turn to all that's organic," by Samantha Critchell, Associated Press, August 25, 2006.

Information about the impact pesticides used on cotton can have on food and drinking water came from "King Cotton—pesticide residue is common in cotton by-products used in agriculture" by Daniel Imhoff, *Sierra*, May 1999, and "Pesticides used in cotton contaminate our drinking water," October 18, 1994, statement of Carol M. Browner, administrator, U.S. Environmental Protection Agency on pesticides in drinking water (www.pmep/cce.cornell.edu/issues/pesticides-water.html).

Much of the information on the impact of gold mining on the environment came from the "No Dirty Gold" campaign website (www.nodirtygold.org); "The Environmental Impacts of Gold Mining in the Etowah," by Candace Stoughton, Nature Conservancy; "Behind Gold's Glitter: Torn Lands and Pointed Questions," by Jane Perlez and Kirk Johnson, *The New York Times*,

October 24, 2005 (www.nytimes.com/2005/10/24/international/24GOLD.html); "New World Gold Mine and Yellowstone National Park," CRS Report for Congress, by Marc Humphries, August 27, 1996.

The information on "conflict" or "blood" diamonds came from Global Witness (www.global witness.org/pages/en/conflict_diamonds.html); "Conflict Diamonds: Sanctions and War," United Nations website (www.un.org/peace/africa/Diamond.html); "Blood Diamonds," by Greg Campbell, *Amnesty* magazine (www.amnestyusa.org/amnestynow/diamonds.html).

Information on alternatives to perc as a dry cleaner came from the Environmental Protection Agency's cleaning guide (www.epa.gov/dfe/pubs/garment/gcrg/cleanguide.pdf); Greenpeace (www.greenpeaceusa.org/multimedia/download/1/544231/0/424); *Consumer Reports:* Dry-cleaning Alternatives (www.consumerreports.org/main/detailv2.jsp?CONTENT%3C%3Ecnt_id=299609& FOLDER%3%3Efolder_id=162695); and "Wet Cleaning and Dry Cleaning Alternatives," by Joanna Howard (www.greenbiz.com/news/columns_third.cfm?NewsID=28417).

Women spend $1,069 ($246 more than men do) on clothing every year, according to the Bureau of Labor Statistics 2004–2005 Consumer Expenditure Survey. "Lay Off, Suze Orman," by Anita Hamilton, *Time* magazine, April 5, 2007 (www.time.com/time/magazine/article/0,9171,1607265,00 .html), provided additional background on women's spending habits.

Information on nanotechnologies was sourced from "Tiny particles promise much, but could pose big risk," Natural Resources Defense Council (www.nrdc.org/health/science/nano.asp); "Nano-technologies and the Precautionary Principle," by Jennifer Sass, Ph.D., Natural Resources Defense Council, The Woodrow Wilson International Center for Scholars Project on Emerging Nanotechnologies; and The 2005 EPA Draft Nanotechnology White Paper prepared by the Science Policy Council of the Environmental Protection Agency.

Information about the impact of leather tanning came in part from "Adoption of Clean Leather Tanning Technologies in Mexico," by Alan Blackman, Resources for the Future (www.rff.org), August 2005.

Ideas for places and ways to recycle clothing were inspired by the clothing recycling list published by Stanford University (www.recycling.stanford.edu/5r/recycledproducts.html#clothing).

Chapter 9. Garden of Eden: Lawn, Garden, and Patio

Facts and information pertaining to the environmental and health impacts of pesticide use on lawns and gardens came from "Reported Residential Pesticide Use and Breast Cancer Risk on Long Island, New York," by Susan L. Teitelbaum et al., American Journal of Epidemiology Advance Access published online on December 13, 2006, *American Journal of Epidemiology*, doi:10.1093/aje/kwk046; "Our Children at Risk: The 5 Worst Environmental Threats to Their Health," Natural Resources Defense Council, November, 1997, "Childhood Pesticide Poisoning" (www.nrdc.org/health/kids/ocar/chap5c.asp) for information on incidence of fatality in childhood pesticide poisoning, including pesticides used on lawns and gardens; and U.S. Fish and Wildlife Service, Division of Environmental Contaminants, July 6, 2000, "Homeowner's Guide to Protecting Frogs—Lawn & Garden Care."

It was staggering to learn that 60 percent of water consumed on the West Coast, and 30 percent on the East Coast, goes to watering lawns. *U.S. News & World Report* states that a one-thousand-square-foot lawn (for example, 20 by 50 feet) requires 10,000 gallons of water per summer to maintain a "green" look. In the West, whole rivers are bled dry for watering. From www.plant native.com.

Data documenting that "some 40 million acres of America are covered in lawns, making turf grass our largest irrigated crop" came from "Could the Grass Be Greener? Lawn Turf Is America's Biggest Crop—and a Mixed Bag for the Environment," by Thomas Hayden, U.S. News & World Report, May 8, 2005.

"There are 10.5 million households spending $3 billion on lawn care." www.scottslawnservice.com/ index.cfm/event/franchses_scottsRep.

"A 2005 survey of 2,000 adults by the Natural Marketing Institute found 20 percent of consumers had bought some kind of environmentally friendly lawn-and-garden product. According to CNN, market researchers Freedonia Group estimate a 10 percent annual growth for the organic fertilizer market, twice the projected growth for all lawn and garden goods," reported the Beyond Pesticides *Daily News* blog, August 15, 2007.

Information on the ability of corn gluten to reduce Chesapeake Bay pollution came from "What You Put on Your Lawn Affects Waterways," December 20, 2005, 10:15 A.M., www.WTOP News.com.

Homeowners use an estimated 100 million pounds of pesticides each year in their homes and gardens, according to Beyond Pesticides (www.beyond pesticides.org/dailynewsblog/?p=136).

Much of the information on the environmental impacts of maintaining a monoculture lawn came from the Environmental Protection Agency: GreenScaping: The Easy Way to a Greener, Healthier Yard, the U.S. Environmental Protection Agency (www.epa.gov/GreenScapes) and "Healthy Lawn Healthy Environment" (www.epa.gov/oppfead1/Publications/lawncare.pdf).

Tips on hiring a lawn service were adapted from Healthy Lawn Care Program for Watershed Protection, Michigan Green Industry Association for Lawn Care Professionals of Michigan, and Nutrient Management for Lawn Service Companies. Authors: James H. May, research associate, Crop and Soil Environmental Sciences; David R. Chalmers, associate professor and extension agronomist, Turfgrass Management; and John R. Hall III, professor and extension agronomist, Turfgrass Management; Virginia Tech Publication Number 430-400, Posted June 2004.

Data on the impact of lawn mowing came from the EPA's John Millett, from the news release "Small Engine Rule to Bring Big Emissions Cuts" 04/17/2007, from the EPA's Lawn and Garden (Small Gasoline) Equipment website (www.epa.gov/otaq/equip-ld.htm) and from *E Magazine*, which wrote that 54 million Americans mow their lawns every weekend; 5 percent of the nation's total air pollutants are generated by gas-powered lawn mowers. Lawn mowers are used mostly in hot months when ground level ozone, or smog, is most intense, making life more difficult for people who suffer from asthma and other respiratory illnesses. (*E Magazine*: Buzz cut: Electric Lawn Mowers Beat the Gas Guzzlers at Their Own Game, by LuAnne Roy, September/October 2007, p. 44.)

"Today, U.S. homeowners spend over $17 billion on outdoor home improvements. More than 26 million households hired a green professional, according to a 2000 Gallup survey and this number is expected to grow," according to "History of the American Lawn," Landscape America website (www.landscape-america.com/history/history_lawn.html).

A 2004 survey by the National Gardening Association reported that 5 percent of households used only organic fertilizers, herbicides, and pesticides, but 9 percent of respondents said they would go organic by 2009. Reported in "Organic lawns slowly catch on," by Dudley Price, *The News & Observer*, August 23, 2007. (www.newsobserver.com/business/story/679743.html).

Some ideas for recycling plastic garden pots and other ways to reduce garden trash originally appeared in "Beauty and the Plastic Beast," by Beth Botts, *Chicago Tribune*, June 10, 2007.

Chapter 10. Kid Stuff: Babies' and Children's Food, Gear, and Toys

Data on when children begin using consumer electronic devices—6.7 years old—came from the NPD Group's third annual Kids and Consumer Electronics Trends Report. "Kids' first exposure to gaming, cell phones coming earlier," by Jacqui Cheng, *Ars Technica*, June 6, 2007 (www.arstechnica.com/news.ars/post/20070606-kids-first-exposure-to-gaming-cell-phones-becoming-earlier.html) and "Kids Are Becoming Exposed to and Adopting Electronics at Earlier Ages," NPD, June 5, 2007 (www.npd.com/press/releases/press_070605.html).

Population trends data came from "This Planet Ain't Big Enough for the 6,500,000,000 of Us," by Chris Rapley, *The Belfast Telegraph*, June 27, 2007; and "Nature's Place: Human Population and the Future of Biological Diversity," by Richard P. Cincotta and Robert Engelman, Population Action International, 2000.

National Wildlife Federation developed the original concept of swapping screen space for green space at www.greenhour.org/section/about.

Information on diacetyl in popcorn came from Liz Borkowski, "Parliamentary Maneuvers Derail California's Diacetyl Legislation Tuesday, September 18, 2007, in Flavoring Workers' Lung, Occupational Health & Safety," The Pump Handle (blog), September 19, 2007 (http://thepumphandle.wordpress.com/2007/09/18/parliamentary-maneuvers-derail-california's-diacetyl-legislation); "FDA set to audit microwave-popcorn safety," by Chris Bowman, *Sacramento Bee* as carried by *Sioux City Journal*, September 19, 2007; "ConAgra to drop popcorn flavoring, Chemical linked to lung disease in factory workers," by Chris Emery, *Baltimore Sun*, September 7, 2007; "Flavoring Suspected in Illness: Calif. Considers Banning Chemical Used in Microwave Popcorn," by Sonya Geiss, *Washington Post*, May 7, 2007 (www.washingtonpost.com/wpdny/content/article/2007/05/06/AR2007050601089.html); "Doctor Links a Man's Illness to a Microwave Popcorn Habit," by Gardner Harris, *The New York Times*, September 5, 2007 (www.nytimes.com/2007/09/05/us/05popcorn.html?ex=1189656000&en=d3196dcf6d692cf8&emc=etal); and U.S. Department of Labor: Occupational Safety & Health Administration Chemical Sampling Information, Diacetyl (www.osha.gov/dts/chemicalsampling/data/CH_231710.html).

Information about how and when toy advertisers target children came from "Six strategies marketers use to get kids to want stuff bad," by Bruce Horovitz, *USA Today*, November 22, 2006.

Dr. Sandra Steingraber, author of *Having Faith: An Ecologist's Journey to Motherhood*, was quoted from her keynote address to the Women's Conference on Health and the Environment.

My understanding of the risks children face from pesticides was based on "organophosphorus pesticide exposure of urban and suburban preschool children with organic and conventional diets." Cynthia L. Curl, Richard A. Fenske, Kai Elgethun, *Environmental Health Perspectives*, October 13, 2002, National Institute of Environmental Sciences, EHP online (www.ehponline.org); Do You Know What You're Eating? February 1999, Consumers Union of United States, Inc. (www.consumersunion.org/food/do_you_know2.htm); Pesticide residues in conventional, IPM-grown and organic foods: Insights from three U.S. data sets, *Food Additives & Contaminants*, May 2002 (www.consumersunion.org/food/organicsumm.htm).

Research commissioned by the Center for Environmental Health (www.cehca.org/lunch boxes.html) in Oakland, California, showed that the lining in some kids' lunch boxes contained high levels of lead. Lead can harm children even in minute amounts. It hinders brain development and can cause a variety of behavior and other developmental disorders. Children may be exposed to the lead in lunch boxes if they eat food that's been carried in them or if they handle the boxes and then put their hands in their mouths.

Chapter 11. Plugged In: Lights, Appliances, and Electronics

Lighting facts came from Home Energy Brief #2, "Lighting," Rocky Mountain Institute (www.rmi.org/sitepages/survF365.php?&surveyId=365&aId=18249).

"Eighty to eighty-five percent of the total energy consumption and CO_2 emissions of a building comes from meeting our energy needs for heating, cooling, ventilation, and hot water use," according to "Energy Efficiency in Buildings: Business Realities and Opportunities," World Business Council for Sustainable Development, a project cochaired by Lafarge and United Technologies Corp. Other participating companies are CEMEX, DuPont, Electricite de France, Gaz de France, Kansai, Philips, Sonae Sierra, and Tepco.

"A staggering ninety-eight percent of electricity in the United States comes from nonrenewable resources such as coal, natural gas, nuclear power, and large hydropower," according to "Your Health" (www.green-e.org). Green-e is the nation's leading independent certification and verification program for renewable energy and companies that use renewable energy.

Tips for buying and using energy-efficient bulbs came from the Environmental Defense site of the same name (www.environmentaldefense.org/page.cfm?tagid=609) and from the Environmental Protection Agency's Energy Star website (www.energystar.gov).

The average home spends almost $1,900 on energy every year. You can reduce your bill 10 to 50 percent a year, says the U.S. Department of Energy, by making several energy-smart improvements.

General Electric provided information on how compact fluroescent lightbulbs work at its website Compact Fluorescent Lightbulb FAQs (www.gelighting.com/na/home_lighting/ask_us/faq_compact.htm#which_bulb).

Information about how much money women spend on electronics came from the Consumer Electronics Association report "Women's Choice in Consumer Electronics at CES 2006" by Jasper Huitink for www.letsgodigital.org, December 4, 2005.

Some ideas for when to repair or replace appliances and other electronics were inspired by "Repair or Replace?" by Amanda MacMillan, *Green Guide* 12, July/ August 2007.

Information on efforts computer companies are making to be environmentally responsible came from "Dell Makes Plans to Be the Greenest Tech Company," GreenerComputing.com (www.greenercomputing.com/news_third.cfm?NewsID=35211); "Google, Intel launch initiative to make computers greener," by Terence Chea, Associated Press Writer, News Fuze, June 12, 2007.

Ideas for how to buy a more eco-friendly computer and dispose of one with minimal impact came from: "Green PC: How to dispose of unwanted tech equipment without hassles, and where to find great new environmentally friendly gear, plus 8 tips for going green," by Jamais Cascio, *PC World*, May 23,2006; "How to Buy a Green PC," Computer Shopper (http://computershopper.com/feature/200704_how_to_buy_a_green_pc); and the Environmental Protection Agency ECycling initiative (www.epa.gov/epaoswer/hazwaste/recycle/ecycling/basic.htm).

big green purse

Chapter 12. Home, Green Home: Furniture, Paint, Flooring, and Fabrics

I gained an understanding of sustainable standards and their importance in greening manufacturing from the Institute for Market Transformation to Sustainability. (http://mts.sustainable products.com). Additional background on the furniture industry was gleaned from the Sustainable Furniture Council (www.sustainablefurniturecouncil.org).

Statistics on the extent that carpeting is used in the U.S. came from Carpeting, Indoor Air Quality and the Environment, www.buildinggreen.com, the website of Environmental Building News (www.buildinggreen.com/auth/article.cfm?fileName=030601a.xml). Information on the environmental and air quality impact of carpet production and installation and the use of carpet adhesives came from Green Seal's Choose Green Report: Carpet, 2001. The statistic noting that the amount of carpet annually sent to landfills covers an area greater than New York City also came from Green Seal's Carpet report. Additional background information on the environmental impacts of carpet was provided by Interface Inc., and its carpet brands, Bentley Prince Street and FLOR.

I got to see many green design concepts in action, thanks to the comprehensive exhibit The Green House: New Directions in Sustainable Architecture and Design, at the National Building Museum in Washington, D.C.

Facts about bamboo came from www.plyboo.com, provided by Smith & Fong manufacturers.

INDEX

ABOUT THE
AUTHOR

Diane MacEachern is a bestselling environmental writer, sought-after public speaker, and founder of www.biggreenpurse.com. She has advised the U.S. Environmental Protection Agency, the World Bank, the World Wildlife Fund, and many other agencies and nonprofit organizations focused on protecting the planet. The author of the bestselling *Save Our Planet: 750 Everyday Ways You Can Help Clean Up the Earth*, she lives in the Washington, D.C., suburbs in the energy-efficient home she helped design and build more than twenty years ago. Diane is a proud supporter of Earth Share (www.earthshare.org), the nation's largest federation of state and local environmental organizations, and the Alaska Wilderness League (www.alaskawild.org), which is leading the effort to protect the Arctic National Wildlife Refuge and other wilderness in Alaska.